Enlightened Bodies

Exploring Physical and Subtle Human Anatomy

Nirmal Lumpkin, *LMT*
Japa Kaur Khalsa, *DOM*

Kundalini Yoga as Taught by Yogi Bhajan®

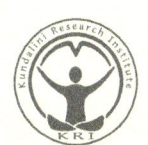

Kundalini Research Institute
Training • Publishing • Research • Resources

ENLIGHTENED BODIES

Exploring Physical and Subtle Human Anatomy

Kundalini Yoga as taught by Yogi Bhajan®

© 2015 Nirmal Lumpkin and Japa Kaur Khalsa

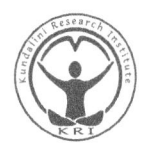

Published by the Kundalini Research Institute

Training • Publishing • Research • Resources

PO Box 1819

Santa Cruz, NM 87567

www.kundaliniresearchinstitute.org

ISBN 978-1-934532-00-3

Creative Director:
Annelise Rampreet Burlett

Production Editor:
Sat Purkh Kaur Khalsa

Copyeditor:
Jane Kupersmith

Consulting Editors:
Sham Rang Singh Khalsa M.D.,
Karta Purkh Singh Khalsa,
Yogaraj (Ayurveda), DN-C, RH, CAP, LMT,
Shanti Shanti Kaur Khalsa PhD, and
Weston Cutter Jr.

KRI Review:
Siri Neel Kaur Khalsa

Illustrations:
Katie Yost
Hector Jara Mukhtiar Singh (Chakra Illustrations)

Design & Layout:
Prana Projects; Biljana Nedelkovska & Ditta Khalsa

Rev. 3.16

© 2015 Nirmal Lumpkin and Japa Kaur Khalsa. All teachings, yoga sets, techniques, kriyas, and meditations courtesy of The Teachings of Yogi Bhajan. Reprinted with permission. Unauthorized duplication is a violation of applicable laws. ALL RIGHTS RESERVED. No part of these Teachings may be reproduced or transmitted in any form by any means, electronic or mechanical, including photocopying and recording, or by any information storage and retrieval system, except as may be expressly permitted in writing by The Teachings of Yogi Bhajan. To request permission, please write to KRI at PO Box 1819, Santa Cruz, NM 87567 or visit **www.kundaliniresearchinstitute.org**.

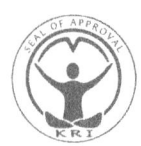

This publication has received the KRI Seal of Approval.

This seal is only given to products that have been reviewed for accuracy and integrity of the sections containing 3HO lifestyle teachings and Kundalini Yoga as taught by Yogi Bhajan®.

The diet, exercise, and lifestyle suggestions in this book come from ancient yogic traditions. Nothing in this book should be construed as medical advice. Any recipes mentioned herein may contain potent herbs, botanicals, or naturally occurring ingredients that have traditionally been used to support the structure and function of the human body. Always check with your personal physician or licensed health care practitioner before making any significant modification to your diet or lifestyle, to insure that the ingredients or lifestyle changes are appropriate for your personal health condition and consistent with any medication you may be taking. For more information about Kundalini Yoga as taught by Yogi Bhajan® please see **www.kundaliniresearchinstitute.org**.

For more information from the authors please see **www.enlightenedbodies.com**.

Book illustrations © Katie Yost, www.katieyost.com. All rights reserved. Reprinted by permission only.

NOTE: Traditional spellings have been maintained in some instances, for example, Pranic Body or Sat Nam Rasayan, even though in the main body of the text the correct transliteration will be applied: praana and Sat Naam respectively.

Contents

v	**FOREWORD**
	Dr. Dharma Singh Khalsa
viii	**A NOTE TO TEACHERS AND TRAINERS**
	Nirvair Singh
x	**FROM THE AUTHORS**
xii	**ACKNOWLEDGEMENTS**
xiii	**ABOUT KUNDALINI YOGA AND YOGI BHAJAN**
1	**Chapter One: THE HUMAN BODY IS AWESOME**
9	**Chapter Two: THE SUBTLE HUMAN BODY**
11	The Chakra System
17	The Ten Light Bodies
21	Ayurveda
24	Humanology
25	Chinese Medicine
26	Plants, Herbs, and Food
29	**Chapter Three: MUSCULOSKELETAL SYSTEM**
30	Physical Anatomy Perspective
50	Subtle Anatomy Perspective
52	Tips and Techniques for a Strong Musculoskeletal System
61	**Chapter Four: CIRCULATORY SYSTEM**
62	Physical Anatomy Perspective
69	Subtle Anatomy Perspective
77	Tips and Techniques for a Strong Circulatory System
85	**Chapter Five: RESPIRATORY SYSTEM**
86	Physical Anatomy Perspective
97	Subtle Anatomy Perspective
100	Tips and Techniques for a Strong Respiratory System

109	Chapter Six: IMMUNE SYSTEM
110	Physical Anatomy Perspective
115	Subtle Anatomy Perspective
122	Tips and Techniques for a Strong Immune System
129	Chapter Seven: NERVOUS SYSTEM
130	Physical Anatomy Perspective
142	Subtle Anatomy Perspective
147	Tips and Techniques for a Strong Nervous System
151	Chapter Eight: ENDOCRINE SYSTEM
152	Physical Anatomy Perspective
163	Subtle Anatomy Perspective
167	Tips and Techniques for a Strong Endocrine System
175	Chapter Nine: DIGESTIVE SYSTEM
176	Physical Anatomy Perspective
181	Subtle Anatomy Perspective
190	Tips and Techniques for a Strong Digestive System
201	Chapter Ten: URINARY SYSTEM
202	Physical Anatomy Perspective
207	Subtle Anatomy Perspective
212	Tips and Techniques for a Strong Urinary System
219	Chapter Eleven: REPRODUCTIVE SYSTEM
220	Physical Anatomy Perspective
228	Subtle Anatomy Perspective
234	Tips and Techniques for a Strong Reproductive System
238	APPENDICES
239	Before You Begin
243	Kriya Analysis
253	Meditations for the Nervous System
256	Chakra Chart
257	10 Bodies Chart
258	Chinese Medicine Concepts
260	Supporting Health Through the Seasons
264	Body Systems Visualization
266	Kriyas for Each System
269	Glossary
272	Resources
277	Index
285	About the Authors

Foreword

SAT NAM.

It is my great privilege and honor to be asked to write the foreword for this book. One thing I can say for sure as you embark on this adventure and journey is that it is a beautiful book written with very clear intentions and a high vibration that will serve you well. I recently saw a woman wearing a tee shirt that read: "Yoga is my health insurance." That's probably true; yoga is an exceptional and time-tested form of preventive medicine. Whether a practitioner or teacher of yoga, it's nice to understand what's going on inside one's body and mind. This lovely book helps you do just that. In my view this is the right book for you right now or you wouldn't be holding it in your hands, or looking at it with your eyes and having it impact your nervous system, or soaking up its vibration with your sixth sense. I've written a number of books myself including the best selling Meditation as Medicine and I am always struck when someone shares with me that, "The book kind of fell out of the sky into my lap," or "The book just jumped off the shelf at me." Perhaps something similar happened to you with this book but, regardless, I know on a very deep level that this is the very best book for you at exactly the right time to fulfill a profound need in your life, known or unknown, or you simply would not be reading it.

Writing a foreword for a book is a big challenge. In the first place it's not your book, which makes it harder to do an authentic job. The most important thing for me was to get to the heart of the matter; why they'd write it? What is the purpose and intention of the authors? To do that, I've read and studied *Enlightened Bodies*. I've also communicated with the authors and interestingly went back into my memory bank to recall my personal experience with one of them, Dr. Japa Kaur, who I first met in Chicago over 15 years ago. My wife Kirti Kaur and I were in the Windy City on a book tour and while visiting the 3HO center there met Japa Kaur. Then she was just getting started on her personal journey of yoga, spirituality, healing, and service to humanity. She was attending college at the time, hadn't yet married and her training in Oriental Medicine was a number of years away. But as I recall, she had the same bright light in her eyes that she has today; a light that signifies her passion to heal and serve humanity. Since then we've seen each other at various gatherings at the mother ashram in

Espanola, and have continued our conversations. When I asked Japa why she was writing this book she shared with me the following thoughts: "This book is a public service for anyone interested in yoga including teachers and practitioners as well as those interested in going forward in the new field of yoga therapy. Also it's for body workers, spiritual people, and even high school students who want to learn more about how yoga can make them smarter and happier."

Now I have to admit that I don't know Japa's co-author Nirmal but I've explored her bio and had an email conversation with her while she completes her studies to take the medical school admission test. I think she is a very intelligent and deep woman who has a lot to offer. She comes from a dance background and from there progressed to a study of anatomy, physiology, massage therapy, and, of course kundalini yoga and yoga therapy. When I connected with her by email she shared the following; "It has always felt odd to me to 'silo' my understanding of the body from a 'scientific' view from the way I understand the body energetically and intuitively. I have longed for a resource that really understood both of these perspectives when talking about the complexity that is the human being. Since there didn't seem to be anything out there that really helped to draw these multiple perspectives together it seemed like the right time and place to write the book. I hope that this book helps to serve as a bridge for people who have a strong knowledge base on one end of that spectrum to begin to see the body in a new light."

In my view they've succeeded. Interest in Kundalini Yoga, as well as other forms of yoga, is growing exponentially. In fact at least 30 million Americans practice yoga today. If you include meditation and other forms of mind-body medicine that number increases. At the same time, according to my colleague, Sat Bir Singh Khalsa, Ph.D. of Harvard Medical School, the development of yoga therapy to help treat illness is also growing. There are more and more research studies being completed and published in medical journals every year. Research on Kundalini Yoga as taught by Yogi Bhajan®, is expanding big time. To date, over two dozen studies have been published on Kundalini based practices such as studying chronic stress, generalized anxiety disorder, PTSD, and children in school settings. According to Dr. Sat Bir Singh, "Given the large breadth of and depth of practices in Kundalini Yoga and their benefits on a wide variety of medical psychological and behavioral issues, this work is likely to progress rapidly."

This book will help you get ready for that knowledge explosion. My own work at the Alzheimer's Research and Prevention Foundation ARPF (www.alzheimersprevention.org) on the practice of Kirtan Kriya, a favorite meditation of Yogi Bhajan, has revealed many positive benefits in people doing it for only 12 minutes a day. Outcomes included a better memory, reversal of memory loss, enhanced mood, less anxiety, less depression, greater feelings of well-being, and improved cellular health such as an up-regulation of good immune system genes and down regulation of inflammatory genes. This means less inflammation and, as you may know, inflammation is associated with just about every disease from heart issues, cancer, and even Alzheimer's disease. Our research has also shown an increase in the end of your DNA called a telomere. Longer telomeres are associated with better health and longer life so simply practicing Kirtan Kriya for only 12 minutes a day has a profound positive effect on your mind, body and spiritual health. You can find the practice of Kirtan Kriya described on page 250.

As the authors state in the beginning of this book, "The Human Body is Awesome!" And in this book you'll discover a multilayered view of health and healing. You'll learn about not only our physical anatomy but also our subtle anatomy, our chakras, which are our subtle energy centers, the proper balance of which is critically important for optimal health. Reading *Enlightened Bodies* has been a tremendously enjoyable experience and I'm sure you will love it too. Much new material is shared, especially in the diagrams and in the concept of how yoga helps you send positive messages deep into your body. You'll also find many artful tips on food, spices, and herbs; cooking tasty and rejuvenating food was a joy of Yogi Bhajan. I'm so happy that this tremendous treasure trove of beautiful work on the anatomy of the physical and subtle body, especially as it applies to yoga, has fallen into your hands. Because of the high vibration that has gone into creating this work, it can only mean that you have great karma and are on your way to fulfilling your ultimate destiny. Enjoy it and use it well.

Best of Blessings.

Dr. Dharma Singh Khalsa, M.D.

President/Medical Director Alzheimer's Research and Prevention FoundationTucson, Arizona
Clinical Associate ProfessorUniversity of New Mexico School of Medicine Albuquerque, New Mexico

drdharma@alzheimersprevention.org

A Note to Teachers and Trainers

Japa Kaur and Nirmal Kaur have been teaching the Anatomy and Physiology segment of our Espanola, New Mexico Immersion Level One Teacher Training in Kundalini Yoga as taught by Yogi Bhajan® for several years. I have watched them use their engaging personalities to convey what can be very dry material to the students. This segment of the course, under their direction, garners great reviews from the students. Their presentations keep getting better and better over the years and I think there is a good reason why the students enjoy the presentation and are really able to understand this information in a very practical way. Integration is the key reason. When anatomy and physiology is taught in isolation from the etheric and energetic parts of Kundalini Yoga as taught by Yogi Bhajan® it is relevant but not very interesting. It is the blending of the two that holds the student's interest and is actually truer to the holistic nature of the yoga. There is a larger context to what Japa Kaur and Nirmal Kaur have done in their class presentations and in particular for this book. This book is attuned to the change of the times and is important for that change. The essence of this is explained by Yogi Bhajan in a lecture he gave July 12, 1992.

"Oh my mind you are a light of God, understand your own principle, in your own light, the problem which we are facing right today. In the exchange of Piscean to Aquarian Age is that you want somebody to do it for you. You want somebody to give it to you. The problem now is that you should give it to somebody, you should come out. You know how dreadful a human life is who said I don't know? You publicly confess it. You have no shame, you have no self-respect, you have no self-esteem. You just say, I don't know. What are you asking for, mercy? You don't know. What are you projecting? Escapism, because you don't know. What are you doing? Face to face you are lying. If you don't know, try to know and know it, assess it and then talk."

In short, Yogi Bhajan said, "This is the Aquarian Age. I know, therefore I believe. In the Piscean Age it was I believe therefore I know" (from July 15, 1981). Traditionally, the relationship between Yoga Teacher and student was one of acceptance and confidence in the teacher for the veracity and the relevance of the teachings. Now students want to know why it works, how it all fits together, what it means to them personally and mostly, they want to have a deep experience of consciousness in their yoga practice. As a reference book for teachers and students of Kundalini Yoga as taught by Yogi Bhajan® this book is invaluable. It explores Western and Eastern anatomy and blends in the subtle aspects of anatomy, chakras, bodies, meridians and flow of *praana*. A Teacher can use this information to inform and inspire their students. Having this knowledge will increase the awareness of a yoga student in their practice and deepen their experience and appreciation for the teachings.

   Nirvair Singh Khalsa, CEO
   Kundalini Research Institute

From the Authors

SAT NAM.

My fascination with the human body began on an experiential level. I loved to move and dance from an early age. I was in baby exercise classes with my mom before I could even walk!

By the time I started college my love of the body had deepened into a desire to explore the human experience through human movement. What I didn't expect was how much I would also enjoy the scientific study of the body through my anatomy and kinesiology classes. I loved learning about the details of the body and starting to see beneath the skin into the depths of our physical beings. As my interest in the human body expanded from artistic and experiential into inquisitive and scientific I found joy in the common ground that is human anatomy. In a rapidly changing world, I find it comforting that I am living in the same structure as my ancestors from thousands of years ago. Of course, anatomy and physiology is not a dead science; we're learning all the time about undiscovered structures, functions of organs, and the subtle relationships within the body. For me the study of the human body is the perfect balance of comforting familiarity and expanding understanding.

The practice of yoga brought me full circle by combining a direct experience of my body that complimented and enhanced my scientific study. It always bothered me that I had to separate my subtle experience of my body from my intellectual understanding of it. We are talking about the same thing after all: the human body. But my anatomy teachers had no interest in my subtle perception of organs, nor did my yoga teachers understand the specificity of the scientific view. I spent the next several years studying these different modalities in metaphorical silos but never found a source that brought them together as I experienced them. I knew that there had to be a way to hold these discrete perspectives in a single, global view of the human body. And so this book was born. I hope that it inspires in you a deep love and appreciation for your amazing human body.

Nirmal Lumpkin, LMT
St. Paul, Minnesota, USA

SAT NAM.

I believe the body is a treasure house of messages about your own path and truth. When I started my practice of Kundalini Yoga, I discovered that my body was my true friend and that it was always here in service. It is our soul's friend in this lifetime, and I have always wanted to help people develop a greater friendship with their human body, so that they suffer less and experience more joy. If the body is the friend instead of the enemy, it creates ease and grace in life. My hope is that this book will help different kinds of people learn new ways to have positive relationships with their own bodies.

In my role as a Doctor of Oriental Medicine, I help people cover the gaps in their lives physically, emotionally, and in realms that may not be visible to the naked eye. Because of my connection to the subtle realms through my work as a healer and yoga teacher, I wanted to share what I see as ways to access more of the body's power. When I adopted my son early in my process of writing this book with Nirmal, I felt that he helped strengthen my connection to intuition and vision through his Native American roots. My prayer is that this book helps you to believe and experience the possibilities for expansion by understanding both the physical and the subtle realms of being.

Blessings,

Japa Kaur Khalsa, DOM
Española, New Mexico, USA

Acknowledgments

We wish to thank the following people for their inspiration and encouragement: Yogi Bhajan, for the technology of Kundalini Yoga and Meditation, and so much more; Sat Purkh Kaur Khalsa, our friend, for the inspiration and encouragement to begin this project and take the first steps to actualize it; Sham Rang Singh Khalsa, MD, Shanti Shanti Kaur Khalsa, PhD, and Weston Cutter Jr. for reading early drafts and offering feedback and support; Nirvair Singh Khalsa, Shiva Singh Khalsa and Shabad Kaur Khalsa, Kirn Kaur Khalsa, Pritpal Kaur Khalsa, Sadh Bakshish Boyd, Hari Charn Kaur Khalsa and Arjan Kaur Khalsa for mentoring and guidance.

We are also grateful to Dharma Singh Khalsa, MD for his continued efforts and research in support of the teachings that inspired this book. And to our Ayurvedic friend and mentor Karta Purkh Singh Khalsa, Yogaraj (Ayurveda), DN-C, RH, CAP, LMT.

Thank you to our families: Harpal Singh Khalsa, Joyce Paxton and Weston Cutter, and Anne and Jim Weaver for logistical support, encouragement and faith that we could do it.

About Yogi Bhajan and Kundalini Yoga

YOGI BHAJAN:
Healer, Teacher, Master

Yogi Bhajan was a master of Kundalini Yoga and Meditation, but he was also a master healer in his own right. During his lifetime, Yogi Bhajan taught a multilayered view of health and healing. He shared with his students and other healers a wealth of knowledge related to energy healing and plant medicine.

On a daily basis, healers and students from all over the world joined Yogi Bhajan to discuss and practice various techniques. His expansive vision of health and healing drew from a wide range of approaches to health care including: medical doctors, indigenous healers, chiropractors, acupuncturists, bodyworkers, and energy workers. Yogi Bhajan believed in an integrative approach to wellness and encouraged healers to work together to create healing for the public.

His teachings included a deep understanding of acupuncture points, meridians, chakras, light bodies, herbs, as well as physical anatomy. His hands-on healing techniques included innovative ways for bodyworkers to manipulate and adjust the body. His understanding of Ayurvedic and Chinese medicine is evident in the breadth of information woven throughout his lectures. His understanding of the body's capacity to heal itself is intertwined in the actions of the thousands of yoga kriyas that were delivered through his life's work. His vision of healing included the world of plants, herbs, and food. He gave his students many opportunities to experiment in culinary herbalism and to use household remedies to support the body.

Kundalini Yoga as taught by Yogi Bhajan®

Kundalini Yoga was developed thousands of years ago by enlightened yogis in India. It was considered to be such a powerful practice that it was kept secret. Only after students had proved themselves worthy would a master begin to teach them the kriyas and meditations. Yogi Bhajan became a master of Kundalini Yoga when he was 16. He came to the United States in 1969 and realized that the time had come for these teachings to be made available

ENLIGHTENED BODIES

YOGI BHAJAN'S KITCHEN: Sat Sangat Singh's Story

Yogi Bhajan was blessed with an experimental and creative mind. His students would sometimes experience situations like this: Walking into Yogi Bhajan's Los Angeles home, they would be so happy to see yummy sandwiches laid out on a table. Imagine their surprise as they bit into the layers of bread, cheese, and veggies and realized that the sandwiches were dripping with the healing oils of camphor, eucalyptus, and other potent but smelly plants. "Eat it, these are good for you," he would bellow. This experimental approach to helping people experience the powerful world of plant medicine embodied the trial-and-error practice of a master with a true love of botanicals.

---

to anyone who wanted to learn. He spent the next 35 years teaching the technology of Kundalini Yoga and Meditation, Humanology, and Sikh Dharma.

Kundalini Yoga as taught by Yogi Bhajan® is a dynamic system including postures, breathing exercises, chanting, relaxation, and meditation. Kundalini Yoga sets are called kriyas and often focus on achieving a particular result such as helping a specific organ, body system, gland, chakra, clearing negative emotions, stabilizing the mind, or balancing energy in the body. Kundalini Yoga gives you the technology to understand and expand yourself on many levels.

In Kundalini Yoga as taught by Yogi Bhajan®, the 'seed mantra' is *Sat Naam*, which can be translated as "truth is my identity". This mantra allows you to tap into and develop a deep inner knowing. You come to realize the truth of who you are. You can also develop your intuition about your body and your experiences as a human being. When you realize *Sat Naam* you become the expert in every aspect of your life, including your body. And, if you think about it, no one else has had the opportunity to be with or study your body more than you—so you should be the expert! The technology of Kundalini Yoga helps you align with your own inner expert, effectively and quickly.

Kundalini Yoga Is A Wellness Yoga

When Yogi Bhajan taught Kundalini Yoga kriyas, often he would say that a set was for a particular thing (the liver or circulation, for example). It is tempting to use these sets as a prescription for someone with a particular disease or disorder. However, most kriyas that he said are "for something", he intended as prevention, not treatment. *We cannot emphasize this enough, unless you have specific advanced training, instructing a kriya that was "for something" to a person with that "something" would be an inappropriate application of Kundalini Yoga.*

Kundalini Yoga practice is meant as a way for people to maintain good health, and increase their awareness of their own lived experience. In fact, it is often advised to *avoid* kriyas targeted at a particular issue when the system is compromised in any way. It is possible that the intensity of a specific kriya could exacerbate the condition (Khalsa, SSK 2010).

Conversely, when Yogi Bhajan taught meditations, those are typically quite helpful to practice in support of what they are "for".

What to do as a Kundalini Yoga teacher? If you are teaching Kundalini Yoga to a person with a particular condition, the recommendation would be to instruct more general wellness and gentle healing yoga sets that provide support without exacerbating the issue. The meditation you instruct could be one that supports recovery from the condition. Pathology, diagnosis, and prescription are beyond the scope of this book.

Our intention is to provide information and tools for those who are relatively healthy to maintain and increase their sense of understanding of the body and their practice of wellness. If you need more information about the application of Kundalini Yoga for a particular pathology contact the Guru Ram Das Center for Medicine and Humanology. See *www.grdcenter.org* for more information.

The Human Body Is Awesome

This book will help you understand what a healthy body looks like when it functions properly. It will give you a broad perspective of the human body from both the physical and subtle perspectives. It will give you tools and techniques to keep a healthy body. And it will give you an understanding of how Kundalini Yoga specifically creates a state of balance, allowing for a sustained experience of health, vitality and expansion. This sets the stage for enlightenment, not as a lofty or far away goal, but a daily practice of being a source of light for oneself and others at any given moment.

Perspectives on the Body

The study of the human body, approached from several angles and perspectives, provides a richer understanding both of the body itself and of the human experience. To understand this mode of studying the human body, let's begin with an example: when you look at a statue if you stand in one place, you only see a small representation of what the artist created. When you walk around and experience the statue from various angles, you begin to appreciate the full extent of the artist's vision. The goal of looking at a statue is not to integrate the many different perspectives into a unified vision of the statute. That is to say, you are not trying to find the *one, right way* to see the statue. Rather by seeing the work from all sides you are able to appreciate and understand the complexity and subtle beauty of the whole in a new way. Each perspective is as much a part of the experience of the statue as any other. Seeing each side serves to inform the view from all other sides.

The goal of this type of seeing, whether it's applied to a statue or the human body, is to appreciate the complexity of the various perspectives and their individual contribution to the experience of the whole. By studying the body from a variety of perspectives you begin to appreciate and understand your own humanness on a more profound level. The goal is not to synthesize all of these perspectives into one vision or to be able

Our hope is that the knowledge of how the body works will reveal the inner secrets of power and peace you already hold within.

"Be the Lighthouse."
© The Teachings of
Yogi Bhajan, April 14, 1987

Exploring Physical and Subtle Human Anatomy

1.0 The David Statue

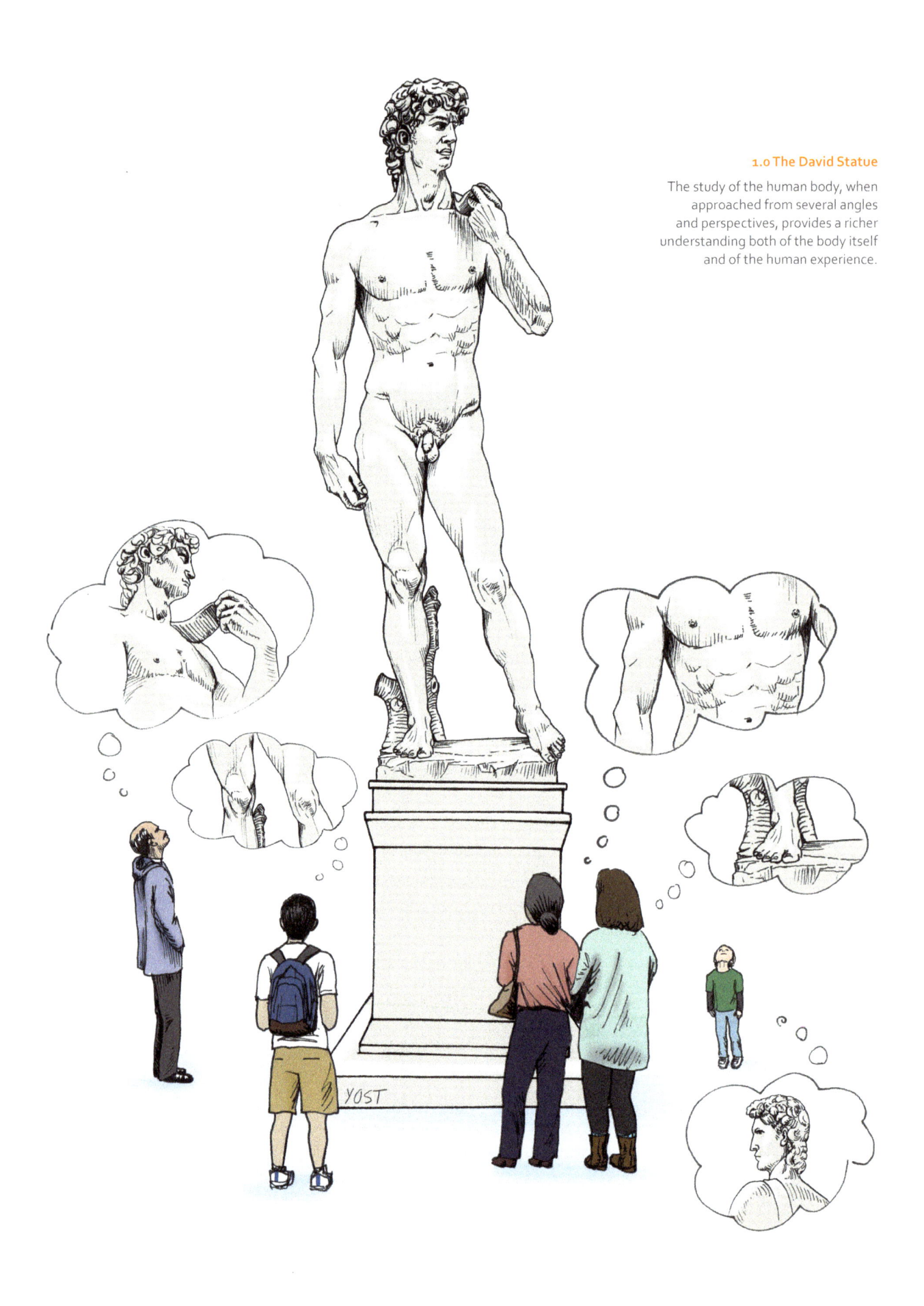

The study of the human body, when approached from several angles and perspectives, provides a richer understanding both of the body itself and of the human experience.

to point to the *one, right way* to know the body. Instead the goal is to see, experience and appreciate the full extent of the human experience, in all its simplicity, complexity and coarse beauty.

Physical anatomy and subtle anatomy are merely different angles on the human body. They work together in intricate ways to create your experience of this human life. There is no single cell, organ or energy center in the body that you could point to and say, "There! That spot is where I am." Existence is a much more complicated network of physical components, empty space, consciousness, and soul. The physical body without the animation of the soul is an empty shell. The *praana*, without the lungs to take it in, is formless. By understanding the human body's physical and subtle structures from a cognitive *and* experiential perspective, we create a deep well of knowledge that allows us to heal and uplift ourselves.

The Human Body in Harmony

The human body is a physical vessel for experience and links to both the earthly plane and the infinity of the heavens. The body, a universe within itself, each system of the body, each organ, every cell work together to complete a vast number of tasks on a daily and even momentary basis. The rhythms of each system work in harmony to create the baseline of your body. Being in this particular body at this particular moment is a complicated symphony of physical and subtle systems working together.

In the study of the body, the whole is greater than the sum of its parts. Magical things happen when all of the systems are working in rhythm, together, which aren't necessarily understood by looking at a part individually. Understanding the physical and subtle structures and how they work together serves to enhance your practice of yoga and meditation. Appreciation of the complexity of your human anatomy inspires living a light-filled life.

THE SUBTLE AND PHYSICAL BODY: A Vehicle for Experience

When we apply a yogic perspective to anatomy and physiology, the elaborate design of our bodies can be seen as more than just a composite of chemicals, structures, and processes. We begin to understand the physical body as a vehicle to experience life. Knowledge about your body will open

> *"The body is a sacred garment: it is what you enter life in and what you depart life with, and it should be treated with honor, and with joy and with fear as well. But always, though, with blessing."*
>
> —Martha Graham, dancer, choreographer and author

The study of the body inspires appreciation for its elaborate design. When moving through life, take a moment to reflect on all the activities happening in each moment and be inspired.

Right now, happening in your body without conscious effort:
- *Breath*
- *Heartbeat*
- *Digestion*
- *Postural balance*
- *Sight*
- *Proprioception (Awareness of Body Position)*
- *Hearing*

you up to greater awareness and take you to new depths in your practice of yoga and meditation. In turn, practicing yoga develops awareness and present-moment consciousness by tuning you in to the physical body and cultivating attentiveness to sensations in the body in each moment of the practice. Take, for example, a simple forward fold. As you come in to the posture you may feel tightness or unease. These sensations are your body's request for you to pay attention. Often as you continue with the exercise the sensation changes, the hamstrings release and you experience the feeling of letting go. Through this experience we come in to a deeper relationship with the capacity to soften into resistance. As you continue to practice, there will be thousands of these valuable moments to cultivate awareness.

The human body has an incredible capacity for divine states like pleasure and joy, and it is ultimately the vehicle that brings us to liberation. It is not *in spite* of your humanness that you can experience divine truth it is *because* of it. Your body, and your experience within it, is your guide. While it is important to learn about and understand the vehicle, don't make the mistake of forgetting the value and depth of your own experience of humanness.

Nirmal's Practice Story

I use my anatomical knowledge to stay grounded during my practice. I may have done a particular exercise hundreds of times, so it would be easy to let my mind wander away. In those moments I reconnect to my physical body, asking myself, *What muscles are active?* and *What organs are being stimulated by this pose?* These questions keep me focused. Working with and from my physical body is one way I have found that helps me to go more deeply into and stay more present in my practice.

Cultivating that small awareness develops the skills to experience the big awareness that is the goal of a meditative path.

The Messages of the Body

The physical and subtle design and structure of the human body are filled with messages, gifts, and lessons that can bring expanded awareness to life. When we look to the body to find those messages, all types of metaphors, reminders, and reassurances that this human life has meaning are revealed. Choose to look carefully at the body; hear its messages for they will bring you closer to your spiritual path.

Physical anatomy is dense, palpable, and visible. When you start paying attention, its messages are like giant flashing billboards. Although a microscope can't see the subtle aspects of anatomy, and your hand may not be able to feel them, they are still there. The messages of the subtle anatomy are softer, more intuitive, and more fluid. All of these lessons help create meaning and balance in our existence. Feeling lost or directionless is part of being human. The complexity of life cannot have it any other way. When you feel lost or directionless on the path, stop and listen, let the body point the way. Observe your breath and be comforted by the remembrance of your place within the scheme of the universe. Or when you feel isolated and lonely, feel your heart beat and remember the heart's lesson to serve and help others as a means of fulfilling a higher destiny.

"Recognize that the other person is you."
—Yogi Bhajan's First Sutra for the Aquarian Age

All of Us Are Human

The study of anatomy and physiology reveals our shared human experience. While there is a certain amount of variation in physical and subtle structures in individuals, the more dominant theme is one of similarity. Across races, cultures, and religions we are more similar than we are different.

You share the same anatomy and physiology with the billions of others on this planet, so while you may believe your experience is unique, those billions of others are having similar experiences. When you connect more deeply with your own body, you begin to appreciate and feel resonance with all those other souls.

Tapping into the shared structures and the common experience of being human is a cornerstone of a spiritual practice. When we think of the great lights in human history (Dr. Martin Luther King Jr., Mahatma Ghandi, Mother Theresa, or Buddha) we recognize that they, too, were human. We have every tool and capacity that they had. Feeling commonality with the lives of these great masters is an inspiration to become the lighthouse for spiritual awakening for yourself and for others.

When we look into the structure of our bodies we realize we carry with us our very own road map to living an elevated life.

"Blessed are those who bless themselves. Gracious are those who put their grace in front of all... Truthful are those who explain things to the best of their knowledge. And highest are those who pick up the lowliest with all their effort. This life is a test of polarity and its composition is based on one's action. Those who love themselves can share the love with others. That's the bliss. Those who redeem themselves and lead the people to the path are blessed ones in the eyes of God. And those who keep in mind the happiness and the grace of others are blessed Gods living in human bodies.... May you all be virtuous and your values... be so beautiful and attractive that they can give a message by itself and may Almighty God give you the strength. Sat Naam."

© The Teachings of Yogi Bhajan,
February 3, 2000

2.0 Bridge Pose with Chakras and Organs

Bridge Pose is a balancing and grounding posture with the palms of the hands and soles of the feet touching the ground. This posture activates all the major muscles in the back, brings energy to the internal organs and opens the chakras.

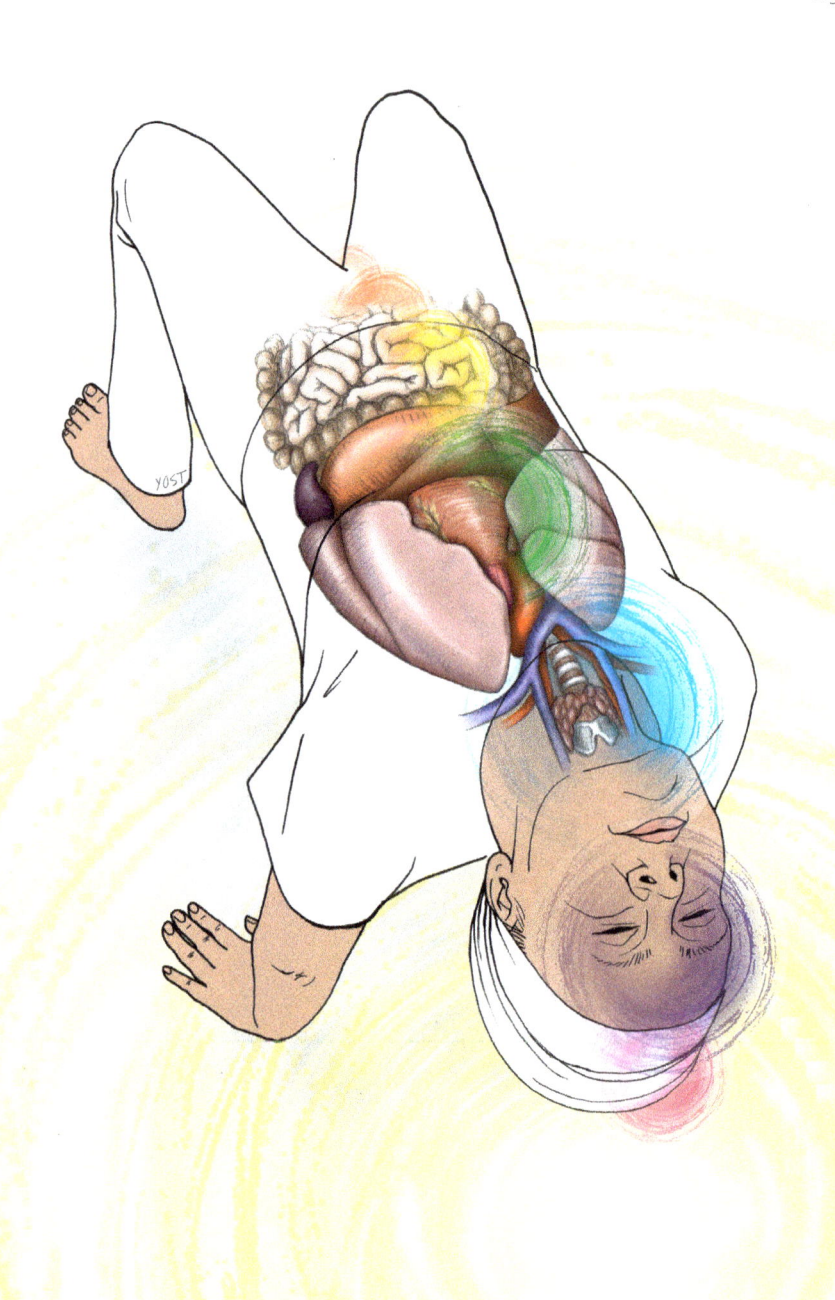

The Subtle Human Body

A yogi experiences her body with creativity and refinement. In her mind's eye she travels through veins and organs, sensing, feeling, and knowing her body intimately. In meditation she deeply listens to the messages of the chakras and meridians, spontaneously knowing where there are blocks, or which areas need more investigation. The yogi, in quiet stillness, opens her awareness and finds the physical and subtle structures of her perfect human body continually pointing her toward her goals: balance, expansion and self-realization.

What do we see when we walk around a human figure and view it from a subtle anatomy perspective? We see all types of energetic, yogic, mystical, esoteric, or metaphysical anatomy, structures, vortexes, and pathways of energy in the human body. The structures in subtle anatomy are not necessarily seen with the physical eyes, but they are still potent factors in being human and being in your body.

What Is *Subtle Anatomy*?

- Yogic Anatomy, Chinese Medicine, Ayurveda, Humanology
- Consciousness, Emotion, Feeling and Intuition: subtle energies that are often unseen or unobserved
- Pervading and underlying visible and mechanical anatomy and physiology

Just like in the physical anatomy there are messages and metaphors within the subtle structures of the body. Where the lessons of the physical anatomy often relate to and support our journey of humanness, the lessons of the subtle anatomy serve as a compass on the soul's journey toward its destiny. Practices like yoga, meditation, and contemplation expand the capacity for witnessing subtlety and finding the soul lessons placed within the energy pathways, emotional experiences and metaphysical components of the human body.

Exploring Physical and Subtle Human Anatomy

2.1 Camel Pose with Chakras

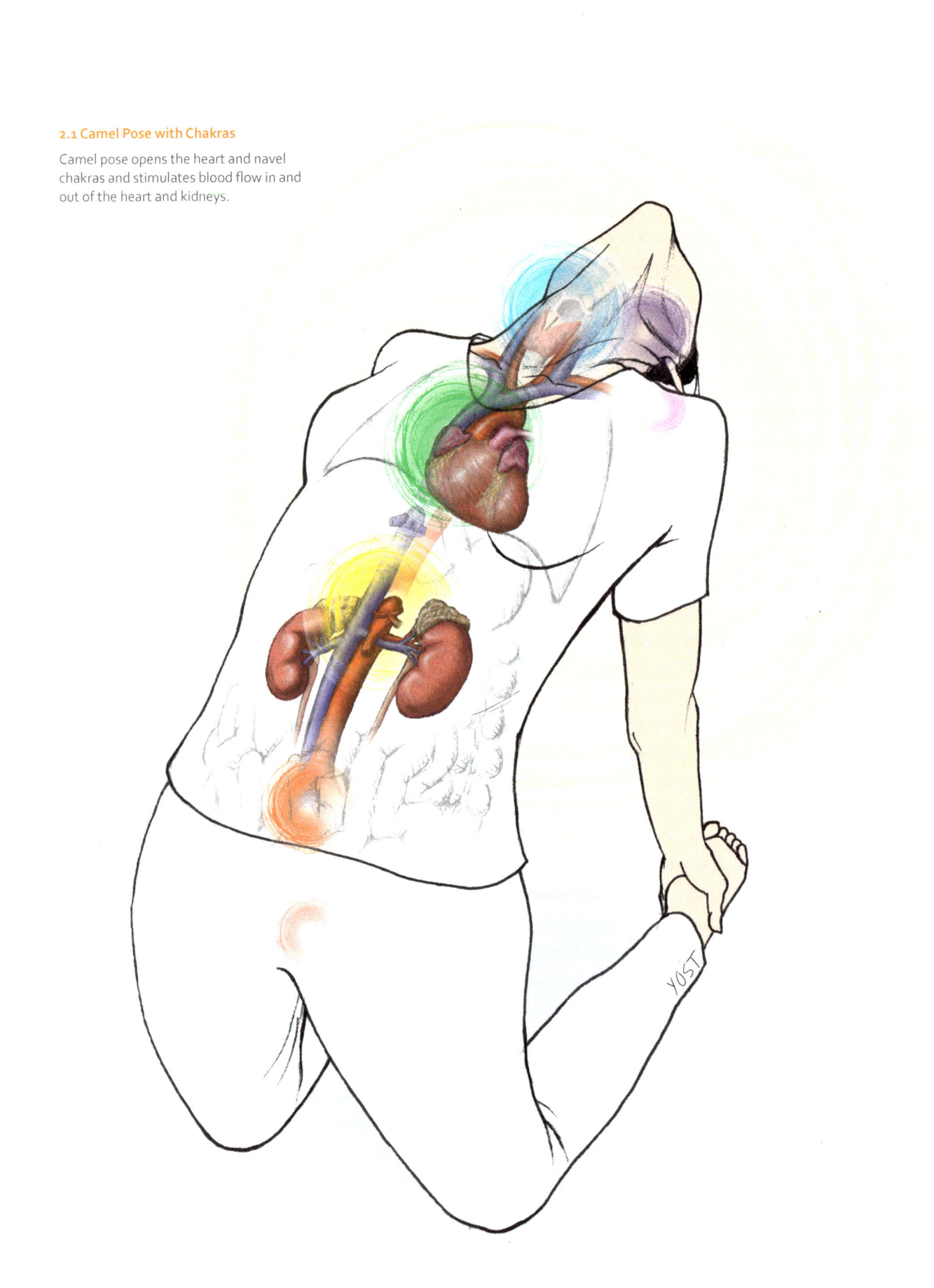

Camel pose opens the heart and navel chakras and stimulates blood flow in and out of the heart and kidneys.

Because the subtle anatomy can't be touched or seen with a microscope, the messages are sensed differently. They may show up as dreams, longings, visions, or flashes of insight. They may also present themselves in one's personal astrology or numerology, repetitive patterns of behavior and recognizing when something feels imbalanced.

Your higher self has certain soul contracts that are part of the core destiny that you came here to serve. Your body is the vehicle for doing this destiny work. Your physical and subtle anatomy connects you to your soul's vast capacity for spiritual learning. The signals and cues that it gives are reminders of the karmas that you have come here to pay and the higher destiny that your body and soul are here to serve.

Knowing how the body is working, in its most subtle levels, deepens your understanding of health and disease. Familiarity with how your body works allows you to make adjustments and take preventive measures to support a better quality of life. At the level of physical anatomy there is concern for how things *function* mechanically. At the level of subtle anatomy there is concern for how things *feel* intuitively.

The Chakra System

The word *chakra* refers to the four dimensional, circular energy centers in the body. They exist beyond the three dimensional physical structure of the body and include the etheric realms. This traditionally Hindu way of looking at the body developed many thousands of years ago in India and has become a common perspective across many schools of yoga and meditation. Most schools talk about seven chakras (see the appendix for a detailed chart and look for chakra spotlights throughout the book). In Kundalini Yoga the aura is considered the Eighth Chakra.

Each chakra relates to a physical area of the body, to specific body systems, and to a particular emotional or energetic capacity of a human being. Ideally, the chakras are in balance and working to support us throughout life. However, due to a variety of reasons, personal or impersonal history, one's karmas, or traumas, the chakras can become out of balance. When a chakra is either too weak or too domineering, it expresses what is known as the *shadow emotion* of the chakra. In this book we use the chakras as a teaching tool to find the crossroads between the physical and subtle anatomy. However, the relationship is not a one-to-one ratio, some body systems correlate with more

Your body is one of your primary teachers in life.

The goal is not to find the one right way to view, understand or work with the body. The goal is simply to see it from multiple perspectives and allow the information to coexist and lead to a deeper relationship with our bodies, our health, and ourselves.

2.2 The Chakra System

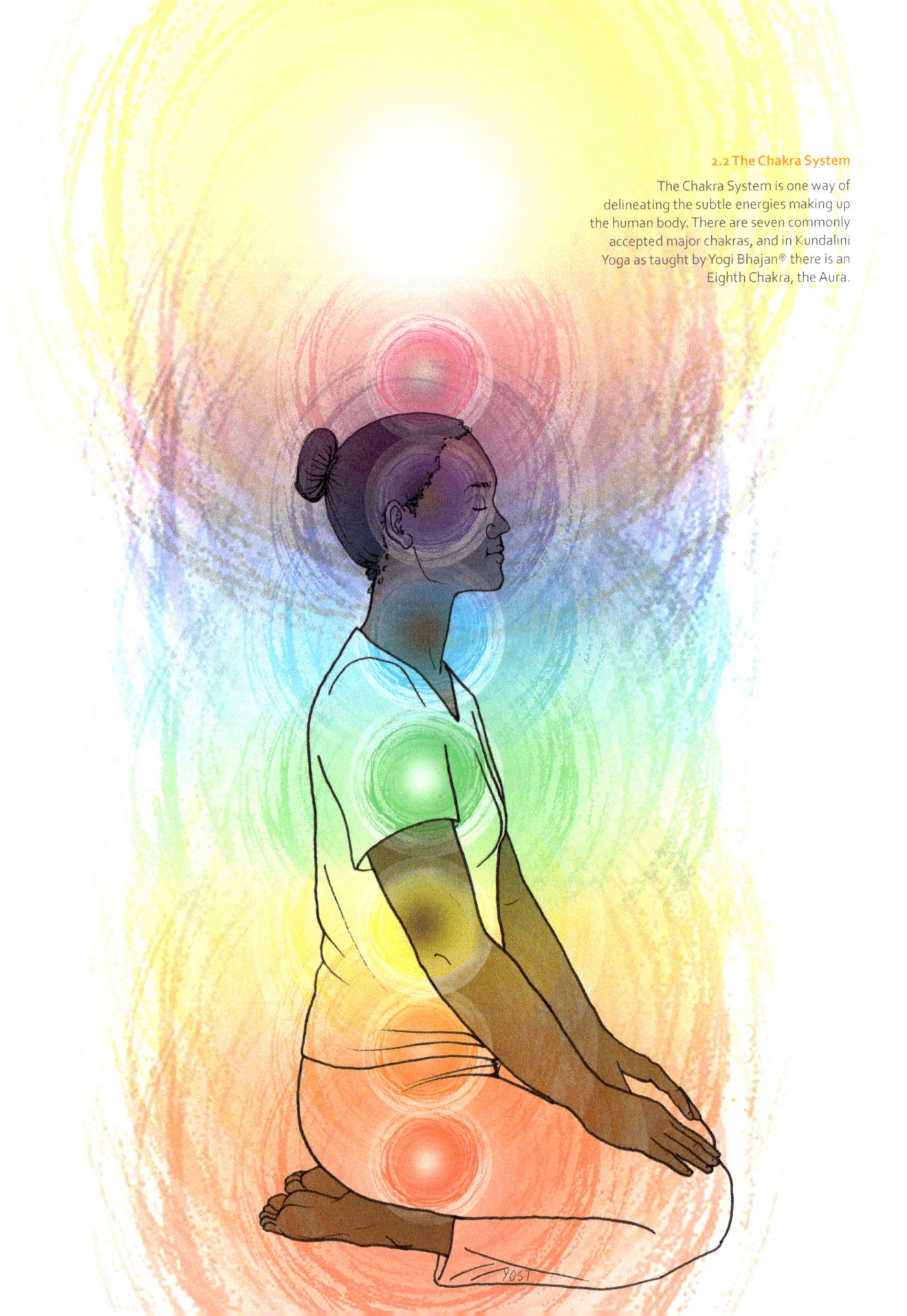

The Chakra System is one way of delineating the subtle energies making up the human body. There are seven commonly accepted major chakras, and in Kundalini Yoga as taught by Yogi Bhajan® there is an Eighth Chakra, the Aura.

than one chakra, some chakras with more than one body system. Because the chakras support physical reality but exist in a subtle reality, this is not an exact science but our exploration of how the physical systems intersect with the chakras, and we hope you find it useful in your practice.

The first three chakras, known in Kundalini Yoga as the "Lower Triangle", are primarily concerned with the energy of living in a human body: processing food and energy, reproduction and elimination. The remaining chakras, called the "Upper Triangle," begin to tap into the energy that moves us beyond physical survival and into our humanity, uplifted consciousness, and connection to something larger than ourselves.

People often mistakenly believe that the goal of a yoga practice is to learn to live completely in the upper chakras. Instead, it is important to balance the entire chakra system and to learn to direct the energy centers rather than to completely disregard the lower triangle. First, it is not possible while still living in human form. And second, we are in this human body for a reason; this human body is a vehicle for true liberation of the soul. We use our bodies to heal, serve, and uplift others.

The flow of energy through the chakras begins from the Navel Center, or Third Chakra. When activated, the energy moves down and pools in the Root Chakra. The **First Chakra,** or **Root Chakra,** encompasses the tailbone, legs, feet, colon, and urinary system. It is the base of stability in life and links the soul to the physical body. When energy circulates freely here, a person will be steady and calm. That calmness can even pass to others and create more steadiness in an entire group.

The confidence that comes from stability in the Root Chakra allows for an easy grace of letting go of what isn't needed. During times where the Root Chakra is unbalanced, there will be feelings of doubt, anxiety and an overwhelming feeling of lack (Bhajan, 2010). These feelings can be enhanced or shifted as the energy moves upward into the Second Chakra and beyond. In Chapter 10, we study and use the Root Chakra to inform our understanding of the urinary system, see page 209.

As energy shifts upward and flows into the **Second Chakra,** or **Sacral Chakra,** feelings of creativity, passion and pleasure are initiated. Here, the reproductive organs and the human desire for connection are sheltered. The ability for balance in sexuality is held in the area of the sacrum, hips and pelvis.

A healthy Sacral Chakra fosters creativity in many forms, including: artistic pursuits, sexuality and a life with purpose. Without the right amount and

> *"Our bodies are like complex worlds within worlds. We know where they begin and end, and yet they are vast and full of mysteries, which we may never understand. No machine has ever been devised by a human that is as complex or artful as our own human body. The ancient system of the chakras is a way to understand ourselves. There is an incredible amount of subtle interaction going on all the time."*
>
> —Gurumukh Kaur Khalsa, *The Eight Human Talents*

intensity of energy flow here, a person may become frigid or hypersexual (Bhajan, 2010). In Chapter 11, we study and use the Second Chakra to inform our understanding of the reproductive system.

Individuality begins to emerge as energy moves up to the **Third Chakra,** or **Navel Chakra**. This chakra is located in the center of the body and comprises the solar plexus, digestive organs, abdominal muscles, and mid-back. When the navel is strong, we experience a spark of willpower and a zest for life. Supported by a strong First, Second, and Third Chakra, a person can follow through on commitments and become known for leadership. When the navel energy is not flowing, the shadow of depression, lethargy, and apathy arise. Power struggles with others crop up and as the energy tries to right itself, and anger and harshness can leak into communication. An extremely unbalanced Navel Chakra results in the abuse of power (Bhajan, 2010). In Chapter 9, we study and use the Navel Chakra to inform our understanding of the digestive system.

The energy of the Navel Chakra is power. But the hope of living from a more elevated state lies in the movement of energy up toward the Heart Chakra. Compassion-based leadership arises as the navel's power is filtered through the **Fourth Chakra,** the **Heart Chakra**. The Heart Chakra's position between the lower triangle and the upper triangle gives it a special role in transformation. As the Heart Chakra's energy activates, alignment with love and forgiveness emerges, which influences the entire chakra system.

The Heart Chakra contains critical organs such as the heart, lungs, ribs, and thymus gland, as well the extremities, the shoulders, arms and hands. A well-developed Heart Chakra allows for the experience of love, compassion, service, and forgiveness. A weak heart center creates a sense of neediness, becoming a doormat, or burning out by giving beyond one's capacity to give (Bhajan, 2010). In Chapter 3, we study and use the Heart Chakra to inform our understanding of the circulatory system.

The energy continues its upward movement as it circulates in the **Fifth Chakra,** or **Throat Chakra**. The ability to speak the truth and influence with the power of the word is invoked by a strong Throat Chakra. The physical area includes the trachea, esophagus, vocal cords, thyroid gland, and cervical vertebrae. When the flow of energy is strong and supported by an expansive Heart Chakra, one can authentically connect with other people through the voice. An unsupported Throat Chakra will reveal the shadow emotions of

> *"Power without love is reckless and abusive, and love without power is sentimental and anemic. Power at its best is love implementing the demands of justice, and justice at its best is power correcting everything that stands against love."*
>
> Dr. Martin Luther King Jr., minister, civil rights activist, Nobel Peace Prize winner

being overly harsh with the word or being afraid to speak up or live your truth (Bhajan, 2010). In Chapter 4, we study and use the Throat Chakra to inform our understanding of the respiratory system.

The energy, propelled by the power of the word, continues upward until it concentrates at the **Sixth Chakra,** or **Third Eye Point**, the seat of intuition. The Third Eye shares the physical space of the pituitary gland, brain, forehead, eyes, ears, eyebrows, upper palate and sinuses. When activated, the Third Eye opens up deep and meaningful insights. The Third Eye must be supported by all the lower chakras in order to be awakened. Otherwise its shadow emerges: spiritual dullness, indecisiveness and lack of depth (Bhajan, 2010). In Chapter 8, we study and use the Third Eye in more depth to inform our understanding of the endocrine system.

The final activation for the energy pathway within the physical body is the **Seventh Chakra,** or **Crown Chakra**, sometimes referred to as the thousand-petal lotus. In meditation one of the primary goals is to awaken the Crown Chakra and to experience the blossoming of the lotus flower. At the very top of the head it encompasses the pineal gland and the skull and its energy extends upward and around the entire body. The Crown Chakra is known as the seat of the soul and activating it awakens the soul's connection to the Divine. Its influence is most clearly revealed after the energy reaches its apex and turns downward, dripping the nectar back down through the chakras, healing and uplifting them all. An inactivated Crown Chakra can lead to unexplained or unrelenting grief and a sense of disconnect from other people and the Divine (Bhajan, 2010). In Chapter 8, we study and use the Crown Chakra to inform our understanding of the endocrine system.

In some traditions the understanding of the major chakras of the human body ends with the Crown Chakra. In Kundalini Yoga, however, Yogi Bhajan talked about the aura, which extends out around the entire physical body, as the Eighth Chakra, or Aura, one of the Ten Light Bodies in the teachings of Yogi Bhajan and will be discussed in-depth here. Read more about the Aura in the endocrine system chapter.

Viewing the human body from diverse perspectives expands the understanding of the self, deepens the practice of yoga and meditation, and expands the capacity for wellness.

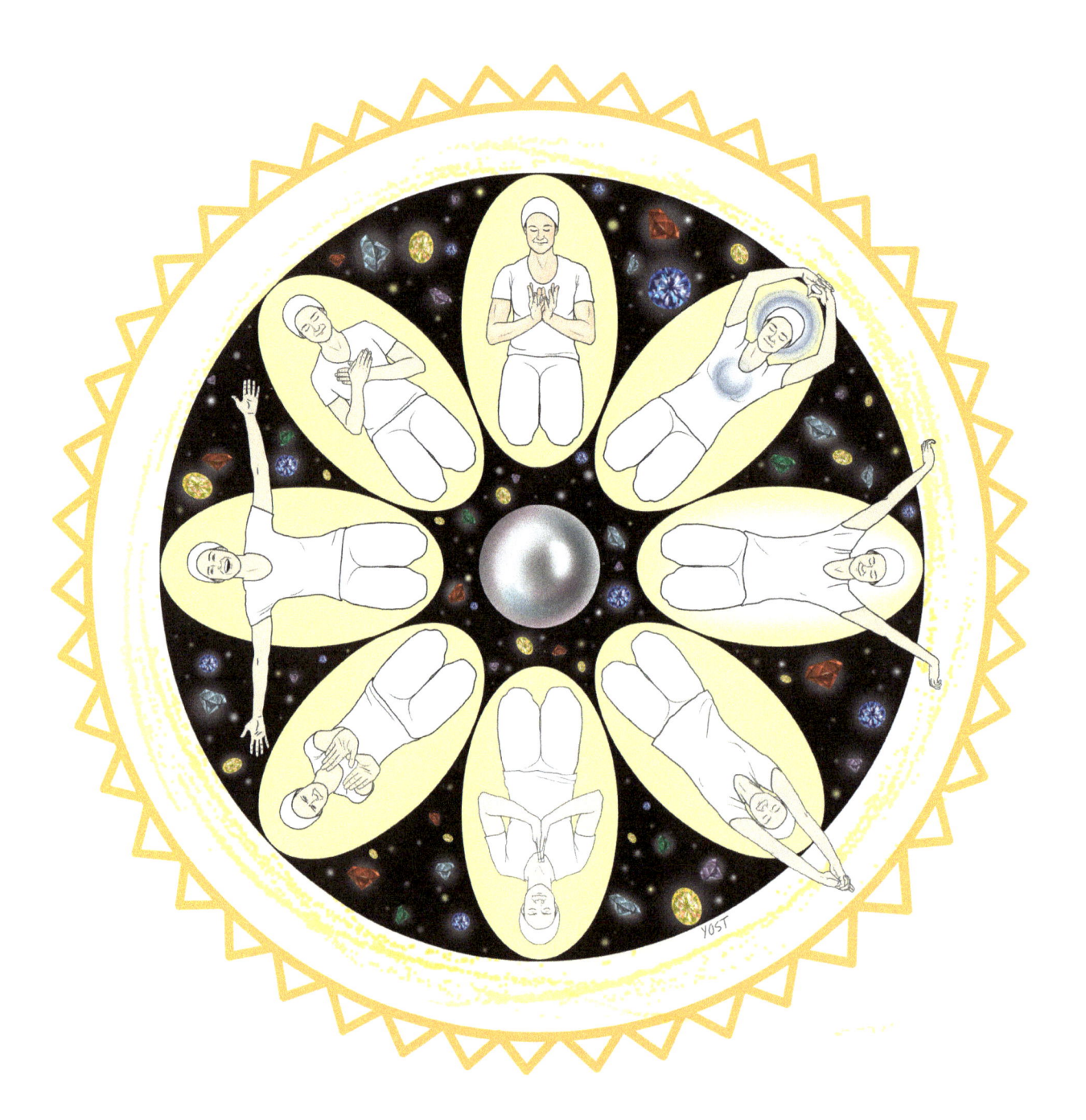

2.3 The Ten Light Bodies

The authors' symbolic representation of the Ten Light Bodies as taught by Yogi Bhajan. Distinct from the chakra system, the Ten Light Bodies adds subtlety and nuance on the Kundalini yoga path.

The First Body—the Soul Body—is represented by the pearl in the center of the drawing; the Tenth Body—the Radiant Body—is represented by the Golden Circle. The other Light Bodies are represented by the mudras and their energies.

The Ten Light Bodies

Yogi Bhajan taught another way of understanding the subtle anatomy, which he called the Ten Bodies. As human beings, we primarily identify with the physical body. But in this way of looking at the body, the physical form is only one tenth of our entire existence. The Ten Bodies should not be misunderstood as a hierarchy, but rather as ten powerful and available tools. As understanding develops around each of the Ten Light Bodies, we have the ability to harness and direct each of their capacities to live with more awareness (Bhajan, 2010).

Tantric Numerology

One way to work with the Ten Light Bodies is through tantric numerology, the study of your individual numerology through birth date analysis. Your personal numbers provide a window into understanding your own gifts and challenges as you interact with the surrounding world. They can also reveal insights into how you are interlocked with a greater and more expansive cycle of time and alignment with the stars and heavens (Khalsa, 1994).

Like the more familiar chakra system, we use the Ten Light Bodies as a teaching tool to find the crossroads between the physical and subtle anatomy. The relationship is not one-to-one and some systems correlate with more than one Body, and some Bodies with more than one system. The parallels drawn here are for you to use to enrich your own understanding.

THE FIRST LIGHT BODY: The Soul Body is the essence of *you* contained within each cell of your body; it is your own embodiment of the infinite. The Soul Body is one of the Ten Bodies that travels with you throughout multiple lifetimes. When balanced you feel connected to your purpose and destiny. You express wisdom, faith and grit. The Soul Body *is* you. A strong connection to the Soul Body allows you to self-initiate on the path of awareness, contemplation, or personal growth. When out of balance, you feel lost or tend to overanalyze everything (Bhajan, 2010). In Chapter 3, we study and use the Soul Body to inform our understanding of the musculoskeletal system.

THE SECOND LIGHT BODY: The Negative Mind gives you discernment and protection, which is why it is also sometimes called the protective mind. When balanced, the Negative Mind warns of potential dangers, both real and imagined. When out of balance it makes you scared of, or stressed by everything, and you can only see the down side of any situation (Bhajan, 2010). In Chapter 10, we study and use the Negative Mind to inform our understanding of the urinary system.

THE THIRD LIGHT BODY: The Positive Mind opens you up to the possibility in every moment. When balanced, the Positive Mind acts like the cheerleader within. You always see the silver lining and are willing to take the risks necessary to live the life you're here to live. When out of balance you think everything is okay even in the face of overwhelming evidence to the contrary, and you become ineffective (Bhajan, 2010). In Chapter 10, we study and use the Positive Mind to inform our understanding of the urinary system.

THE FOURTH LIGHT BODY: The Neutral Mind finds the win-win in any situation. When balanced it is meditative and exists beyond the polarity of "good" and "bad." Decisions made from the Neutral Mind always bring alignment with destiny for the self and your community. When out of balance or weak there is an obsession with weighing the pros and cons and a lack of ability to make decisions (Bhajan, 2010). In Chapter 4, we study and use the Neutral Mind to inform our understanding of the circulatory system.

THE FIFTH LIGHT BODY: The Physical Body is the nucleus of the other nine Light Bodies. It contains aspects of the Mental, Soul, and Subtle Bodies. It is surrounded by the Arcline, Aura, and Radiant Body. The Pranic Body exists inside and outside of the Physical Body. When it is balanced, the other bodies can flourish and there is strength to comfortably share with others in the role of a teacher. When overly expressed, there can be narcissism and too much concern with perfection of the Physical Body (Bhajan, 2010). In Chapter 3, we study and use the Physical Body to inform our understanding of the musculoskeletal system.

THE SIXTH LIGHT BODY: The Arcline is a line of energy that extends over the head from ear to ear (imagine halos in medieval religious paintings). Women have a second Arcline that extends in front of the body from nipple to nipple, which creates the safe nurturing space necessary if they choose to have children and breastfeed. A strong Arcline gives the power of prayer—the power to take the desire to serve humanity out of the theoretical and into every day action. With a weak Arcline, it is easy to feel overexposed to other people's misery or sadness; and when overwhelmed by all the pain in the world, one is unable to act effectively (Bhajan, 2010). In Chapters 6 and 11, we study and use the Arcline to inform our understanding of the immune system and the reproductive system.

THE SEVENTH LIGHT BODY: The Aura is an electromagnetic field around the human body. It extends up to nine feet (3 meters) around the body, and when balanced creates a sense of presence and charisma. When this field is weak, a person might try to take energy from other people or things. Addictions can be a problem as the person is reaching for a false sense of expansion of the Aura (Bhajan, 2010). In Chapters 8 and 9, we study and use the Aura to inform our understanding of the endocrine and digestive systems.

THE EIGHTH LIGHT BODY: The Pranic Body shifts the energy of the body with each breath. With a strong Pranic Body one is able to shift gears between action and relaxation with ease. A weak Pranic Body leads to shortness of breath, panic that there won't be enough, and greediness (Bhajan, 2010). In Chapter 5, we study and use the Pranic Body to inform our understanding of the respiratory system.

THE NINTH LIGHT BODY: The Subtle Body notices everything in stillness and creates through the power of silence. The second of the Light Bodies that travels with you across lifetimes, the Subtle Body exists beyond time and space and is known for carrying the soul to liberation. Cultivated through steady discipline, which leads to mastery, a person whose Subtle Body is developed without the intention to apply that mastery to serve or support others can be perceived as high maintenance, difficult, or overly picky (Bhajan, 2010). In Chapter 11, we study and use the Subtle Body to inform our understanding of the reproductive system.

THE TENTH LIGHT BODY: The Radiant Body energetically contains all of the other Light Bodies. It creates the seal of the entire system, like the cherry on top of the sundae. The first nine Bodies are about individual perception of the world; the Radiant Body is about their projection *into* the world. A strong Radiant Body creates a clear projection, authentic interactions with others, and an overall well-balanced life. An underdeveloped Radiant Body leads to absolutist black-and-white thinking and a "my way or the highway" attitude (Bhajan, 2010). In Chapter 7, we study and use the Radiant Body to inform our understanding of the nervous system.

Naadis

Naadis are channels of subtle energy flowing through the body. They pulsate through and affect all layers of the physical and subtle anatomy. *Naadis* are a subtle web linking together the various energy centers and structures in and around the human body. *Naadis* carry energy and support the interplay among the chakras, Light Bodies, physical organs, consciousness and karmic energies. When all of the *naadis* are active and flowing there is a sense of overall health, lightness and expansive potential.

Yogis teach that there are 72,000 of these *naadis* or currents starting at the Navel Point and flowing in and around the body, ending at the hands and feet. The three principle currents are the *ida*, the *pingala* and the *sushmana*. The *sushmana* is known as the silver cord and is the central and most important channel. Activation of the *sushmana* during meditation cleanses all of the other *naadis.* Since all *naadis* meet at the Navel Point, this gives us yet another good reason to cultivate a strong navel center (Bhajan, 2010).

When the *naadis* are blocked, imbalanced or lack flow, problems will inevitably arise. Imagine your *naadis* like a network of garden hoses. If there is a kink in a hose, the water cannot flow to its intended destination easily. Yoga, breathwork and meditation help to open up the flow of energy through the *naadis*. When *naadis* unblock there can be a buzzing, or pulsing feeling, much like the gush of water when a kink is let out of a garden hose.

The *naadis* are akin to the meridians of Chinese medicine. They are essentially the same structure viewed through a different historical and cultural lens. The *naadis* are from the Ayurvedic system and are connected to the chakras. The meridians are from the Chinese medicine system and are connected to acupuncture points and internal organs.

The Subtle Human Body

Japa's Yogic Kitchen

Years of living in a yogic kitchen have made me comfortable adding spices and herbs to my cooking. I notice that when I start to get a cold I gravitate towards onion soup with garlic and ginger or when I'm feeling depleted I make myself mung beans and rice. Over the years, I realized I was practicing the wisdom of Ayurveda and the tradition of cleansing and rejuvenating the body through healing foods.

Ayurveda

Yoga has a sister science known as Ayurveda. Yogi Bhajan often taught the principles of Ayurveda, without directly referencing it as the science of Ayurveda. Considered the mother of the healing arts, Ayurveda is one of the earliest documented systems of healing that exists today. Ayurveda awakens healing potential for the individual as it addresses the roots of illness and the body-mind-spirit connection.

The herbs and plants in *Enlightened Bodies* are from both the Chinese and Ayurvedic traditions. Our goal is to present you with a simple and likely familiar body of herbs that you can use for yourself and your family.

The Elements in Ayuvedic Medicine

ETHER
AIR
FIRE
WATER
EARTH

Tattvas

In Yoga Philosophy, the *tattvas* are the elements that form the universe; they are earth, water, fire, air and ether. They interact in continual cycles of activity and rest, and their interplay makes up our reality, both subtle and physical.

The *tattvas* support both material existence and the ephemeral experience of life in the human body. There are many ways to define the *tattvas* and slight differences in their understanding depend on the different perspectives. The Ayurvedic or yogic system has roots in Vedic philosophy and strives for balance in the *tattvas*. The Subtle Anatomy perspective sections of this book speak mostly of the Ayurvedic or yogic understanding and presents how the *tattvas* are affected by and affect the Physical Anatomy.

Each physical system has a dynamic mix of all five *tattvas* (Bhajan, 2010). The energetic essence of a particular *tattva* can be strongly correlated to one system and working on balancing that *tattva* can bring harmony to that system.

The Elements in Chinese Medicine

EARTH
METAL
WATER
WOOD
FIRE

In Chinese medicine the five *Elements* form an interdependent cycle of support. They are the core of the body's ability to change or shift physical health, mental states, or emotional experiences. See the Chinese medicine *Element* charts in the appendices (page 259) for a wonderful visual diagram explaining how these *Elements* tie in to various meridians, body systems and even times of the day.

Doshas

In Ayurveda, the mix of *tattvas* in a person is said to determine their constitution. The three main types of constitutions, called *doshas*, are *Vata*, *Pitta* and *Kapha*.

- *Vata* is a mix of air and ether (space)
- *Pitta* is fire with some water
- *Kapha* is earth and water

Each person's constitution includes a combination of these *doshas*, and usually has a tendency toward one. In this model, understanding your natural *dosha* and working to create a more balanced relationship between the elements supports health. You can increase or decrease the effects of each *dosha* by lifestyle practices and diet (Lad, 2009).

Vata

A person with a predominantly *Vata* physique will express the qualities of air and ether. They will be fast-moving, creative, thin and a free spirit. A *Vata* will become imbalanced through stress, overwork, overwhelm or eating dry and hard to digest foods on the run. When they tip too far into their airy nature they will start to appear fragmented or flaky to others. When a *Vata* type is out of balance, it is necessary to nurture the earth and water elements to help restore balance in the body (Chopra, n.d.).

Some current standards of living contribute to chronic *Vata* imbalance (see the Nervous System chapter, page 129). Because of this, techniques for balancing *Vata* can be a great place for anyone to begin a regimen of Ayurvedic self-care.

Techniques to Balance *Vata*

- Establish a regular schedule, including timely meals and gentle exercise
- Eat grounding foods (warm, moist foods with sweet, dense, warming spices)
- Massage the body with oil

Pitta

A person with a predominantly *Pitta* physique has qualities of fire and water. Someone with a Pitta type has a dynamic personality with a big heart. They tend to be leaders and can be known for the ability to create positive change. They often are strong, muscular and of medium build. When a *Pitta* type gets too much *Pitta* they will be angry, short-tempered and generally inflamed. When a *Pitta* type gets out of balance he or she needs to nurture the earth and water and reduce the air and fire elements in their life (Chopra, n.d.).

Too much *Pitta* can also be an indication of too much wind (*Vata*). Think of a forest fire that is raging out of control because there is so much wind (*Vata*) blowing it. When the wind calms, the fire calms, and burns at a more controlled, less threatening pace. From a doshic perspective, to calm the wind, *Vata* must be supported with a regular schedule that includes plenty of time to unwind and relax. Oil massage, especially with cooling oils like coconut or olive, is an essential balancing routine for a *Pitta* constitution.

Techniques to Balance *Pitta*

- Eat cooling, sweet, bitter or astringent foods
- Avoid spicy food
- Make time each day to relax, spend time in nature (especially moonlight)

Kapha

A person with a predominantly *Kapha* type embodies earth and water elements. *Kapha* types tend to be nurturing, loving and stable. A *Kapha* constitution often has a larger build, big eyes, and a mellifluous voice. *Kaphas* tend to be loyal and devoted; remaining dedicated to jobs and relationships even when they no longer serve their best interest. With an overabundance of *Kapha,* a tendency towards stubbornness, resistance to change and laziness reigns. When a *Kapha* type is out of balance it is key to reduce water and earth elements and increase air and fire in their life (Chopra, n.d.).

Techniques to Balance *Kapha*

- Moderate to vigorous physical exercise every day
- Warm water with every meal
- Warming and spicy foods
- Clear clutter, give away unneeded and unused items

Humanology

Yogi Bhajan taught much more than just yoga classes. He came to the North America in the late sixties at a time of significant cultural change: redefinition of gender roles, complete social reformation, and major splits with traditional thinking. He brought with him an ancient understanding of human existence and taught many lifestyle practices including how to care for the body, and how to work with Kundalini energy to uplift others and ourselves and improve many aspects of our lives. His teachings include information about the polarities, the differences between males and females, and ways to foster better understanding and conscious communication. Yogi Bhajan's Humanology teachings, as he called them, were given to support the personal changes and transformation that occur as a result of a steady practice of Kundalini Yoga (Bhajan, 2010). Humanology teachings relating to the body systems will be covered throughout this book in the *Yogic Lifestyle* section of each chapter.

Chinese Medicine

Chinese medicine has been practiced for thousands of years and is growing in popularity around the world. The Chinese way of understanding the body is based on experience and careful observation of human beings and our relationship to the world around us. Yogi Bhajan brought an awareness of this medicine into the kriyas that he taught and would often mention a particular acupuncture point or meridian while he was teaching a posture.

In Chinese medicine when discussing a specific body part or organ it is often in-between the physical and non-physical realm. For example, in Chinese medicine the *Kidneys* (referred to in this book with a capital K) do not necessarily refer to the physical kidney organs. Instead, it refers to the energetic processes that they embody and how they influence the soul and emotions. The Chinese *Kidneys*, for example, are located in the mid-back (like the physical kidneys) but some of their energetic processes are buried deep beneath the Navel Point. Knowing the energetic essence of an organ can inform the subtle effects of a particular posture.

In Chinese medicine, every organ has a meridian that extends from the internal organ to the surface of the body. This energetic pathway is not a physical structure but an energetic opening to influence the health of the organ. Points along the meridian can be stimulated to influence the corresponding organ. The meridians were discovered thousands of years ago in ancient China when it was illegal to cut or operate on the body. Doctors had to treat a patient completely from the outside. They discovered ways to influence the health of the internal organs through touching the body and stimulating the nerves via the acupuncture points. Recent studies of the physical body reveal a nexus of small branching nerves at many acupuncture point locations, which begins to deepen our understanding of how acupuncture influences pain.

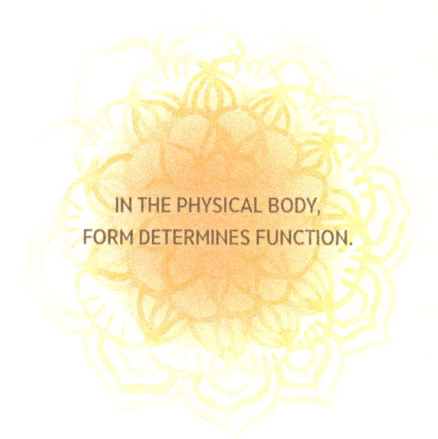

> IN THE PHYSICAL BODY, FORM DETERMINES FUNCTION.

Distinguishing Chinese Medicine Concepts

For clarity, throughout this book, references to organs or body parts within the Chinese medicine system will be capitalized and italicized. For example, *Kidneys* refers to the Chinese energetic processes distinct from the anatomical kidneys.

Imagine holding a flashlight against the body at an acupuncture point. The energy of this light would travel along the meridian creating an energizing, healing effect. In this tradition of healing, these points are pathways of connection, spreading light and healing to the internal organs and throughout the whole body. Using a specific yoga posture to apply pressure to an acupressure point is a way to open up the flow of a meridian and direct light and energy to an internal organ.

Plants, Herbs, and Food

Plant medicine can play a dramatic role in the overall healing of the body. The nutrients in herbs are more potent and quickly available than those in food. The properties of plant medicine have been known for centuries; they help build or tonify the health of the body quickly while dietary changes create slower, sustained changes in health.

When we say "an apple a day keeps the doctor away" we mean that an apple has so much nutrition that it serves as a tonic for the body. In herbalism, there are many substances that can tonify the body (details on plant medicine are included in each chapter; look for the heading, Plants, Herbs, and Food). Herbs are often taken in capsule, powder, or tea form and have many different properties that can directly affect the body at physical and subtle levels. Even some common household substances, like black pepper or onions, have special properties suitable to herbal medicine applications. Weaving plant medicine into everyday cooking is often a keynote feature of a yogi's kitchen.

Tonifying herbs are plants that are rich in minerals and generally build the strength of the body.

"Doctors diagnose, herbs heal and God cures."

© The Teachings of Yogi Bhajan, November 18, 1988

SUBTLE AND PHYSICAL:
A Functional Distinction

Delineating physical and subtle is helpful for explanatory purposes, but in reality distinguishing where physical begins and subtle ends is less concrete and potentially not even possible. Modern physics is showing us that everything is energy, which is a game-changer for how we explore the human body in energy and in form. Learning about both the energies and the forms (the visible and mechanical aspects) is important to our evolving understanding of the human body.

There is great value in learning about the body by closely observing the structure and function of specific parts. This kind of mechanical observation has served as the basis of general anatomy and physiology for most of recorded history. But it only takes a brief glimpse at that recorded history to realize that popular scientific understanding of the physical body has changed drastically over time and across different cultures. In Western medicine, for hundreds of years the only way the body was known was through external observation, extrapolation from animal dissection and educated guesses as to what lay beneath the skin. Early explorations into human dissection began in the 14th century. It wasn't until the rise of science and the rejection of religious superstition that marked the historical period referred to as the Enlightenment that doctors began dissecting cadavers, which opened the door to a whole new way of observing, understanding and working with the body. Over the years these observations formed the basis for modern anatomy and physiology. Increasingly advanced technologies have since developed, allowing us to peer inside the living human body (e.g., CT scanners, MRI machines) and observe a myriad of processes, allowing us to learn more and more about how our bodies work, including developing an understanding of minute biochemical reactions, genetics, and brain functions.

Gaining an understanding of the physical anatomy enhances your experience of the subtle anatomy. And learning to perceive the subtle anatomy enhances your connection to the physical. These systems when taken together form complementary views of the same work of art, the human being.

"The beauty of a living thing is not the atoms that go into it, but the way those atoms are put together."

—Carl Sagan, scientist, author

3.0 Archer Pose

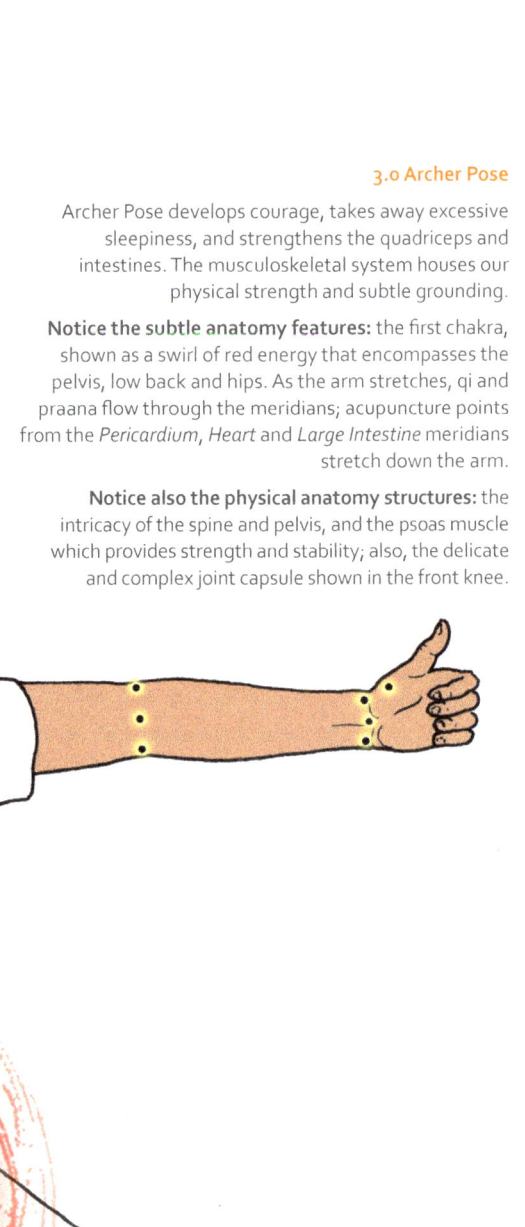

Archer Pose develops courage, takes away excessive sleepiness, and strengthens the quadriceps and intestines. The musculoskeletal system houses our physical strength and subtle grounding.

Notice the subtle anatomy features: the first chakra, shown as a swirl of red energy that encompasses the pelvis, low back and hips. As the arm stretches, qi and praana flow through the meridians; acupuncture points from the *Pericardium*, *Heart* and *Large Intestine* meridians stretch down the arm.

Notice also the physical anatomy structures: the intricacy of the spine and pelvis, and the psoas muscle which provides strength and stability; also, the delicate and complex joint capsule shown in the front knee.

The Musculoskeletal System

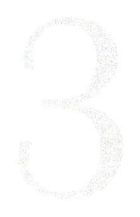

The musculoskeletal system could be seen as one of the least subtle systems of the body while, from a mechanical standpoint, one of the most obvious systems involved in the practice of yoga postures and exercises. Bones, muscles, and joints communicate messages about balance, efficiency, and resilience. The body skillfully maintains only those processes it needs. If a part of the body is not used regularly, that skill or strength will not be maintained. Use it or lose it! In an interesting paradox, even when muscles do go unused they don't lose actual muscle cells, just strength. Barring trauma or surgery, you have the same number of muscle cells in your body today as you did at birth. Individual muscle cells can hypertrophy (get stronger) or atrophy (get weaker) but the total number of cells generally doesn't change. Muscles always hold the potential to get stronger with determined and purposeful use (Tortora, 2006).

> *"Every disease is the outcome of structural change. You may not like this idea but I am telling you the oriental, ancient way of looking at it, what they feel that this body, bones, all over my body, all over this has no screw and bolt, nut and bolt. It is held by muscles. By working and living my life, by doing my things, I change my movements in a certain way.*
>
> *Certain muscles get acted upon and certain don't, and then certain muscles are stronger, they hold the skeleton in a different way than the other muscles. That is why I have my sexual problem, I have my sensual problems, I have my vision problems, I have my hearing problems, I have my computer brain problems, I have my heart problems, my circulation problems, my stomach problems, my sex problems, my elimination problems, my walking problems, my knee problems, my ankle problems and my toe problems…*
>
> *The whole body structure is responsible for my elevation, for my beingness."*
>
> © The Teachings of Yogi Bhajan, July 2, 1984

PHYSICAL ANATOMY PERSPECTIVE

Components of the Musculoskeletal System

- Bones
- Joints
- Connective Tissue (fascia, ligaments, tendons)
- Muscles

Benefits of a Strong Musculoskeletal System
A strong musculoskeletal system allows for the exploration of the full range of experiences in life.

Primary Purpose
The primary purpose of the musculoskeletal system is to provide structure and movement for the physical body.

Bones

THE LAST BONE TO STOP GROWING IS THE CLAVICLE OR COLLARBONE. IT TYPICALLY GROWS UNTIL AGE 25.

Bones are the scaffolding for the body. Their primary function is to support the soft tissue structures of the body: muscles, organs, and blood. They protect the delicate organs: the skull protects the brain, and the pelvis protects the reproductive organs. They also act as levers for the muscles to pull on in order to create physical movement. Finally, bones are a living tissue and play a role in the chemistry of the blood and formation of red blood cells.

Bones adapt to whatever situation gravity presents to them. At birth the bones are mostly made of cartilage. When the crawling and walking stages begin, these activities put stress on the bones. The body realizes the cartilage won't be strong enough for these new activities, so it signals for the building of cartilage into a more durable substance, bone. Bone density develops over many years, primarily during adolescence. Girls develop their density the most markedly between the ages of 11 and 13, and males develop the most from 11 to 17 years of age (Kröger et al, 1993). During the aging process, the body slowly loses bone density. Bone-building activities and eating a whole-food diet can mitigate this loss.

Bones and the Yogic Cycles of Consciousness

Yogic philosophy lays out several cycles that individuals undergo during their lives: the 18-year cycle of life, or physical-energy cycle; the 11-year cycle of intellect; and the 7-year cycle of consciousness. These cycles help to frame the significant changes in physical and subtle aspects in individuals as they move through their lives. Specifically, being familiar with the 18-year physical-energy cycle helps to frame the shifts we experience in our bodies as we age. (Bhajan, 2010).

The bones are an excellent representation of this cycle. During the first 18 years of life, the bones grow in density and size. In the first physical-energy cycle, the body's focus is on growth and expansion. Everything you eat and all your habits during the first 18 years contribute to this metabolic furnace, which builds and shapes the physical body. The next cycle, from 18–36 years, moves into a time of physical stability and maintenance. This phase for bone health means a slowing down and stopping of growth without a significant loss of bone density. It is a very steady time for the body and bones. After the age of 36, a very slow process of decline in energy and physicality begins and gently accelerates as the body moves closer to the next cycle. After age 54, greater care must be taken to protect the health of the bones and the entire body.

Often bones are thought of as hard and rigid. And while they are strong and sturdy, they aren't completely unyielding. Bones are, in fact, very responsive and adaptable to what happens in the body. The bones are constantly built, broken down, and rebuilt by special cells called osteoblasts and osteoclasts. This happens every day in response to physical activity and the chemistry of the body. Weight-bearing activity conditions the bones to stay strong by increasing osteoblastic activity. Yoga is an example of a weight-bearing activity.

The bones also act as a calcium reserve for the body. There must be a certain amount of calcium in the bloodstream in order for muscles to contract, including the heart muscle. If blood-calcium levels get too low, the body will decide to take calcium out of the bones to keep the heart pumping. While this is an important adaptive solution on a short-term basis, it is not a good long-term solution for overall bone health as it can weaken the bones. Therefore, it is important to get enough vitamins and minerals in the diet and to make weight-bearing exercise a part of your daily routine for bone health.

Bones also contain a special substance called bone marrow, which is responsible for creating the platelets and red blood cells that make up the blood. The dynamic creation of billions of red blood cells happens deep within the bones of the musculoskeletal system every day (Myelodysplastic, 2012).

Bones: Use 'em or lose 'em!
Bones need to be put under a degree of stress and used in order to build and maintain strength.

An Overview of Some Key Bones of the Skeleton

The Pelvis

The pelvic bone is a large and complex structure in the body. The pelvis creates the junction of the legs to the torso in a way that allows upright movement. It is also the foundation of the spinal column and provides a protective basin for internal organs. Three fused bones form each half of the pelvis. They are the pubis, ilium, and ischium.

Many people hold tension and experience tightness in the hips. Physically this is caused by daily activities of sitting in chairs, driving cars, leaning over computers, and a lack of walking and squatting. From a subtle perspective tension in the hips, low back, and buttocks comes from constantly trying to control life. Human beings are inclined to control or manage the experience of life. And when the universe doesn't cooperate, we subconsciously try to create stability and

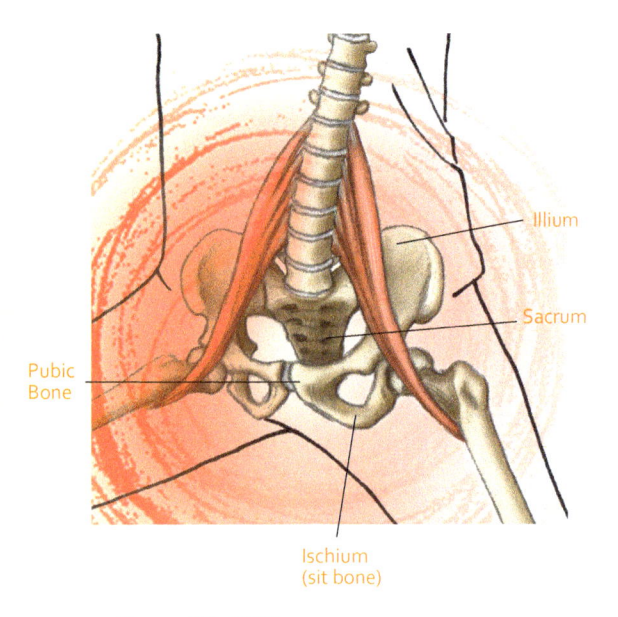

3.1 Bones of the Pelvis
The pelvis is made up of the Illium, Pubis and Ischium.

A Hands-On Exploration of the Pelvis

This is a hands-on exercise. Follow along; use your hands to identify the landmarks described.

First we'll find the ischium, the bone at the bottom of the pelvis. To find the ischial tuberosities, commonly called sit bones, sit on the hands and rock the pelvis back and forth. The pointy bones you feel as you move are the sit bones. In an ideal sitting position the sit bones are pointing straight down. Next, we'll find the back crest of the pelvis, called the ilium or iliac crest. To find the iliac crest, bring your hands to your sides and press in on the space below the ribs. Then press down to feel the curved top edge of the ilium. Follow the bone forward to the points at the front of the body; this point is often referred to as the hip bone. Now follow the ridge back behind your body; it gets harder to feel toward the back, but this bone goes all the way around and meets with the triangular shaped sacrum at the base of the spine.

Finally, we'll find the pubic bone. This bone connects the two sides of the pelvis together in the front of the body. Bring your hand to the lower, front section of the torso. To find your pubic bone, feel for the bony bump just above the genitals.

Men, Women and the Pelvis

Both male and female pelvises are held together by an intricate collection of ligaments. Generally ligaments are not designed to stretch. However, in women the pelvis must be able to open to deliver a baby. The female body produces a special hormone during pregnancy called relaxin, which softens all of the ligaments in the body and allows the pelvic bones to move apart so that the baby can descend through the pelvic opening. Because of the softening of the pelvic ligaments during pregnancy, the pelvis can become unstable and thus more susceptible to injury during and after pregnancy. More information about modifying a yoga practice during pregnancy is available in Chapter 11 (see page 235, the section titled "Yoga restrictions during pregnancy").

Beyond the ligaments, the female pelvis is structured quite differently than a male pelvis. The ilium is at a much wider angle in the female pelvis. This makes the opening at the bottom of her pelvis wider. This evolutionary design allowed human females to give birth to babies with larger heads and therefore larger brains. This is a key factor in the evolution of the human beings. There seems to be a standoff at this point in evolution. If female pelvises were to get wider to make way for babies with even bigger brains, their ability to walk on two feet would be inhibited. This concept is often referred to as the obstetrical dilemma.

Male pelvises on the other hand have been evolutionarily optimized for walking and running instead of birthing. Typically the male pelvis is narrower and taller; when combined with their larger ribcages this makes for a shorter lower back and a more straightforward gait (Boundless, n.d.).

---

control elsewhere. Often this shows up in the physical body as tightness in the hips, which is at the same level as the First Chakra—the energetic center of stability and safety. When we surrender to the divine, tightness in this area can begin to unwind.

The Scapula

The scapula, or shoulder blade, is a triangle-shaped bone that is the primary link between the arm and the torso. The scapula is attached to the body at the clavicle by ligaments and tendons and around the top of the arm bone by the rotator cuff muscles. The inner edge of the scapula is free floating, which allows the scapula to slide around on the back of the ribcage for maximum range of motion of the arm at the shoulder.

A Pelvic Bone By Any Other Name...
- *Os Coxa*
- *Pelvis*
- *Hips*
- *Ilium, Ischium, and Pubis*
- *Innominate Bone*

Rachel's Story of Postural Realignment and Emotional Healing

Rachel showed up at a self-help workshop and could hardly make eye contact with anyone due to her painfully rounded upper back and tucked-in chin. She spoke so softly and guardedly that the teacher frequently asked her to repeat herself. The particular day the group was working on emotional scars carried from childhood. As part of the exercise everyone wrote letters to their parents. The next day, when she arrived at the workshop, Rachel looked very different to everyone in the group. She held her head high, her shoulders were thrown back, and she spoke in a clear voice. The night before, Rachel had called her father and read the letter to him. He was deeply moved and apologized to her. He told her that he had never loved her brother more than her. This opened the door for a deeply healing conversation where he told her he loved having a daughter, and that he loved her. This allowed Rachel to heal an emotional scar that had been shutting down her heart for many years. That subtle shift allowed her to stand up straight physically and emotionally overnight.

The arms and shoulders are part of the energy of the Heart Center. The shoulders, in particular, are another place where many people commonly hold stress. Tightness in the shoulders or the feeling of having to protect oneself from the world or from emotional scars compromises the Heart Center, which leads to a physical armoring by slumping forward or hunching up the shoulders. From a physical standpoint, the many activities that require the arms to be held in front, for example typing at a computer, driving a car, or carrying bags, perpetuate the physical accumulation of tension in the muscles around the shoulders.

This positioning, combined with the emotional defensiveness of the heart, creates tightness in the pectoral or chest muscles, until they become chronically shortened. Because all muscles work in pairs of opposites this also creates a chronic stretch or over-lengthening of the muscles in the upper back. When this posture has been maintained for a long time, these muscles recalibrate, and these over tightened and overstretched positions begin to feel normal. When this happens it actually becomes uncomfortable to sit with correct posture.

The Musculoskeletal System

To correct this issue, we must continually remind and realign the muscles in addition to strengthening and stretching them. Over time, and with the support of yoga and bodywork, the muscles can recalibrate to the correct position, and then sitting up straight with good posture becomes *easier* than slumping or rounding forward. A reprogramming of posture can also begin on the subtle level. By working to heal the scars of the Heart Center and building a sense of connection and love, we can allow subtle restrictions to release and correct posture to return.

The Spine

The spinal column is a series of irregularly shaped bones stacked on top of each other. They have a canal running through the center, which houses the spinal cord. There are three sections of the spinal column. The cervical spine, or neck area, has seven vertebrae. The thoracic spine, or upper area, has 12 vertebrae. The lumbar, or lower back area, has five vertebrae. At the end of the spine is the sacrum, a triangular-shaped bone that joins with the pelvis and is comprised of five, fused vertebrae. And finally the tailbone is at the end of the spinal column and is formed by four fused bones. The coccyx or tailbone actually curls underneath the spine.

There are four curves to the spine. These curves are designed to create stability and strength.

The cervical spine is made of little, delicate vertebrae with a lordotic curve. Thoracic vertebrae are a bit bigger, attach to the 12 ribs, and have a kyphotic curve. Lumbar vertebrae are the thickest, sturdiest vertebrae and again have a lordotic curve. The final curve of the spine is formed by the sacrum and tailbone, and again is kyphotic.

A Hands-On Exploration of the Cervical Vertebrae

This is a hands-on exercise. Follow along; use your hands to identify the landmarks.

The very top vertebra, C1, is up higher than seems possible at the base of the skull. Put your thumbs in your ears and wrap the index finger around the back of your head, the index finger is at the level of C1.

The last cervical vertebra, C7, is at the bottom of your neck. Drop your chin to your chest and run your hand along the back of your neck and feel for a bump that sticks out the most; that is C7.

Why Does Kundalini Yoga Omit Headstands?

Shoulder stand, plow pose, or other core-strengthening inversions have a lot of benefits. Practicing headstands has similar benefits, but with the additional risk of extreme pressure on the cervical spine. The risk of putting the entire body weight on the tiny vertebrae of the neck is not worth the potential benefit of a headstand (Bhajan, 2010 and Sullivan, 2014).

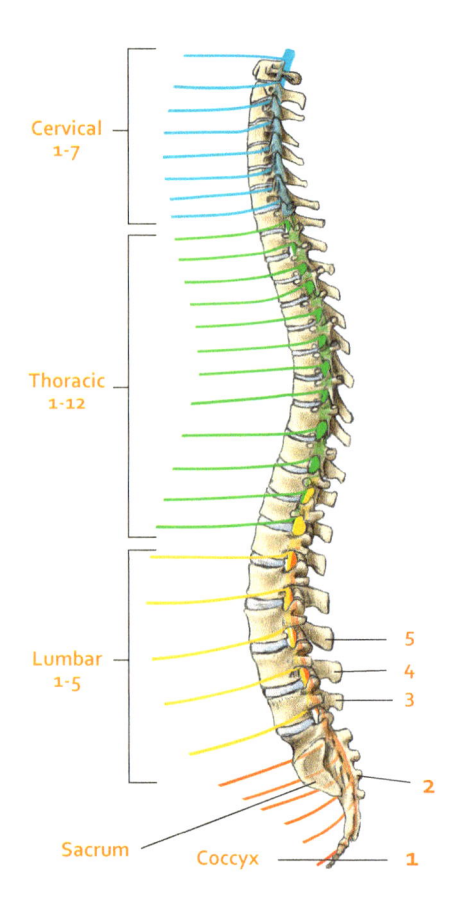

In physical anatomy their curve and sequential number name the vertebrae. Starting at the top the first vertebra is called cervical one, or C1; the numbering continues down to C7. The thoracic section of the spine starts the numbers over, so the first thoracic vertebra is called T1 and continues to T12. The lumbar section consists of L1 to L5, and is followed by the sacrum and coccyx.

Yogi Bhajan sometimes referred to the vertebrae differently. Most often, he started at the bottom of the spine and moved upward so that each vertebra gets just a number. He called the tailbone number one, the sacrum number two and then counted each vertebra up the spine from that point. The vertebra known as L5 in physical anatomy terms would be called number three in Yogi Bhajan's style of counting.

Yogi Bhajan often referred to the seat of the Kundalini as the fourth vertebrae, which in physical anatomy is called L4. One purpose of yoga and meditation practices is to activate this Kundalini energy. Kundalini energy lies dormant in the Navel Point, at the fourth vertebra. When *praana* and *apaana* mix, through the practice of posture, breath, and locks, the energy is stimulated and activated. When the Kundalini energy is activated the soul is awakened.

The Ribcage

The ribcage is a protective structure for the heart and lungs made up of 12 pairs of ribs that curve around and attach to the spine in the back and to the sternum in front. The first seven ribs, called true ribs, attach directly to the sternum. The next three, called false ribs, attach indirectly to the sternum via cartilage attaching to the ribs above them. This indirect connection

3.2 Curves of the Spine

The conventional numbering system is shown on the left. Yogi Bhajan's system for naming areas of the spine, which differed at times from the conventional system, is shown on the right.

The Musculoskeletal System

adds extra flexibility for expansive deep breathing. The last two ribs, called floating ribs, do not attach in the front. In puberty, testosterone causes the male ribcage to expand, generally giving men greater breath capacity.

Yogi Bhajan spoke of the ribcage as the prison of the soul or the dungeon of karma; the shape of the ribs, reminiscent of prison bars, contributing to the metaphor. Between each rib are layers and layers of muscle and connective tissue woven together to create a thick wall. Inside this imposing structure are the delicate and sensitive heart and lungs.

The heart resides in the ribcage; as the soul moves through the challenges of life, grief and pain compound, day-to-day stress and chronic grief can cause restrictions in the ribcage. Through regular yoga and *praanayam* (breathwork), we can begin to soften and expand the physical possibilities of the ribcage. Chronic tension in the webbed muscles of the ribs can be conditioned to unwind. This allows for the ribs to continue their role as a protector but also to soften and expand at the proper moments, which in turn allows for deep healing, energizing, and vitality to manifest for the soul's purpose. A daily practice can train the ribcage to have its full range of motion and that flood of praana allows for an experience of expansiveness and joy. Yet the capacity of our lungs is finite, and the soul must be contained with the limits of the human body. In the experience of death the soul is released from the ribcage and finally freed.

Joints

Bones themselves cannot move. They must create a joint with another bone in order to have the space for movement. A joint is any place in the body where two bones come together. There are a variety of types of joints, with varying load-bearing possibilities, ranges of motion, and stability.

Some joints are designed for safety and stability, like the bones of the skull, while other joints, like the shoulder, sacrifice stability for mobility. The shoulder's vulnerability also allows for its large range of motion, which in turn facilitates all kinds of arm movements like feeding oneself, throwing a ball, carrying a baby, or walking the dog.

The moving parts in any structure are the ones most susceptible to damage or wear and tear. The same is true of the joints in the physical body. Because of the amount of movement and the complexity of the structures involved, joints are susceptible to injury.

A SMALL PERCENTAGE OF PEOPLE HAVE AN ADDITIONAL RIB AT THE TOP, ACTUALLY ATTACHED TO THEIR SEVENTH CERVICAL VERTEBRA

(ScienceForums, 2010–13).

"Your physical body will give you stamina, it cannot give you more than stamina. Your mind will give you caliber and your spirit soul will give you consciousness."

© The Teachings of Yogi Bhajan, October 11, 1993

> A JOINT IS NOT DESIGNED TO STRETCH ON A PHYSICAL LEVEL, YET ON A SUBTLE LEVEL THE JOINTS HOLD THE CAPACITY FOR MAXIMUM TRANSFORMATION

Joints and Subtle Energy Channels

From a subtle perspective, joints are areas where various energy pathways come together, shift, and exchange information. They are akin to major highway overpasses with restaurants and amusement galleries where people can pause and have dinner or change direction and get onto a different highway. This is the function of joints in the subtle energy highways of the body.

These rest stops can also be places of stagnation. There can be a concentration of too much or too little energy in the joints. And just like real traffic, sometimes even small distractions or imbalances create a ripple effect, slowing everything down. Or suddenly a rush comes through and traffic spills out to surrounding streets. When energy moves too quickly or stagnates it can lead to imbalance or injury. Ideally there is a steady stream of easily moving traffic through the highways and joints of the body.

There is also a concentration of acupuncture points located at each joint where the energy channels can most readily be affected. Whether by the placement of acupuncture needles, precise placement of the joints in a yoga posture, or pressure applied to the skin, stimulating these points and pathways has a deep impact on the subtle balances of the body, stabilizing and promoting proper flow of energy for general health.

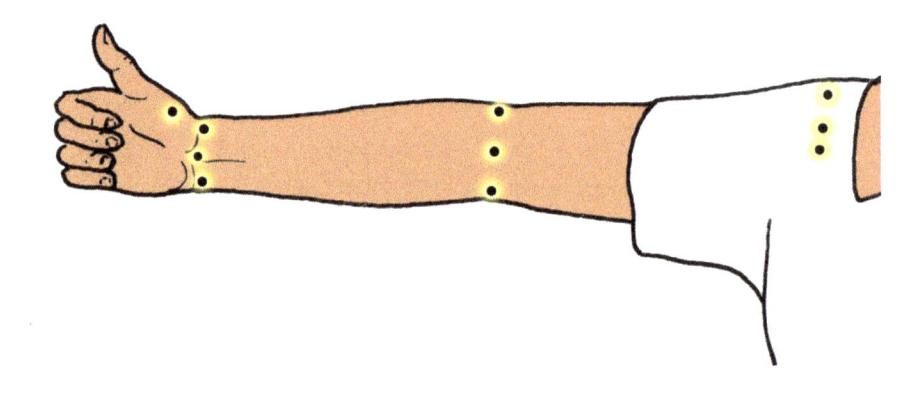

"Each day gives me the message of beauty, of bounty, of prosperity, of flourishing, of blossom. I am going and going and going and going on the path of Infinity, cycle after cycle, prayer after prayer, grace after grace, rosary after rosary, feast after feast, and fast after fast. I've gone through the passage of life, but still I am the slave of the dungeon of the ribcage."

© The Teachings of Yogi Bhajan, December 6, 1982

3.3 Joints & Acupuncture
Acupuncture points tend to be concentrated at the joints; creating a place in the body for focused energy transformation.

Three Classifications of Joints

Synovial Joints

Synovial joints are the joints typically talked about with bodily movements: elbows, hips, knees. All synovial joints have somewhat similar structures.

Two bones come together. At the end of each bone is articular cartilage, which acts as padding. A joint capsule, which is a sack of connective tissue around the joint, surrounds the space between the two bones. The sac is filled with fluid, which lubricates and creates ease of movement in the joint. The bones are held together with ligaments, which run directly from bone to bone. Muscles taper into tendons and cross the joint space.

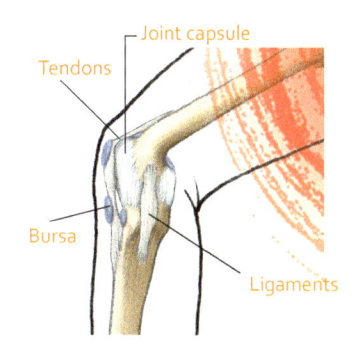

3.4 Joint Capsule
The knee is an example of a synovial joint capsule.

Immovable Joints

Some joints are classified as immovable; they do not create big, obvious movements of the physical body, nor do they have a joint space. But there is still the potential for slight shifts in these spaces, which can affect the functioning of those areas. Immovable joints include the sutures of the skull bones and the bones of the pelvis.

Semi-Movable Joints

The joints between the vertebrae of the spine are classified as semi-movable. The space between each of the vertebrae is filled with a disc. There is no actual joint space, but the disc is flexible, which allows for some movement. There is a very small amount of movement available between any two individual vertebrae. The body adds up these little bits of movement from each vertebra to create the larger range of motion of the spine as a whole.

Connective Tissue

Connective tissue is everywhere in the body; it holds organs together, creates shape and separates structures. All joints are surrounded by connective tissue, from the joint capsule, to the fascia, to the ligaments.

In order to do its job of holding things together; most connective tissue is not designed to stretch. When practicing yoga, the goal is to feel the sensation of stretch in the bellies of muscles, not in the joints. Pain in the

Good Pain versus Warning Pain

A yoga practice may at times feel uncomfortable. Some pain that comes up during your practice is part of the natural process of stretching your body in new ways. This type of pain can actually indicate beneficial growth or healing occurring in your body. Learn to listen to and honor your body's limits in order to avoid injury. Develop a sense of knowing which discomfort you can breathe through from those that call for immediate attention. If you're having trouble distinguishing between the two, err on the side of caution until you can develop a better sense of "good pain" and "warning pain".

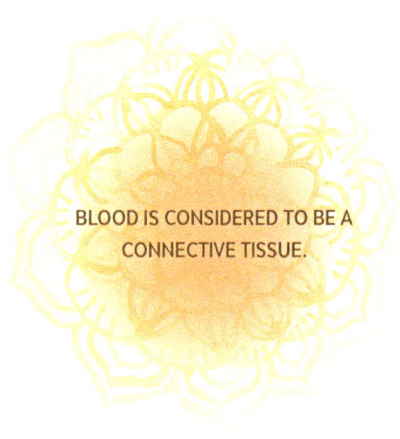

BLOOD IS CONSIDERED TO BE A CONNECTIVE TISSUE.

joints, during yoga or other activities, is generally not beneficial and indicates a problem. Intensity in the middle of a muscle belly can be a healthy and normal part of the process of strengthening or lengthening the muscles. Intense sensations in the joints often indicate stress on connective tissues. One reason to be especially mindful of straining the joints is the relatively slow rate of connective tissue repair. Connective tissue generally does not have a blood supply so it receives the necessary nutrients to regenerate cells at a slower rate.

Fascia

Fascia is a type of connective tissue that is found throughout the entire body; it is a thin, filmy covering that surrounds every muscle, bone, and organ. The purpose of fascia is to create clear boundaries for each muscle, to make structures more slippery so they can move over each other without creating friction, and to create functional connections between distinct muscle groups. Fascia exists in continuous sheets throughout the body; so when one area is pulled or stretched it has a ripple effect throughout the whole musculoskeletal system.

Fascia can hold tension in the same way that muscles do. When people complain of tension or tightness in their upper back both the muscles and the fascia must be addressed to release this tension. To only work with the muscles and ignore the fascia would be like letting a Popsicle melt in its plastic wrapper. The hard block of ice may be gone, but the shape of the container is still intact. Both the muscle and the fascia determine the relative tension of the musculoskeletal system.

Ligaments and Tendons

Ligaments are bands of connective tissue that connect bones directly to each other. The nuchal ligament, for example, runs down the back of the neck directly connecting the skull and each of the cervical vertebrae together.

Tendons are bands of connective tissue at the ends of muscles that cross joint spaces and connect the muscles to bones. The tendons are responsible for transferring the tension of a muscle into an actual pull on the bones, which creates movement. Within each tendon of a skeletal muscle are very special structures called Golgi Tendon organs. These structures provide direct proprioceptive or sensory information to the brain about the position of the body. They are also part of the reflex arc that prevents one from exerting the muscles too forcefully.

Ligaments connect bone to bone. Tendons connect muscle to bone.

Muscles

There are three types of muscle tissue in the body:
- Smooth muscle: This type of muscle is found in the internal organs and acts involuntarily. It assists in moving food through the digestive tract, for example.
- Cardiac muscle: This type of muscle tissue is only found in the heart muscle. It allows the heart to beat without fatiguing. It, too, acts involuntarily.
- Skeletal muscle: These are the muscles attached to your bones. Their purpose is to create physical body movement. Skeletal muscles, generally, have a muscle belly that then taper into tendons at each end. These tendons cross a joint space and attach to a bone. Every skeletal muscle must attach to at least two bones and cross at least one joint space. Skeletal muscle moves both voluntarily and involuntarily.

How Skeletal Muscles Work

When a skeletal muscle is stimulated it wants to make itself as short as possible. Since a muscle is attached to two different bones, when it tries to pull its two ends together, it moves those two bones together. Take the very simple action of a traditional sit-up: lying on the back and moving to a seated position. The brain tells the abdominal muscles to fire, which are

Each action requires a complicated symphony of muscle activation and your experience is the silent conductor.

attached to the bottom of the rib cage and the top of the pubic bone. The abdominal muscles then bring those bones as close together as possible, which results in a sit-up.

In reality, no muscle works alone. When creating even the simplest of physical actions, like picking up a bag of groceries, a complex and well-orchestrated combination of muscle actions are involved.

Each action centers on the agonist muscle, which is also called the primary mover. This muscle is responsible for the main action created. In the example of carrying groceries it might be the *biceps brachii* or upper-arm muscle, which contracts to bend the arm and pull the bag up.

All muscles have an opposing muscle (called the antagonist) on the opposite side of the joint that creates the opposite action. While the primary mover muscle is contracting or getting shorter the muscle on the opposite side of the joint has to get longer in order for the desired action to take place.

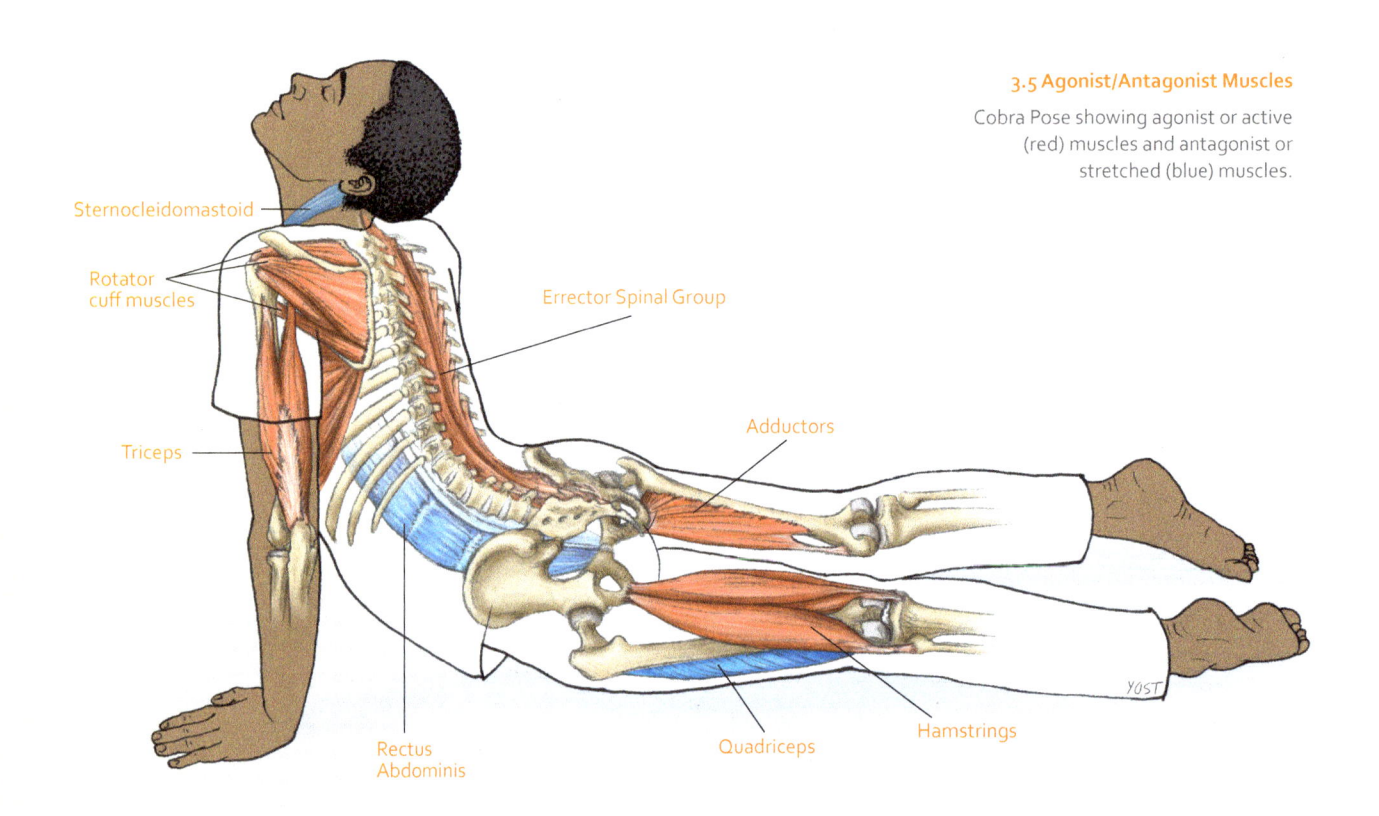

3.5 Agonist/Antagonist Muscles
Cobra Pose showing agonist or active (red) muscles and antagonist or stretched (blue) muscles.

Sternocleidomastoid
Rotator cuff muscles
Triceps
Rectus Abdominis
Errector Spinal Group
Adductors
Quadriceps
Hamstrings

42   ENLIGHTENED BODIES

As one muscle contracts, the opposing muscle *must* stretch. When the biceps contract to flex the elbow, the triceps, on the back of the upper arm, *must* stretch. If they don't stretch, the motion will not happen.

In every action some muscles also act as stabilizers, or fixators. When picking up groceries, the leg muscles must also be engaged so the weight of the bag doesn't pull you over. Other muscles will act as synergists, helping out the primary mover and eliminating any unwanted action of the joint. This allows for the elbow to bend without changing the angle of the shoulder.

Even in a very simple action like picking up a bag of groceries, there is a complex series of contracting, stretching, and stabilizing actions that occur in the muscular system. The body learns over time by trial and error exactly how to create the needed motions without much conscious input.

Muscle Shape Determines Function

In muscles, shape determines function. Those that are closer to the skin tend to be thinner, broader muscles that specialize in moving the body. Muscles that are closer to the center of the body tend to be thicker, stockier muscles that work on creating stability, especially in seated and standing postures.

It is generally easier to access, control, and feel the superficial muscles. But it's a great skill for yogis to develop awareness of the deeper core-stabilizing muscles. Begin postures by engaging these deeper muscles to create a strong foundation on which to build the pose safely. For example, coming into Stretch Pose by just lifting the head and feet puts too much strain on an unprepared lower back. Instead, first engage Root Lock and the abdominal muscles to keep the core steady while lengthening the feet and lifting the head. This makes the posture much easier and safer for the body.

An Overview of Some Key Muscles

Abdominals The abdominal muscles consist of several layers in the mid-to-lower anterior torso. The muscle fiber directions of abdominal muscles vary, creating a strong web of muscle tissue that can move the torso in any direction.

- *Rectus abdominis* is a very thin muscle with fibers that run straight up and down from the pubic bone to the bottom of the ribcage. There are bands of connective tissue that run horizontally across the *rectus abdominis*, which serve to create shorter, stronger sections of pull for the muscle fibers and to create the ridges in classic "six-pack" abs.

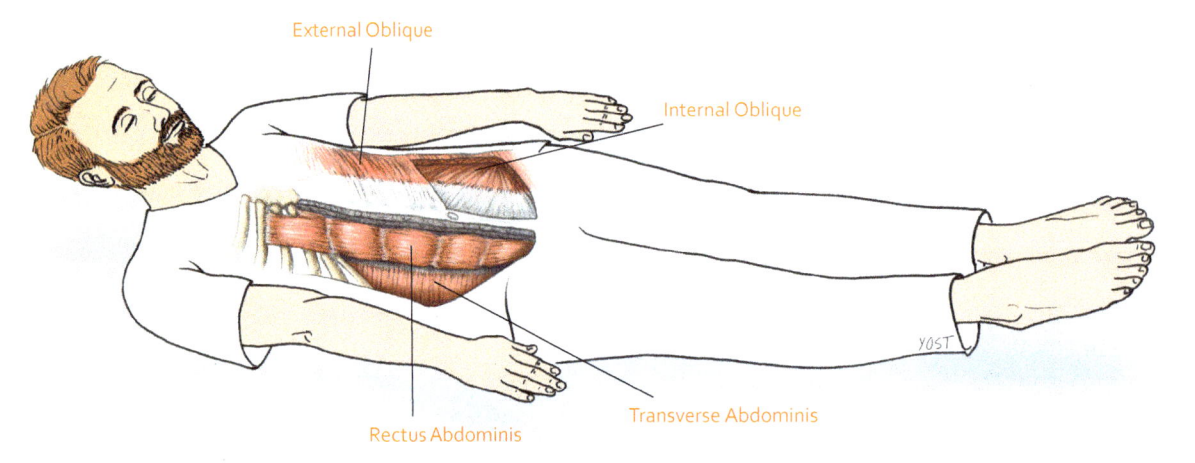

3.6 Stretch Pose
Stretch Pose showing layers of the abdominal muscles.

- *Internal and external oblique* muscles are angled on the sides of the torso from the bottom of the ribcage to the pelvis. They allow for twisting and side-bending movements.
- *Transverse abdominis* is the very deepest layer of abdominal muscles. The fibers run horizontally and surround the belly like a belt or a girdle. The *transverse abdominis* encircles the entire torso, connecting to the fascia of the lower back. When pulling Root Lock, by engaging the muscles of the pelvic floor the *transverse abdominis* naturally and subtly engages, and then strongly locks when the navel is actively engaged.

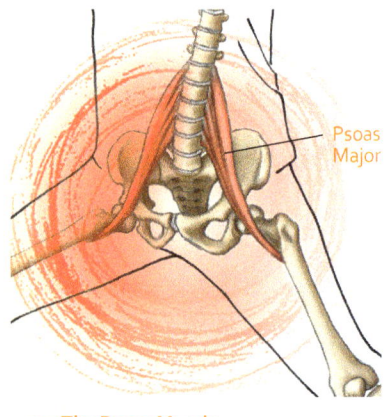

Illiopsoas The *illiopsoas*, which is more commonly called the psoas (pronounced *soaz*) helps with standing and walking. It attaches to the front of the spine at the level of the bottom of the ribcage or T12. The psoas runs parallel to the spine for a while and then angles out and passes through the pelvis and attaches to the leg. This muscle is often overused or chronically shortened in the typical, modern lifestyle. Sitting too long in chairs and not walking enough are the primary culprits of a tight psoas. When the psoas is chronically tightened, it can contribute to low back pain. It can also make back-bending postures (like cobra) uncomfortable or painful, as they create the opposing stretch. Taking the time to relax and stretch the psoas by practicing a forward lunge—every day—creates a healthier relationship between the pelvis and the spine.

3.7 The Psoas Muscle

From a subtle perspective, the psoas connects between the lower centers and the upper centers. When the psoas is tight or in spasm it can be a subconscious way of protecting yourself from the intensity of transformation. Releasing old emotional patterns can help relax the physical tension held in the muscle.

Diaphragm The respiratory diaphragm is a thin sheath of muscle that divides the chest cavity from the abdominal cavity. The muscle fibers attach around the bottom, inner edge of the ribcage, and connect to a central tendon. The diaphragm muscle also has several holes that allow vital structures to pass through, such as the aorta and the esophagus. When the diaphragm contracts, it enlarges the thoracic cavity, which creates a suction force, drawing air into the lungs. When the diaphragm relaxes, the natural recoil of the lungs and abdominal muscles assist the release of air from the lungs.

On a subtle level the diaphragm can store tension related to old fears. This is one of the reasons that when people start yoga, breathing, or meditation practices they may find they are processing experiences from childhood. They are stretching and opening this area of the body where those experiences have been stored. It requires bravery to move past those memories and fears and into a new, expansive way of being.

Pelvic Floor Muscles The pelvic floor muscles hang like a hammock and cover the triangular space between the two sit bones and the pubic bone. This sheath of muscles is important in creating pelvic stability and supporting the pelvic organs. The pelvic floor is in a vulnerable position because it has the weight of the torso resting on it. This vulnerability increases during pregnancy and childbirth; if the muscles of the pelvic floor are weakened they lose the ability to maintain the integrity and safety of the internal organs.

3.8 The Pelvic Floor
Muscles of the pelvic floor create an interwoven tapestry which supports all of the internal organs and the Root Chakra.

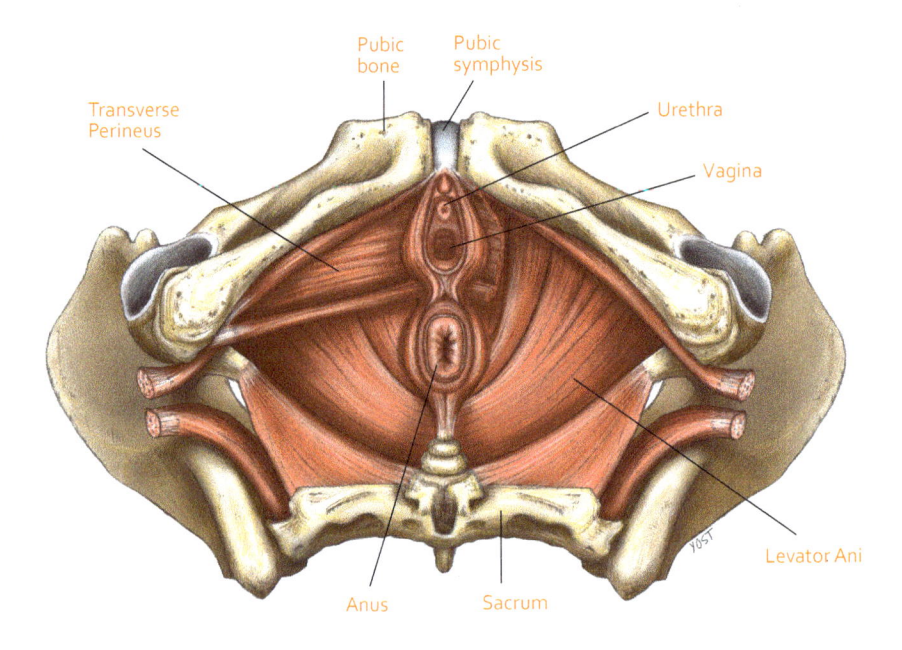

Yogic Root Lock and the Pelvic Floor Muscles

Beginners who learn about Root Lock often incorrectly engage the gluteal muscles (buttocks) instead of the pelvic floor muscles. It takes some diligent practice to be able to isolate the pelvic floor, but it is possible and makes Root Lock much more effective. Find guidelines for performing Root Lock on page 212.

Some Common Challenges to the Musculoskeletal System

Stagnation

Stagnation is a lack of energy flow or blood flow that leads to increased inflammation. There is some amount of inflammation in the body at all times. It becomes a problem when there is too much inflammation, or when it can't stop after its usefulness has been exhausted. Any yoga pose that is upside down or moves the body in a non-habitual way can help to reduce the effects of stagnation. Yoga postures support the reduction of inflammation more than traditional exercise regimens because yoga incorporates *praanayam* (breathwork); the sustained stretch of a yoga posture is synchronized with the breath, which bridges the gap between the conscious and subconscious minds allowing for a healing change to take place. The *praanayam* gently energizes the body allowing for stagnation to clear and a subtle mind-body connection to emerge which supports the body in prevention of disease.

Overuse

Overuse usually shows up as a postural distortion from moving the body in imbalanced ways. It is common to stand with most of the body's weight on one foot or to have a dominant right or left side. Over time the uneven strain on the body leads to habitual weakening or over-strengthening of particular muscles. Sitting at a desk for hours a day can lead to a chronic slumped forward posture. This posture creates restrictions in the fascia and muscular imbalance that perpetuate the slump even when the desk is removed. Yogic exercises can balance these habitual physical patterns by moving the body in new patterns: extensions to balance the constant flexion; standing postures to balance the long hours of sitting.

Injury/Trauma

Accidents of many types are the third source of imbalance or dysfunction in the musculoskeletal system. Always consult with your Physician about your practice of yoga and how it will fit in with your care and recovery. If you are able to go back to yoga practice, be sure to let your teacher know your injuries so he or she can guide you during your practice so that the posture works favorably for your body while you are recovering.

Yoga after an Injury

After an injury, including yoga and meditation as part of the healing process can be an appropriate practice if approached mindfully and with care.

The Healing Process

When the body is injured there are several stages of response. The first step is to create pain, which signals the brain to stop doing whatever it is that is injuring the body. Pain is the body's way of saying, "Please, stop that!"

The next step is to create inflammation, which often gets a bad reputation. Thought of as the enemy or the problem, inflammation is actually a healthy part of the body's response to an injury. Inflammation means that extra fluid is moving into the area and bringing with it specialized cells and chemicals to help repair the torn or stressed tissues. Inflammation also makes it difficult to move the area in question, which helps to prevent further damage.

Inflammation becomes a problem when it continues to linger after having already served its purpose. It can start to create prolonged immobility, which detracts from the later stages of recovery. Ideally, once the inflammation has done its job, fluids are easily reabsorbed by the lymphatic system. After an injury tissues are often tender, weak, or vulnerable, even after the acute phase has ended. The type and location of the injury affect how long that vulnerability can last.

Injured Ligaments

If the injury is to a ligament, the healing process can take weeks to months. Ligaments are thick fibrous bands that are not meant to stretch. Even after they do repair, they are always going to be more prone to injury. Imagine a bungee cord used to hold something together. If that bungee cord gets too stretched out it is never going to be as good at holding things together. If the injury is to a muscle, tendon or fascia there is the potential for a more complete healing. Still one has to go slow in rebuilding strength and listen to the body once returning to activity.

Subtle Perspectives on Injuries

When viewed from a subtle perspective there are often patterns in injuries or traumas that reveal deeper energetic imbalances. The left side of the body, for example, holds the feminine energy, and the right side holds masculine energy. Everyone, regardless of genetic sex or gender expression has the energies of both divine feminine and divine masculine within them. If a person continually has left-sided problems, it may help to look not only at his or her physical strength and flexibility but also at his or her relationships with women, or his or her own femininity. When they start the subtle healing, the physical healing can also begin.

Relationship to Other Systems

Musculoskeletal and Digestive Systems. Food moves through the digestive system by peristalsis, a process where muscles in the intestines contract and relax. This is an involuntary process regulated by the autonomic nervous system. Movement of the abdominal area in yoga supports digestion by helping food to move more easily through the system.

Musculoskeletal and Immune Systems. The musculoskeletal system is responsible for moving the lymphatic fluid in the body, which supports the functioning of the immune system. Lymphatic fluid is moved upward through the body by muscle and joint movements. Unlike the bloodstream, the lymphatic system has no pump to circulate lymphatic fluid. When the body is moved through space, it creates then releases pressure on these vessels, which helps pump the fluid through.

Musculoskeletal and Nervous Systems. At the origin and insertion points of skeletal muscles Golgi tendon organs connect them to the nervous system. This is one of the feedback mechanisms between the nervous and musculoskeletal systems. In a particular situation it is possible to have strong muscles and a weak nervous system or vice versa. Think of a muscular strong athlete (strong muscular system) who passes out at the sight of a drop of blood (weak nervous system), or the skinny mother (weak muscular system) who pushes a heavy boulder off of her child (strong nervous system); for ideal function we want a strong nervous system which helps us control strong voluntary muscles. We are, as in all things, striving for balance between the two systems.

SUBTLE ANATOMY PERSPECTIVE

The musculoskeletal system is situated around the internal organs both to protect and support the function of those organs. Muscles that are located directly above an organ can be pressed or massaged to bring vitality or healing to that organ. The impact is subtle but powerful. Consider constipation. Pressing on the abdomen directly with the fingers often helps to ease constipation. An easy way to support the internal organs is by massaging, moving, and compressing the muscles around them.

Pull one thread in a woven tapestry and the whole image changes. In the musculoskeletal system the limbs act as the threads. By moving or exerting pressure on the limbs it effectively pulls on and massages the organs. A repetitive yoga exercise, such as a leg lifts, impacts digestion by creating pressure on the abdomen with the movement and activation of the legs. Likewise there is a subtle effect on the lungs, heart, and other organs covered by the rib cage when the arms are moved. The ripple effect begins with muscle action, either in the core or the limbs, and the effects expand to the vital organs in the body.

The Musculoskeletal System and the Soul Body

The musculoskeletal system aligns with the frequency of the Soul Body. The soul is the essence of a human being. It stays with the body throughout this life and beyond. In the same way that muscles initiate action throughout life, the soul holds the capacity to initiate self-realization. When life is lived from the wisdom of the Soul Body, it is a life leading toward authentic and expansive consciousness.

Like a rock thrown into still water, the ripple effect of the Soul Body permeates through all the organs, chakras, and Light Bodies. The Soul Body is unchanging, infinite, and the lynchpin to an ability to lead and achieve in a way that is truthful to the soul's purpose.

The Musculoskeletal System and the Physical Body

The Physical Body may be the easiest of the Light Bodies to understand, because it is the most concrete and correlates to the musculoskeletal system so directly. The Physical Body is the vehicle that allows for a complete experience of life. It is said that the angels are jealous of the human in the Physical Body, because liberation is possible only in human form.

"We worked and we worshipped and then we got this human body. Angels worship this body, because this body is the way to salvation. What a waste, when we neither recognize nor reconcile with the sacredness of our own existence."

© The Teachings of Yogi Bhajan, March 25, 1985

The extremes in emotion from ecstasy to sorrow can be felt through a Physical Body. The Physical Body also allows for a grounded experience of a spiritual path. The Physical Body reminds a person to *do* the practice. A strong Physical Body keeps a person grounded even when tempted by the far-out, esoteric aspects of spiritual growth. Leading a balanced life of healthy physical practices leads to satisfaction, a sense of soul connectedness, and a connection to all creation.

Connect deeply with the Physical Body. Learn to appreciate it and move it in ways that feel good.

Earth Tattva and the Musculoskeletal System

Earth nourishes, provides for life, and is extremely stable and dense. These qualities are manifested in the subtle aspect of the earth *tattva* and revealed in the body. Of all the *tattvas*, the earth *tattva* is the most grounded and stable. It represents the ability to tend to worldly pursuits and needs in a steady fashion. Because earth is literally and metaphorically the support of human life, this *tattva* is by nature supportive; in this same way, the muscles and bones support the body.

Being attentive to physical posture is one way to build the earth tattva and strengthen the musculoskeletal system.

A person with balanced earth *tattva* will be reliable, steady, and sweet. Someone with too much earth energy can be bullheaded or stubborn, like a tight muscle that is bound up and unable to move, while someone with too little earth becomes flighty and unreliable. The slow and steady physical practice of yoga unwinds and balances the earth element.

In the pursuit of precision in our postures it is important to release any grasping for perfection. The idea of a spiritual practice is not to become perfect; it is to continue to practice even with the awareness that we will never be perfect. To continue to nurture, heal, and serve ourselves and others because it is the right thing to do not because it is going to give us something or make us into something else. We will always be beautiful and flawed, physical and spiritual, perfectly imperfect humans.

"Nothing is perfect except your soul and its beauty."

Yogi Bhajan in a letter written to Japa Kaur Khalsa, March 7, 1999

TIPS AND TECHNIQUES FOR A STRONG MUSCULOSKELETAL SYSTEM

The body operates at a very sophisticated level of subconscious performance. There is no conscious thinking about blood calcium levels or the many other processes that keep the body alive. The body is designed with built-in systems to catch and correct potentially dangerous internal situations. Through the skillful application of self-care techniques one can increase the stability, strength, and vitality of the musculoskeletal system.

Meridians, Acupuncture and Yoga

Each joint has six major meridians flowing through it. The legs and torso contain the receptive yin meridians of the *Kidney*, *Spleen* and *Liver* as well as the yang meridians *Stomach*, *Gall Bladder* and *Urinary Bladder* that help with growth and movement. Yoga prevents energy from getting stuck by applying pressure to the multiple acupuncture points located in the joints. Large leg movements, for example, support transformation of consciousness through the subtle shift of the energy of the meridians.

The arms and upper body contain the yin meridians *Lung*, *Heart* and *Pericardium* while the arms, upper body and head hold the yang meridians *Large Intestine*, *Small Intestine* and *Triple Burner*. Upper body movements of yoga transform the consciousness through the flow of *Praana* or *Qi* through these energy pathways.

Aasanas and Exercises

Upper-body, Weight-bearing: Build arm strength; pressurize meridians in arms; strengthen all core muscles.
Examples: Triangle, Shoulder Stand, Platform, Cobra, Bridge
Expansive Postures: Counteracts the habitual rounded shoulder posture. Stretches overly tight pectoral muscles and engages weak upper back muscles, and/or opens pelvic tightness.
Examples: Camel, Kundalini Lotus, anything with arms up
Bent-Knee, Weight-Bearing Poses: Strengthens quadriceps, gluteus, and low back and aligns pelvis. Weight bearing puts healthy pressure on bones.
Examples: Archer, Crow Pose or Squats, Frogs

The Musculoskeletal System

Transformational Energy Points

Gallbladder 21: Shoulder Well

Location: Top of the shoulder, point is usually tender

Effects: Releases energy that is trapped in the head and neck, a confluence point of many energy pathways.

Yoga for this Point: Shoulder shrugs, Sat Kriya, Vigorous arm movement

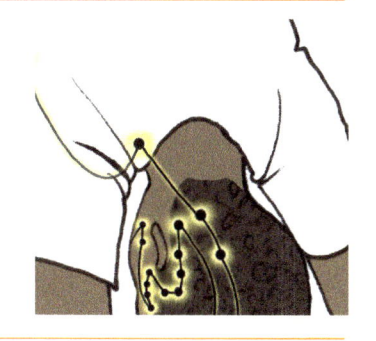

Yogic Locks *(Bhandas)*

A foundational element of practicing physical yoga postures is correctly engaging the locks, or *bhandas*.

Root Lock is typically cued as pulling up on the rectum, sex organs and navel. Learning to correctly apply this technique creates a powerful experience. The physical purpose of Root Lock is to create stability in the pelvis for the safe execution of postures. The core muscles used to apply Root Lock are the short, stocky muscles of the pelvic floor that are designed to help maintain posture and stability. Begin by isolating and engaging the muscles of the pelvic floor; this will allow for engagement of the anal sphincter without squeezing the gluteal muscles. Then, gently engage the deepest layer of the abdominal muscles, the *transverse abdominis*, which is the muscle that runs horizontally across the abdomen. When engaged the *transverse abdominis* creates a cinching action at the waist. In a correctly applied Root Lock, it is these deeper muscles in the body that are activated.

Yogi Bhajan said that a properly executed Neck Lock, combined with pressing the teeth together and the tongue into the roof of the mouth, will make the neck so strong that even a sword cannot cut through it!

©The Teachings of Yogi Bhajan, May 13, 1986

Keeping Up as You Age

The oldest living man to complete marathons, Fauja Singh, became famous in 2000 for carefully training and completing the grueling London Marathon at age 89 in record time. He is now over 100 years old and continues to beat records for his age group. He credits his success to careful training, a simple vegetarian diet, and surrounding himself with positive people. Speaking about the marathon, he said, "The first 20 miles (32 km) are not difficult. As for last six miles (9.5 km), I run while talking to God."

Subtle Effects of the Bhandas

- Root Lock redirects the *praana* and *apaana*. Mixing them to create *tapas*, or transformative fire.
- Diaphragm Lock enhances the power of the navel energies.
- Neck Lock seals and distributes the energies to the upper centers.

Diaphragm Lock is engaged by specific, meditative exercises, and it changes the inter-abdominal pressure. See the respiratory system for more on the Diaphragm Lock (page 93).

Neck Lock is important to engage correctly in a yoga and meditation practice. The purpose of Neck Lock is to create space and alignment in the neck and head which supports energy flow. To engage Neck Lock, sit or stand with a straight spine and gently tuck the chin. By lifting the base of the skull away from the neck and letting the chin pull in slightly this also lifts the chest and creates the desired neutral posture. A common mistake is to see beginners lifting their chin high because they are given a verbal cue to sit up straight. This action disrupts energy flow by creating a kink in the line of the spine and is not conducive to meditation. Teachers can remind new students to lift the spine *and* shorten the distance between the chin and the collarbone.

Plants, Herbs, and Food

Greens or Dairy Sufficient calcium intake is crucial for maintaining bone density. In many cultures, it can be easy to fall into thinking dairy products are the best way to add calcium to your diet. However, there are many excellent sources of calcium besides dairy, including dark leafy greens (e.g., spinach, kale, and Swiss chard), herbs (e.g., basil, thyme, rosemary, and dill), sesame seeds, Brazil nuts, tofu, almonds, and flax seeds, which have more calcium per gram than whole milk or yogurt.

Many people have allergies or sensitivities to dairy that lead to sinus problems, skin irritations and digestive distress. For these people the removal of dairy from their diets can lead to reduced symptoms and improved health. In Ayurveda, dairy is considered a cooling and mucus-building substance. The Ayurvedic way of preparing milk involves scalding it, which breaks down milk proteins and allows it to be a more digestible source of protein

The Musculoskeletal System

for all doshas (Khalsa, Tierra, 2008). When used in moderation it can be beneficial to balance the heating or drying aspects of an intense Breath of Fire practice and the spicy herbs of Indian cooking. In the Ayurvedic system, your individual constitution, or dosha, determines the amount of dairy that may be beneficial for you.

Got (something else besides) Milk?

Healthy bones are developed over many years of eating healthy, whole foods. Nuts, seeds, whole grains, and all brightly colored vegetables supply crucial amounts of magnesium, calcium, and vitamins. Vitamin D acts as a type of hormone to regulate bone density and should be supplemented as food sources and inadequate exposure to sunlight do not typically provide enough vitamin D for optimal health (Khalsa, 2009).

Turmeric helps lubricate joints, is good for skin and mucus membranes, and cleanses the blood and reduces inflammation. It is commonly used to ease joint or muscle soreness. It also aids digestion by clearing bad bacteria from the gut. Yogi Bhajan recommended turmeric as a way of supporting the stomach and intestines, which in turn supports the entire body by reducing inflammation (Bhajan, 1984). It is also recommended for the prevention of Alzheimer's because of its ability to reduce inflammation systemically (Duke, 2007). Including large quantities in the diet daily can do wonders in preventing the onset of inflammatory disorders. Turmeric is economical when purchased in powdered-spice form and can then be cooked with water to make it more readily available to the body. Create turmeric paste and treat the body to one to two teaspoons or more a day.

Corydalis is a well-known Chinese herb known for its analgesic or pain-killing properties. Related to the opium plant, it is sedating in nature and beneficial for headaches, back pain, and overall muscle pains. It has been used since the eighth century in China and is the main ingredient in a formula called Sudden Smile Powder, which eases the pain of menstrual cramps. The root of the plant can be purchased at herb stores or take it in capsule form. Even small quantities will help to relieve muscle pains. It should be taken only for short periods of time and under the supervision of a health care practitioner.

Magnesium Adding magnesium at night can be very soothing to the musculoskeletal system and can lead to a deeper sleep that allows for recovery and repair to take place. It is especially helpful if there are hypertonic (weak) muscles that are unable to relax even after a good workout or massage. Magnesium restores proper blood chemistry, which allows the muscles to relax.

Bodywork

There are many types of supportive bodywork that can help with the overall health of the musculoskeletal system. The stresses of life and gravity can lead to wear and tear and chronic misalignment in the body. A yoga practice, balanced exercise, or physical therapy may help to repair and correct some of these imbalances, but support from bodyworkers can be another very beneficial way to improve overall postural health.

Chiropractic Care focuses on realigning the joints to allow optimal flow of energy and optimum function of the nerves. There is often a special focus on spinal alignment in chiropractic care, but work on hips, feet and other areas of the body is not uncommon.

Therapeutic Massage helps to release tension in the muscles and fascia, allowing for a greater range of motion and quicker recovery from injury or stress.

Acupuncture stimulates energy flow in meridians, nerves, and blood to promote the release of past trauma and pain and to stimulate proper alignment.

Energy Healing works to release blockages or imbalances in the subtle anatomy, thus allowing the bones, joints and muscles to work with greater ease. Practitioners of Reiki, Touch for Life, and other healing touch modalities fall into the category of energy healing.

YOGI BHAJAN'S TURMERIC PASTE AND RECIPES

YOGI BHAJAN'S TURMERIC PASTE

Warms digestion gently, but is cooling in all the tissues. Balances all doshas.

- ✓ 1/4 cup (60 ml) powder
- ✓ 1 cup (240 ml) water

Prepare turmeric paste by combining ingredients in a saucepan and cooking on a low simmer for five minutes, until a thick paste is formed. Keep adding water if it gets too thick. After the paste is made, store in an airtight container and refrigerate. It can be stored for up to forty days. Optional: add some honey, cinnamon or cardamom to taste.

GOLDEN MILK

- ✓ 1 cup (240 ml) milk, rice milk, or other alternate milk
- ✓ 1 tsp t (5 ml) turmeric paste
- ✓ 1 tsp (5 ml) almond oil, ghee, coconut or sesame oil

Combine paste and milk in saucepan, on low heat. Bring milk to just short of boiling point while stirring. Remove from heat. Add oil. Add honey to taste. The mixture may be blended to make a foamy drink.

GOLDEN YOGURT

Take 1–2 tablespoons (15-30 ml) of paste, mix with a little yogurt or cottage cheese and eat.
Follow with a glass of water.

GOLDEN RICE

Take 1–2 tablespoons (15-30 ml) of paste and add it to your rice as it is cooking.

GOLDEN TOAST

Spread butter onto toast and slather 1–2 tablespoons (15-30 ml) of paste on top of melted butter.
Drizzle honey on top.

Shopping List for the Musculoskeletal System

- ✓ Avocados
- ✓ Coconuts
- ✓ Nuts
- ✓ Turmeric
- ✓ Leafy Greens

Balance the Root Chakra

When the Root Chakra is out of balance, we become spacey, forgetful, confused, and unfocused; we have a hard time following through on projects. It can also cause chronic urinary tract infections, constipation, or diarrhea.

To Balance the Root Chakra
- Walk on the ground barefoot
- Practice crow pose
- Eat a diet high in plant based foods
- Wear red
- Wear or meditate with black tourmaline
- Tap or massage the lower abdomen

Affirmations for the Root Chakra

I trust myself and the Divine to cover me with infinite protection. I love and nurture myself as I am right now, and I enjoy the flow of life.

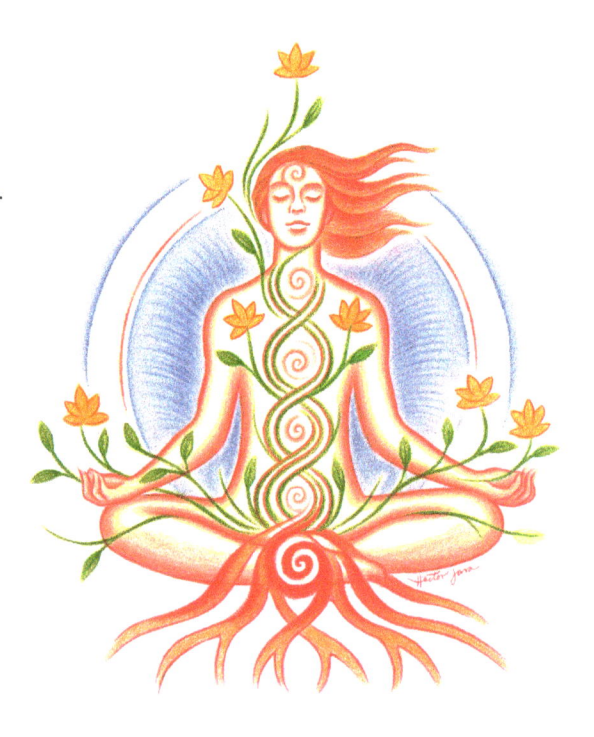

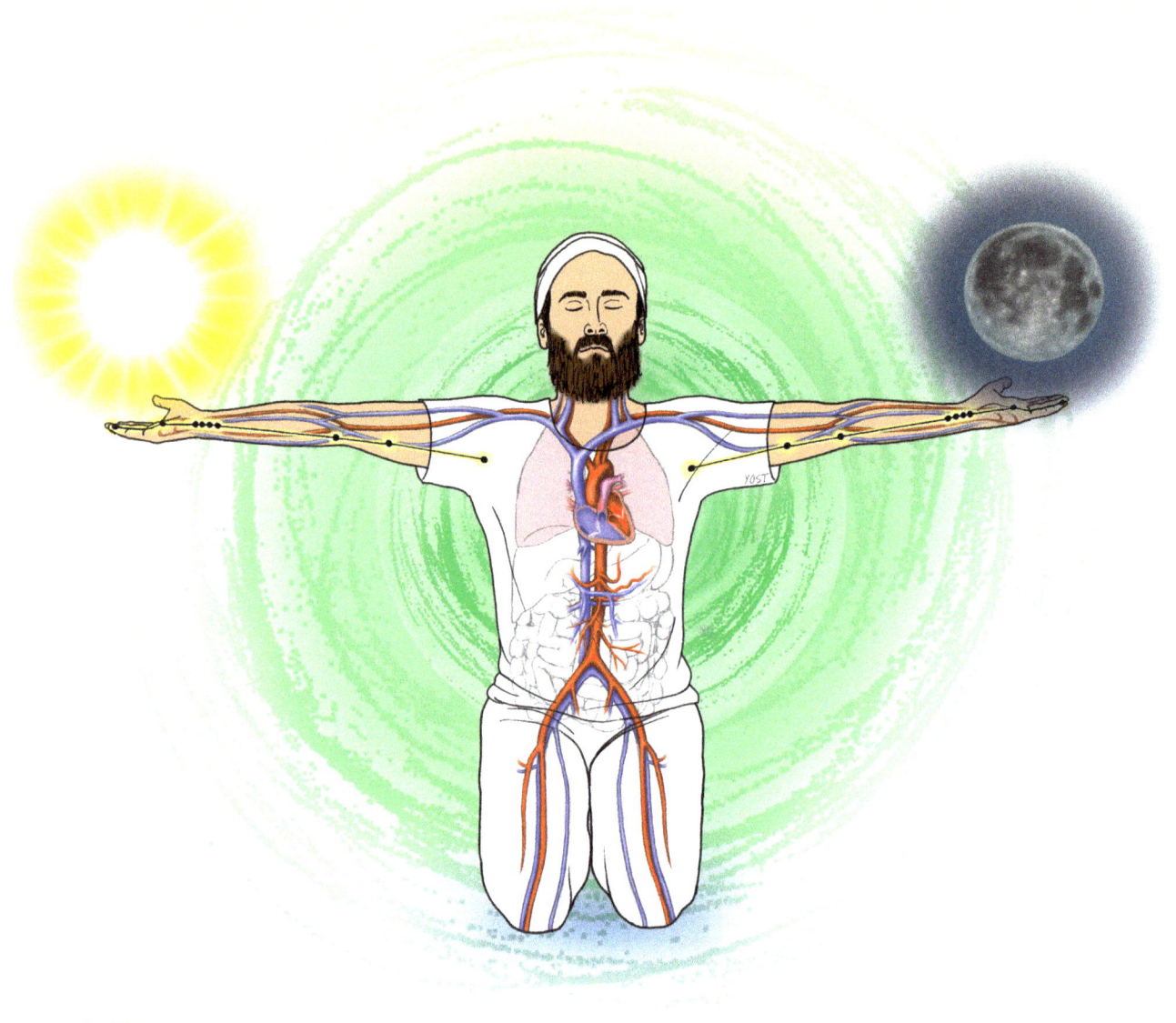

4.0 Rock Pose

Rock Pose (sitting on the heels) is helpful for the digestion through the pressure on the *Stomach* meridian in the legs. Any posture with the arms extended opens the heart space. The *Heart* meridian and its origin in the armpit are stimulated by all arm exercises. The circulatory system is all about the give and take involved in the flow of life.

Notice the subtle anatomy structures: the green swirl background represents the loving, giving energy of the heart chakra, the sun and moon represent the negative and positive minds which are balanced in the neutral mind of the yogi.

Notice the physical anatomy features: the powerful muscle of the heart a constant and essential force of life and the complexity of veins and arteries reaching throughout the body.

The Circulatory System

The circulatory system is one of the primary avenues of exchange in the body. Our bodies are in a constant state of flux. They are perpetually in the process of breaking down food or old blood cells and rebuilding things like bones and the stomach lining. A large number of chemical reactions and energy exchanges are happening in the body at any given moment. The heart and blood vessels are in a continual process of giving nourishment and energy to the body and supporting the release of used-up elements.

In the subtle realm, the circulatory system offers a message about incorporating service into our lives. An important part of a spiritual path is the act of service. Service on the spiritual path may mean volunteering to serve meals at a soup kitchen, hosting a visiting teacher in your home, or just listening to the concerns of a person in need. These selfless acts burn karmas and offer healing to both the giver and the recipient. The design of the heart or the circulatory system is a reminder to constantly be in a service mindset. There is nothing overly romantic about the physical organ of the heart. The heart is a tough chunk of muscle that works and serves the body at all times. It is the most continuously giving structure in the body. The heart teaches us about love through service.

PHYSICAL ANATOMY PERSPECTIVE

Components of the Circulatory System

- Blood
- Arteries
- Capillaries
- Veins
- Heart
- Lungs

Benefits of a Strong Circulatory System
Developing a strong circulatory system allows us to have the strength to give and receive in our daily lives. It creates an efficient exchange of oxygen, carbon dioxide, and energy.

Primary Purpose
From a physical perspective the primary purpose of the circulatory system is to carry oxygen and nutrition to the cells through the bloodstream. The circulatory system also assists in the removal of waste from the body. From a subtle perspective the circulatory system works to carry and balance the *praana* and *apaana* in the body.
The circulatory system is like the postman of life, constantly dropping off oxygen, and picking up carbon dioxide. At the center of that system is always the heart.

Blood

Blood is the medium for carrying energy, fuel, and water to every cell in the body. The cells of the body are constantly building things up, breaking down old cells, removing waste from the body, and creating new life. All of these processes require energy. There are two critical fuels that must be present for all of these processes to take place: glucose and oxygen.

In addition to providing cells with fresh energy, the blood is equally important in removing waste products. Most cellular processes result in extra carbon dioxide, or other waste products, which must be removed from the body. From a chemical perspective oxygen is needed for almost every reaction or process in our cells. From a subtle perspective, *praana* is needed in order for the body and consciousness to function and thrive.

The overall purpose of the circulatory system is the exchange of oxygen and carbon dioxide throughout the body. But the functions of blood are even more complex and varied than that. When the blood flows through the body, it is carrying lots of *praanic* building blocks beyond just oxygen. The blood transports hormones, waste products and toxins, nutrients (proteins, vitamins, minerals), white blood cells (immune response), and clotting factors. Blood is also critical for maintaining balance and homeostasis in the body. Specifically, it helps regulate pH and water balance.

"Inhale a little more, hold it tight; give your circulatory blood a chance to totally consume the entire oxygen which is there."

© The Teachings of Yogi Bhajan, May 27, 1990

Praana and *Apaana*: Primary Forces of Life

Praana is life-force energy or vitality. *Praana* governs all restorative and building functions, like inhaling and absorbing oxygen or eating and absorbing food. When our bodies are full of *praana*, we feel energized and content. *Praana* comes from every single thing in life; from the people around us and the clothing we wear to the joy or sadness felt in any given moment. A myriad of thoughts, emotions and physical experiences contribute to our *praanic* levels. The two largest sources of *praana* are food and air. Food and air are the primary energy sources in both the subtle and physical view of the body.

Apaana is the eliminating or destructive energy that regulates all elimination of waste in the body. Everything—from purging old clothes from the closet, a bowel movement, or even a complete exhalation—is governed by the eliminative energy of *apaana*.

Gas Exchange

The actual exchange of oxygen and carbon dioxide happens in two places. In the tissues of the lungs the blood absorbs oxygen and releases carbon dioxide. And in the tissues of the body the reverse exchange takes place. Both parts of this equation must be in balance to provide consistent, usable energy to the body.

In Kundalini Yoga, the suspension of breath on the inhale or exhale is a dynamic moment for blood chemistry. According to the Teachings of Yogi Bhajan, the blood chemistry changes at the moment of suspension and allows for a transformation that protects the body from disease (Bhajan, 1990b). During the suspended breath, the blood is able to fully absorb the praana and oxygen, and perhaps this pause allows for a shift in the blood chemistry. When the blood chemistry is adjusted it impacts the entire being (Bhajan, 1990b).

GOD

Yogi Bhajan taught that GOD is the generating (G), organizing (O), and delivering (D) force that pervades everything. This play of GOD is constantly present in the human body. The metabolic processes of the body constantly create, organize, and deliver its cells, mirroring the play of GOD happening in the universe all the time. God is the infinite and beautiful capacities within each person's physical and subtle anatomy (Bhajan, 1995, a.).

The Subtle Exchange of Energy

The energy exchange happens in a more subtle way. There is more *praanic* energy available on an inhale and more *apaanic* energy available on an exhale. However, the actual exchange is not a literal swapping, like the exchange of oxygen for carbon dioxide. In every moment there is absorption of *praana* and *apaana* through not only the lungs but every cell of the body. *Praana* is used to create every aspect of life and experience, and *apaana* is used to release what is no longer of service.

Blood Pathway Through the Body

Blood flows into the right side of the heart (at this point it does not have oxygen, and is known as oxygen poor or hypoxemic blood). Then the heart pumps and the blood is forced out and goes to the lungs where the oxygen/carbon dioxide exchange takes place. The, now oxygen-rich blood flows back to the heart. This time it enters the left side. The next time the heart beats, the blood pumps out to the body.

It starts its journey through the body in the aorta, the artery with the largest diameter. The blood then flows down smaller and smaller arteries until it is dropped into a rich cellular feeding space called the capillary

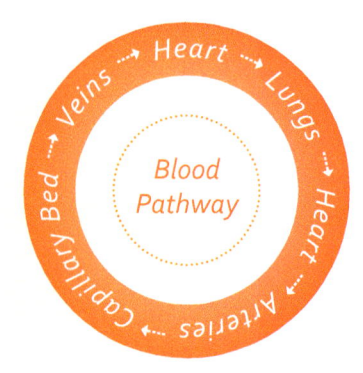

The Circulatory System

bed. This is where the other half of the oxygen/carbon dioxide exchange happens. Once all the oxygen has been dropped off and carbon dioxide picked up the blood flows into the veins. It travels in larger and larger veins until it reaches the heart, where the cycle repeats. This cycle happens continuously in every moment.

Arteries are tubes that run out from the heart to the body. They begin with a huge tube called the aorta that runs down the center of the body. The aorta is about one inch (2.5 cm) in diameter when it starts its pathway down the body. Other tubes branch out from it and decrease in diameter as they reach the body's extremities. They carry blood rich with oxygen and nutrients away from the heart and out to body tissues.

Arteries operate in a high-pressure system. The powerful contraction of the heart as it forces blood into the arteries, combined with the smooth muscle cells in the walls of the arteries themselves, creates the high pressure that moves blood through the circulatory system. As the arteries become smaller they lead into what are called arterioles, which become even smaller and lead into capillaries. The diameter of a capillary is so small that only one blood cell can pass at a time.

Capillaries Transactions and exchanges of energy and nutrition take place in the capillary bed. This is the microscopic exchange site. Oxygen and nourishment move into the body cells here and plasma oozes out of the blood and turns into lymph. Once the blood has dropped off its nutrients and picked up waste products it continues on and enters the veins.

Veins are a series of tubes bringing oxygen-depleted blood back to the heart. Veins are structured in the opposite way as the arteries; they start with tiny tubes called venules, and gradually grow larger in diameter as they lead to the heart.

The veins are a low-pressure system: they are so far away from the heart that they aren't getting the force of the heart's pump, also they do not have muscle cells in the walls to help with blood flow. The veinous system has the added challenge of having to work against gravity to return blood from the legs.

> THE BODY IS BEAUTIFULLY DESIGNED TO PROTECT ITSELF. THE BODY PUTS THE ARTERIES DEEPER IN THE BODY TO PROTECT THE VALUABLE OXYGEN-RICH BLOOD.

Exploring Physical and Subtle Human Anatomy

Chapter 4

4.1 Circulatory Family

Major players in the blood pathway: Oxygenated blood in the arteries is shown in red, while deoxygenated blood in the veins appears blue. The veins and arteries create a closed circuit which is continually moving through the body bringing oxygen and nutrients and carrying away waste and toxins.

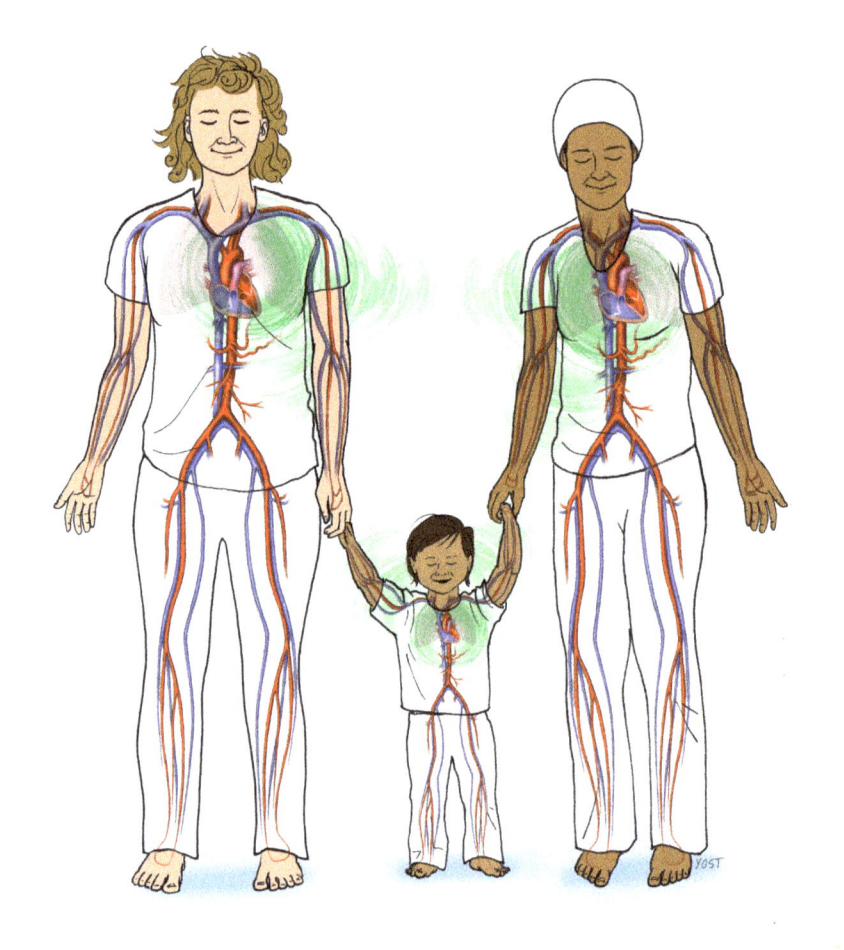

To combat these challenges and prevent blood from backing up or pooling the veins have a system of valves. The blood is forced forward through the vein by skeletal muscle action and then a valve closes behind it, which prevents it from flowing backward. In effect, the skeletal muscles function as the pump to move the blood back up to the heart. Veins rely on the structure of the valves and the movement of our bodies to do their job.

The Heart

The heart is composed of four muscular chambers; two atria that receive blood and two ventricles that push blood back out. There are specialized valves between each chamber that control the direction of blood flow. The heart is about the size of a human fist and is located slightly left of the midline of the body. It is protected by the breastbone and ribcage. The muscle tissue of the heart itself is supplied with blood via the coronary arteries. These act as a special supply loop to bring fresh oxygenated blood to the heart muscle.

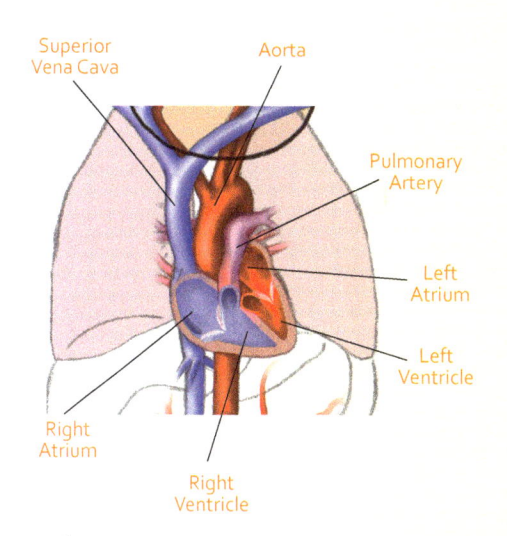

What Is Blood Pressure?

Blood pressure readings measure the pressure blood exerts on the walls of the large arteries. Systolic pressure, the number usually listed on top of a blood pressure reading, is the peak of the pressure generated when the heart contracts. Diastolic pressure, the number on the bottom of a blood pressure reading, is the pressure exerted when the heart is relaxed.

The Lungs

The lungs collect fresh air and through a system of smaller tubes and arterioles, supply oxygen to the blood. They act as a dropping off point for carbon dioxide, which is then exhaled out of the lungs. The diaphragm muscle acts as a bellows, expanding the lungs on the inhalation and compressing the lungs on the exhalation.

Relationship to Other Systems

Circulatory and Immune Systems The lymph is sometimes considered the second circulatory system because of its cooperative role in moving fluids around the body. The lymphatic vessels generally run parallel to the veins and arteries. They have slightly different structures; arteries have more rigid, muscular walls, while lymph vessels have softer, collapsible walls.

EVERY DAY THE HEART BEATS OVER 100,000 TIMES AND MOVES 8,000 LITERS OF BLOOD THROUGH THE BODY.

Plasma and lymph fluid are the same substance though occurring in different systems and serving unique functions.

Plasma is the clear part of blood. In the capillary beds some of the plasma moves into the spaces between cells where it is called interstitial fluid. Some of that fluid gets picked up by open-ended lymphatic vessels. Once it enters the lymph vessels this fluid is considered lymph. The lymphatic fluid moves through the lymph vessels until it is deposited into the blood through a large vein in the chest.

The tubes of the circulatory and lymphatic systems act as the transportation highways of the body. The lymph system supports the function of the circulatory system by getting rid of the waste products of cellular activities and other toxins. Blood and lymph work synergistically to move nutrients and immune cells, which protect the body from viruses or bacteria, into the body.

The Circulatory System

SUBTLE ANATOMY PERSPECTIVE

The Heart Chakra

The Heart Chakra is the wheel of energy located at the level of the sternum, or breastbone. It encompasses the heart, lungs, sternum, clavicle, shoulder blades, breast tissue, thymus gland and rib cage. The arms and hands are also extensions of the Heart Chakra. The Heart Chakra relates to the ability to feel compassion and love. It encompasses the ability to heal yourself and others. It is enhanced by a life of service, because selfless service comes from the strength and integrity of unconditional love.

When the Heart Chakra is balanced and open there is an experience of compassion, love, selflessness, and healing. If the Heart Chakra becomes too weak or too guarded, there is a lack of trust and sense of disconnection from other human beings. If the Heart Chakra is too open or unsupported we are easily overwhelmed by sympathy for others to the point of losing perspective of our own needs or becoming an emotional doormat.

The shadow emotion of the Heart Chakra is imbalanced attachment or detachment. Over-attachment shows up when we think there is not enough love or protection in life. We start grabbing at everything in sight, trying to force people into relationships, or a feeling of desperation for love, regardless of the cost. The opposite of this is complete detachment, when there is a purposeful cultivation of aloofness as a way of protection from the potential pain of loving. People in this state will say, "I don't *need* anyone in my life. I can do it myself." They push people away rather than risk being vulnerable. To pretend that other people aren't necessary might temporarily feel better, but in the end it is lonely and unsustainable. The solution to both of these issues is to trust that the need for love and compassion will be met. This allows the Heart Chakra to be open and balanced.

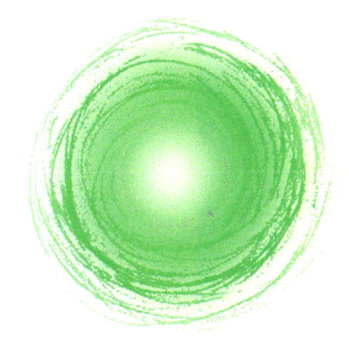

4.2 The Heart Chakra

"*We need people in our lives with whom we can be as open as possible. To have real conversations with people may seem like such a simple, obvious suggestion, but it involves courage and risk.*"

—Thomas Moore, psychotherapist, author

The Heart as a Model of Service

"Only a life lived for others is worth living."

—Albert Einstein, theoretical physicist, Nobel Prize winner

The physical muscle of the heart embodies the capacity to work hard, deliver, and be of service. The heart pumps all day long, every day, our entire life and creates the capacity to be steady, to sacrifice and ultimately to be happy. The heart creates the steady rhythm of life. It reminds us to serve steadily and to sacrifice in the service of others.

Yogi Bhajan's Seven Steps to Happiness

Commitment *In every life you are meant to commit. That is why the word is commit-meant. Commitment gives you* **character**.

Character *Character is when all your characteristics—all facets, flaws and facts—are under your control. Yin and yang meet there, totally balanced. Character gives you* **dignity**.

Dignity *People start trusting you, liking you, respecting you. Dignity will give you* **divinity**.

Divinity *Divinity is when people see no duality about you. They trust you right away. They have no fear of you. Divinity gives you* **grace**.

Grace *Where there is grace, there is no interference, no gap between two people, and no hidden agenda. Grace gives you the power to* **sacrifice**.

Sacrifice *You can stand in any pain for that person. That sacrifice gives you* **happiness**.

Happiness *Happiness is when you can be thankful for the chance of being these seven things* (Khalsa, 1996, Bhajan, 2010).

A Yogic Concept of Love

In Yogic philosophy love is a verb; a powerful active force rather than the emotional phenomenon that is typical of society's fantasy-oriented ideas of love and romance. In many cultures, love is portrayed as a gooey, hot, sentimental experience with candlelight, love songs, and sexual arousal. While this is a very exciting and fantastic sensation, it is not sustainable. Statistically, this *in love* feeling is most dramatic for the first two years of a romantic relationship and can be largely attributed to a primal mechanism that encourages a couple to create, cooperate, and cohabitate. Being *in love* is part of your body's mechanism to make sure the human race continues. The challenge of love *in action* is to sustain this feeling through the grind of daily life after those initial two years. True love is the daily choice to wake up and serve another person, sharing your divine, deep and true qualities. This type of love extends beyond the primary romantic interest in a person's life and is a way to be in service and relate in kindness to all people (BBC News, 2006).

The Heart Nourishes Itself First

How can the heart maintain this never-ending service? This requires a two-part answer. The heart is made of a unique type of muscle tissue called cardiac muscle. This allows the heart to beat without getting tired or losing effectiveness. Cardiac muscle has a higher percentage of mitochondria—the power sources of the cells—than skeletal muscle and does not fatigue, because the mitochondria quickly produce energy for the heart. But this tireless service cannot happen unless the heart itself is nourished—first. When the oxygen-rich blood leaves the heart it travels through the aorta and out to the body. The first branch off of the aorta superhighway of blood is back to the muscles of the heart itself, via the coronary arteries. The first thing the heart does is nourish itself. It serves the entire body tirelessly every day, for our whole life, but it will *always* take care of its own needs first.

Here, the heart has another important message: you can't really be of service to humanity if there is no self-care. As a yogi, if all the focus is on serving students and teaching, but you neglect your own practice, there will be stress and possibly even burnout. With a mother, if the focus is on taking care of the children's needs, and the mother never takes a quiet moment to relax and do what nourishes and recharges her, both the mother and the children will suffer. As a doctor, if the long hours of treating patients aren't accompanied by enough rest, the price may be mistakes or resentment. It is important to hear this message of the heart: Be steady in service and practice self-care. This allows for a balanced heart and a balanced life.

"*It's time for you to serve people—humanity… Our main job is to be together and inspire each other to reach for the golden light… Let us be one in the oneness of each other; love and reach out, make life happy. I hope you'll carry the day with these words in your hearts.*"

© The Teachings of Yogi Bhajan, republished in Aquarian Times, April 18, 2002

"*Love isn't a state of perfect caring. It is an active noun like struggle. To love someone is to strive to accept that person exactly the way he or she is, right here and now.*"

—Fred Rogers, *The World According to Mister Rogers*

> BE STEADY IN YOUR SERVICE AND TAKE CARE OF YOURSELF FIRST. THIS ALLOWS YOU AND YOUR HEART TO BE MUCH MORE EFFECTIVE IN SERVICE TO ALL.

Healthy Heart = Calm Mind and Spirit = Strong Neutral Mind

Yoga and Meditation cultivate a peaceful Heart Center, the foundation for the Neutral Mind, so that a person can exist as a soul that is firmly grounded and at peace.

Developing the Neutral Mind

The Neutral Mind is the fourth of the Ten Light Bodies. It works with the Negative Mind and Positive Mind to observe life and guide the decision-making process. When a thought or idea comes into the Light Bodies, it is first processed through the Negative Mind, then the Positive Mind. Ideally, the thought flows into the Neutral Mind where we accept the situation and then follow with appropriate action. The Neutral Mind is not about weighing pros and cons (that is what the Negative and Positive Minds are for). The Neutral Mind operates beyond the polarity of good and bad. When decisions are made from the Neutral Mind they move us toward righteous action. This capacity of the Neutral Mind is deeply rooted in the Fourth Chakra. When the Heart Chakra is balanced it creates the sense of safety and expansiveness that allows for movement away from duality and toward neutrality.

If a person is in a state of deep trust with the Infinite, she moves beyond the ups and downs of life and accepts what *is*. The energy wasted by constantly questioning and doubting—*Should I do this? Should I do that? Why didn't this happen? Why did that happen instead?*—is transformed into a state of acceptance and trust. This state of consciousness is not affected by the good or bad in life, but instead allows for and exists in a state of constant, neutral acceptance.

This neutral acceptance of what is allows for a closer alignment with the great Masters. Cultivating a connection to Guru Ram Das, Christ Consciousness, or Buddha Consciousness is an important part of many spiritual traditions. Their mental state is desired because it leads to a balanced heart, calm mind, and expansive spirit. The goal of many spiritual traditions is to take a person to a place of oneness, where there is no duality between heart and mind, and where they can experience neutrality. This is accomplished by a steady practice of prayer, yoga, or contemplation.

Just as the circulatory system serves the whole body selflessly, a strong Neutral Mind serves the entirety of a person's destiny. Cultivating the Neutral Mind is an act of service because by walking on your own destiny path, you also bring everyone around you a little closer to their truest, most authentic, and highest path. Having a daily spiritual practice is the surest way to support both the heart center and the Neutral Mind. It allows for the release of pent-up anger and negativity and releases toxins from the Physical Body. A consistent practice at any time of day is deeply valuable, but many traditions suggest an early morning practice, before or during sunrise.

Early Morning Spiritual Practices

Ayurveda Waking up before the sunrise is a time to dwell in the peaceful, deeply healing aspects of nature. This gives more time for cleansing Ayurvedic routines that nourish the body-spirit-mind connection.

Christianity In many branches of Christianity, there is a recognition of the special blessing that is early morning prayers and reading the Bible in the quiet hours at the dawn of day. The Benedictine tradition, for example, has an early morning prayer, called *Matin*, which is recited between 3:00–6:00 a.m (Weaver, 2014).

Islam *Fajr* is the first prayer of the day, offered at the beginning of dawn. It is sometimes known as God's favorite prayer since many are still asleep.

Judaism The *Modeh Ani* is recited in bed immediately upon waking up; it roughly translates to "I offer thanks before you, living and eternal King, for You have mercifully restored my soul within me; Your faithfulness is great" (Wikipedia, n.d.).

Kundalini Yoga and Meditation The two and a half hours before sunrise, called the *Amrit Vela,* are the most potent hours of the day for yoga and meditation. The Aquarian Sadhana, practiced during the *Amrit Vela*, is the recitation of sacred prayers, physical yoga postures and 62 minutes of mantra meditation.

Lakota Songs are sung to the early morning star and sunrise is a special time to appreciate living in the moment and being part of nature (Black Elk, 2014).

Tibetan Buddhism His Holiness the Dalai Lama sets the standard for his followers by rising at 3:30 a.m., showering, and doing prayers, meditations, and prostrations for two hours.

> *"There is nothing either good or bad, but thinking makes it so."*
> —William Shakespeare, *Hamlet*

> *"Getting up in the morning for sadhana is totally a selfish act for personal strength, for personal intuition, for personal sharpness, for personal discipline and above all for personal absolute prosperity."*
> © The Teachings of Yogi Bhajan, May 14, 1989

Chinese Medicine and the Heart

In Chinese medicine the spirit lives and sleeps in the *Heart*. The four thick muscular chambers of the human *Heart* hold the spirit. The strength the *Heart* carries through a person's lifetime allows for their soul to grow and expand and face the challenges of life.

A calm and integrated spirit manifests through the health of the *Heart*. When the *Heart* is healthy we experience energy, creativity, and feelings of joy. When a person is balanced and healthy, the spirit can rest there comfortably, and they sleep well at night because of this inner sense of peace.

When a person is going through a challenging time, the unease in the *Heart* prevents the soul from resting peacefully. Bad dreams or fear and anxiety about life may torment them. This is seen as a separation between *Heart* and spirit. These symptoms can be worse at night, because in Chinese philosophy it is said that the disturbed soul wanders at night in the ethers, unable to settle in the *Heart*.

The wandering of the soul and lack of deep rest creates duality, confusion, questioning and self-doubt. Many great saints and sages over the years are known as much for their times of suffering and doubt as for their divinity. Joan of Arc, Christ, and Buddha all deeply questioned themselves and their missions at various times in their lives. Perhaps the questioning and doubt are a necessary part of the spiritual life and part of the preparation of the *Heart* for great things. As yogis there are tools to use during the times of questioning to move out of the duality and into the expansive, balanced, peaceful spirit. Meditation and *praanayam* balance the energy of the *Heart* and bring about a state of calm and ease.

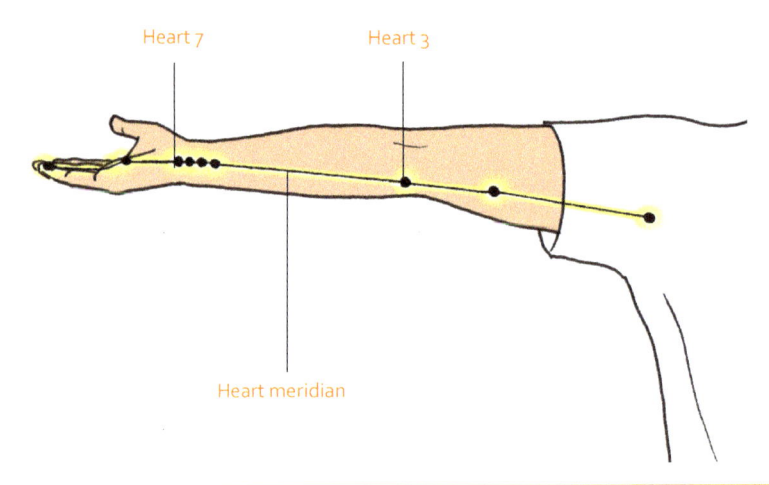

4.3 The Heart Meridian

The *Heart* meridian stretches from the armpit out to the pinkie. Pressure on this meridian through yoga postures helps to support a calm mind, deep sleep and creativity.

The *Heart* Meridian

The *Heart* meridian is located on the inner aspect of the arm stretching from the armpit all the way to the tip of the pinkie. Mudras that move the wrist or fingers and hands impact the *Heart* meridian. Many traditions speak of the hands as an extension of the *Heart*; the location of this meridian reflects that belief.

Challenges to the Heart and Circulation

Healing Through the Power of the Heart Center

Healing from both the physical and subtle perspectives comes from the area of the heart. Physical healing ranges from the immune system fighting off a common cold to the more dramatic healing of traumatic injury or life-threatening illness. The nutrients and cells traveling through the bloodstream are all under the domain of the heart. When the Heart Center is doing the extra work of recovering from injury or illness puts a strain on the whole body which is why during times of healing the body needs more rest and simple foods.

Subtle healing revolves around understanding and shifting emotional patterns or scars. It means jumping from the known attachment to one's story of victimhood or pain to the unknown possibility of health, vibrancy, and personal responsibility. That subtle capacity comes from the loving energy of the Heart Chakra. Subtle healing allows one to live from the light of the soul instead of from the ingrained patterns and scars of the heart. To do this, we must practice forgiveness and acceptance of the past. This work must happen in a space that feels safe. Emotional safety comes from a strong heart center. Emotional safety allows for deep surrender and healing. It would seem that there is a paradox here, you must feel safe to do the healing work of the heart, but in order to feel safe you must have a strong Heart Center. This is one of the challenges of the spiritual path. We must walk on the path while we are laying the paving stones. And this is why healing often happens in waves, years after a wound has healed it may resurface to be soothed again in a new, more profound way.

Healing is both a common human experience and also deeply singular and personal. Healing requires faith that one *can* get better, even in the worst moments. The blending of subtle anatomy and physical anatomy

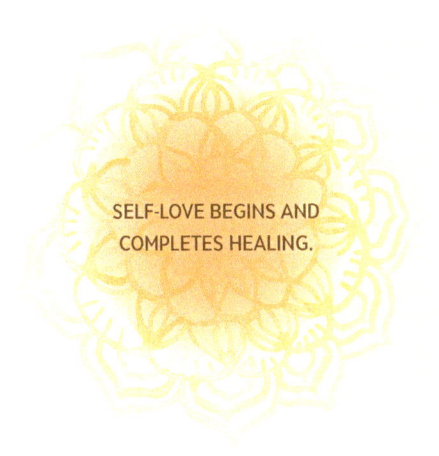

> SELF-LOVE BEGINS AND COMPLETES HEALING.

> *"We cannot ascend in the journey of the soul to our ultimate liberation without being connected to our heart. We can practice mantras and meditations, prayers, do ceremonies, or be a sadhu, but without that connection to the heart we do not have God's blessings."*
>
> —Rajinder Kaur Khalsa

Japa's Fathers Story

My father is a cardiovascular and thoracic surgeon and has cared for many people during his career. He is a scientific and analytical thinker yet he would tell me that he always noticed the people that seemed to do the best in surgery were the ones who would say, "I know I am in God's hands."

> THE PRACTICE OF BOWING PLACES YOUR HEAD BELOW YOUR HEART CENTER. THIS CREATES A PHYSICAL POSTURE OF SURRENDER WHICH ALLOWS FOR DEEP TRANSFORMATION AND HEALING.

in the Heart Center is what creates the possibility for this faith. Because of the unpredictable and mysterious nature of health, healing also requires acceptance. Part of the challenge of disease, illness, or injury is the seeming randomness of it. One person might eat the perfect diet and not survive serious illnesses. Whereas another will drink, smoke, and not do a lick of yoga and live to age 99. Surrendering and having faith also means accepting that sometimes being sick, even terminally, is what is meant to be.

There are many ways to feel trapped and suffer in this body, but if the Heart Center is alive there can be joy. Joy comes from merging the lower aspects of the body—fear, separation, and ego—and surrendering them to a higher good. The merger with the infinite or the unknown allows for transformation and miraculous healing. Life's challenges can be transmuted into a surprise blessing instead of a curse through the forgiving power of the heart.

The Heart Center Is the Healing Center

The Heart Center is where the capacity to heal others and the self originates. Healing professionals use their hands to create the healing exchange of energy from themselves to their patient or client. Doctors use their hands to examine. Nurses use their hands to deliver medication. Acupuncturists use their hands to place needles. Massage therapists use their hands to massage. Chiropractors use their hands to adjust the joints. Energy workers most often use their hands to sense, receive, and transmit energy. People instinctively use their hands to create connections to the people around them. The natural instinct when seeing someone in distress is to give them a hug or a pat on the back. The arms and hands act as extensions of the Heart Center's healing, compassionate and loving energy.

The Circulatory System

TIPS AND TECHNIQUES FOR A STRONG CIRCULATORY SYSTEM

The heart and circulation are a complex and vital component of the physical body. They are also a clear indicator of the overall health of the organism. If the physical body is tended to and cared for, the heart will work much better. And when the heart works better, the *whole body* feels better, more vital, and more alive. When the heart is more efficient, the body feels better and it is easier to engage in activities, such as walking or jogging, that support heart health. It is a health-promoting, *praana*-building, happiness spiral.

Aasanas and Exercises

Inversions: Any posture that puts you upside down takes the pressure of gravity off and helps the venous blood flow back to the heart with greater ease.
Examples: Shoulder Stand, Triangle Pose, Plow, Standing Forward Bend
Heart Meridian Postures: Stretching the arms and the upper ribcage in the heart and chest clears stagnation from the subtle pathway of the heart meridian. The crease of the wrist near the pinkie and the pinkie finger itself are also important parts of the heart meridian. Mudras that pressurize those points can have a calming effect.
Examples: Camel Pose, Bridge Pose, Cobra
Heart Opening Postures: Any posture that stretches or opens the front of the body helps to counteract the common posture of slumped forward shoulders. Moving exercises like arm swings or torso twists will help to clear obstructions from the Heart Chakra.
Examples: Yoga Mudra, Half Wheel, Arm Swings

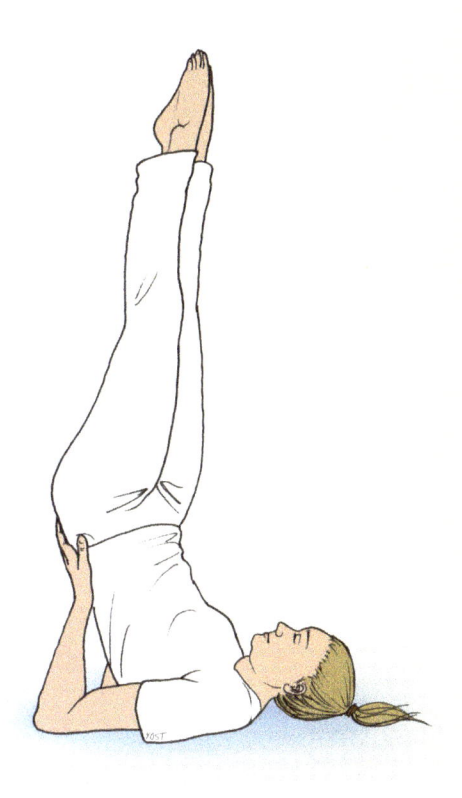

4.4 Shoulder Stand

Shoulder Stand is a classic yoga inversion. Inverted postures reverse the daily stress imposed by gravity, giving the body a chance to restore and heal; supports lymph movement, venous blood return and pressurizes the glands of the neck and head.

Transformational Energy Points

Heart 7: Spirit Gate

Location: Wrist crease, beneath the pinky

Effects: Releases disharmonies in the mind-body-spirit connections. Helps sleep. Soothes anxiety.

Yoga for this Point: Cat-Cow, mudras with bent wrists

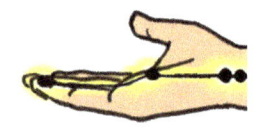

Squeeze the pinkie before going into an important meeting or conversation to activate the energy of the heart.

Cardio Workouts

What is the best way to improve the health of the circulatory system? *Move the body.* It is important to put the circulatory system under a little bit of stress on a regular basis. This helps the circulatory system stay tuned up and efficient throughout life. Kundalini Yoga has a variety of kriyas, and some involve aerobic, sustained activity specifically intended for building the heart and circulatory system. A variety of activities involving sustained movement and generating sweat can be considered 'cardio workouts', including hiking, dancing, cycling, and more. Find activities that you enjoy and practice them regularly to keep the heart, veins, and arteries healthy.

Praanayams for the Heart

Blood nourishes every cell in the body and *praanayam* adds *praana* to the blood. Increasing the *praanic* life force brings health, energy and efficiency to every cell. Breath techniques, especially Breath of Fire, are the easiest and quickest way to increase overall vitality (Bhajan, 2010).

The tongue is also used during certain breathing exercises, like Lion's Breath or *sitali*, to help balance the heart. The vagus nerve is stimulated when the tongue sticks out. Stimulating the vagus nerve has a calming influence on the heart rate. In physical anatomy, there is a connection between oral health and cardiovascular health with studies showing the benefit of proper oral hygiene. In subtle anatomy, the tongue is considered an organ of detoxification. Practices that cleanse or physically cool the tongue are helpful in maintaining a balanced heart-spirit-mind connection (NIDCR, 2014).

Sitali *Praanayam*

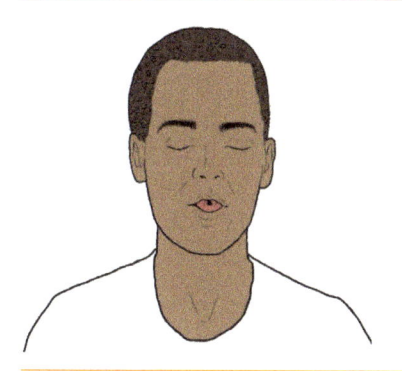

Sit in a comfortable meditative posture with the spine straight. Curl the tongue and protrude it slightly past the lips. Inhale deeply and smoothly through the mouth, as if you are sipping the air in over the tongue. Exhale through the nose, keeping the tongue extended. Feel how cool your tongue gets during this meditation. The coolness has an overall benefit by reducing inflammation in the whole body. Continue for three–five minutes (Bhajan, 2010).

Plants, Herbs, and Food

Specific herbs for building the blood are recommended in Ayurvedic and Chinese medicine. Menstruating women who are losing blood, iron, and minerals can use certain teas to replenish the body. Men can also benefit from the following list of botanicals, especially if they have thin, brittle nails or thinning or graying hair.

Amalaki is a restorative herb in Ayurveda used to benefit the blood and circulation. A small, sour fruit high in Vitamin C, it is an excellent remedy to balance *Pitta* dosha and support heart health. This Indian gooseberry supports the skin on many levels, the inner lining of the arteries and the heart, the lining of the digestive tract, and the outer protective layer of the physical skin. It helps to prevent anemia and build red blood cells. It can be taken in the well-known Ayurvedic tonic *triphala*, which works to regulate digestion in all the doshas. Try it in the delicious jam known as *chyawanprash* (Khalsa, Tierra 2008).

Dang Gui is available as thick slivers of dried wood and can be tossed into soup to add flavor and blood-building, nourishing minerals. Take it out at the end of the cooking process because the dried root is not digestible. It is known as the best plant to rebuild the blood, which is especially important for females. Keep a mason jar filled with the herb in the kitchen and when feeling depleted, rundown, or generally weak, boil it and drink the liquid. This herb can also be purchased as a tea or in capsules.

Nettle Leaf grows as a prickly unpleasant plant that can sting when touched. Once it is harvested (with gloves) it can be steamed like any vegetable and eaten safely as steaming destroys the prickly part. It can also be purchased in dried form or in tea bags and boiled into a dark, mineral-rich tea. Like spinach in flavor and purpose, it is one of the densest sources of iron and minerals in green vegetables. It is the best resource for reducing inflammation for seasonal allergies. Nettle leaf works best for allergies when it is not heated as this destroys the anti-allergy property. For best results treating allergies use freeze dried or fresh juice. Nettle leaf tea helps build *Qi* and blood especially in pregnant and menstruating women.

Milky Oat Seed is known as "meditation in a bottle" for its ability to soothe anxiety and calm the mind. Handy for yogis as it helps to transform a racing mind into a Neutral Mind. It works quickly, which makes it especially helpful for those freak-out moments in life when a calm center is needed. Because it is harvested at a particular stage of the growing cycle it is best taken in tincture form (alcohol extract). As an added bonus, Milky Oat Seed can also help to reduce cravings for stimulants, like coffee.

Yogic Lifestyle

Ishnaan

Cold showers are good for the organs and inspire the whole being.

A traditional part of yogic lifestyle, *Ishnaan,* or cold showers, helps to flush and move the blood. This clears toxins by rapidly moving the blood through the body. It also sends fresh oxygen and biochemical information to every cell (Yogiji, 2006).

How Do Cold Showers Work?

"You have to have a cold shower whether you like it or you hate it, doesn't matter. There is no medical human system to open up your capillaries better than a cold shower."

© The Teachings of Yogi Bhajan, September 16, 1993

Normally blood is found at all levels of the body from the skin to the depth of the organs. Jumping into cold water sends the body into a protective response. To keep the vital organs warm all of the blood rushes into the internal organs. Once out of the water the blood rushes back to the skin level. That's why you feel such a rush of being tingly and alive after a cold shower.

Cold water is the best way to open up and invigorate the capillary system. The subtle stress on the body during a cold shower is strengthening for all of the internal organs and increases circulation (Khalsa, 2011).

How to Do *Ishnaan*

1) Massage the body with almond oil.

2) Turn the cold water on in the shower.

3) Put an arm in. Put a leg in. Put the whole body in.

4) Go in and out a few times. While moving in and out of the water, massage the body and chant a mantra to help keep up with the cleansing process. If you wish, tap the thyroid and thymus and for women, tap at the location of the ovaries. Pay special attention to massaging the armpits and breast areas. It is recommended to leave shorts on. The thighbone is the largest and most dense bone and mineral reservoir in the body. It deserves to be buffered from the shock of direct cold water. Do not wash the hair in cold water. No cold showers for women on the heavy part of the moon cycle or who are pregnant. This is not a shower for bathing; it is a hydrotherapy experience (Yogiji, 2006).

Mantra

The vibration of certain mantras are healing for the Heart Chakra. Mantras for the heart include:

Guru Guru Wahe Guru
Guru Ram Das Guru

This mantra is said to awaken the Heart Chakra, create healing miracles, and access the Neutral Mind. This mantra can be chanted anytime and anywhere to bring in the full and purest love of the Heart Chakra without becoming codependent or an emotional doormat.

Guru Ram Das

Guru Ram Das was the fourth Sikh Guru and was known as a teacher, sage, and yogi who humbly served all. Guru Ram Das is believed by many to be a master of the Heart Center.

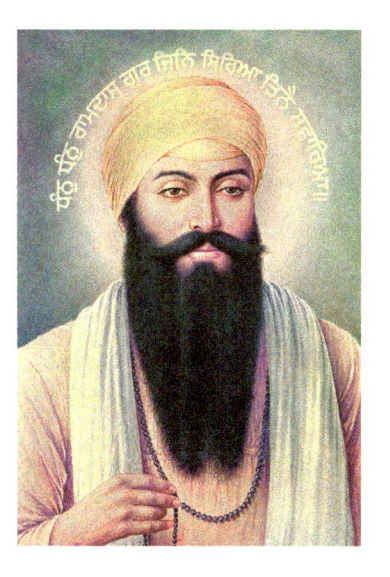

Hammee Ham Brahm Ham

This mantra means, "We are we; we are God." It connects to the expansive energy of the Heart Center and remedies the tendency toward aloofness.

Raa Maa Daa Saa
Saa Say So Hang

This is *the* mantra for healing energy. It calls on the elements of earth, sun, moon, and infinity and consolidates their power into the present moment in time for transformation. It can be used in long-distance healing treatments.

Balance the Heart Chakra

The Heart Chakra is out of balance when we feel overly emotional or emotionally closed off; when we have a lack of boundaries; when we lack compassion or have few close relationships. Physically it is indicated by heartburn, shoulder tightness, chronic injuries to arms, wrists or hands.

To Balance the Heart Chakra
- Wear Green and/or Pink.
- Wear or meditate with rose quartz.
- Practice Ego Eradicator.
- Find a place to serve or volunteer.
- Ensure the faculties of both giving and receiving are balanced in your life.
- Gently tap the Heart Center.

Affirmations for the Root Chakra
I give to myself and others, and I share with grace and ease.

My life is a balanced flow of love, forgiveness, and expansion through my trust in the Divine.

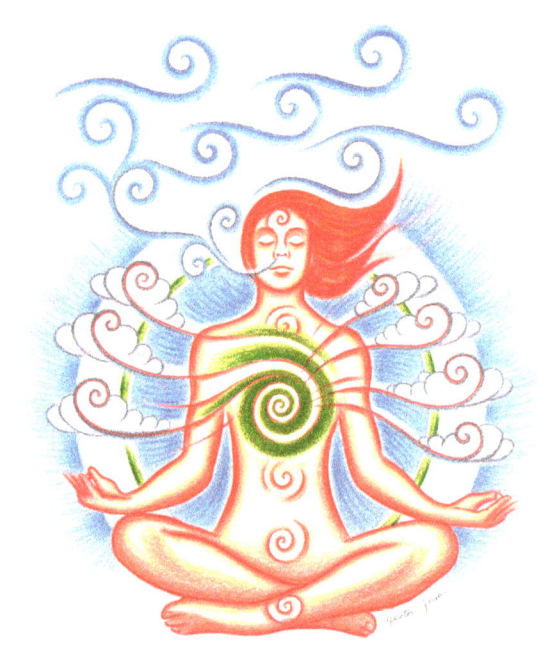

5.0 Ego Eradicator

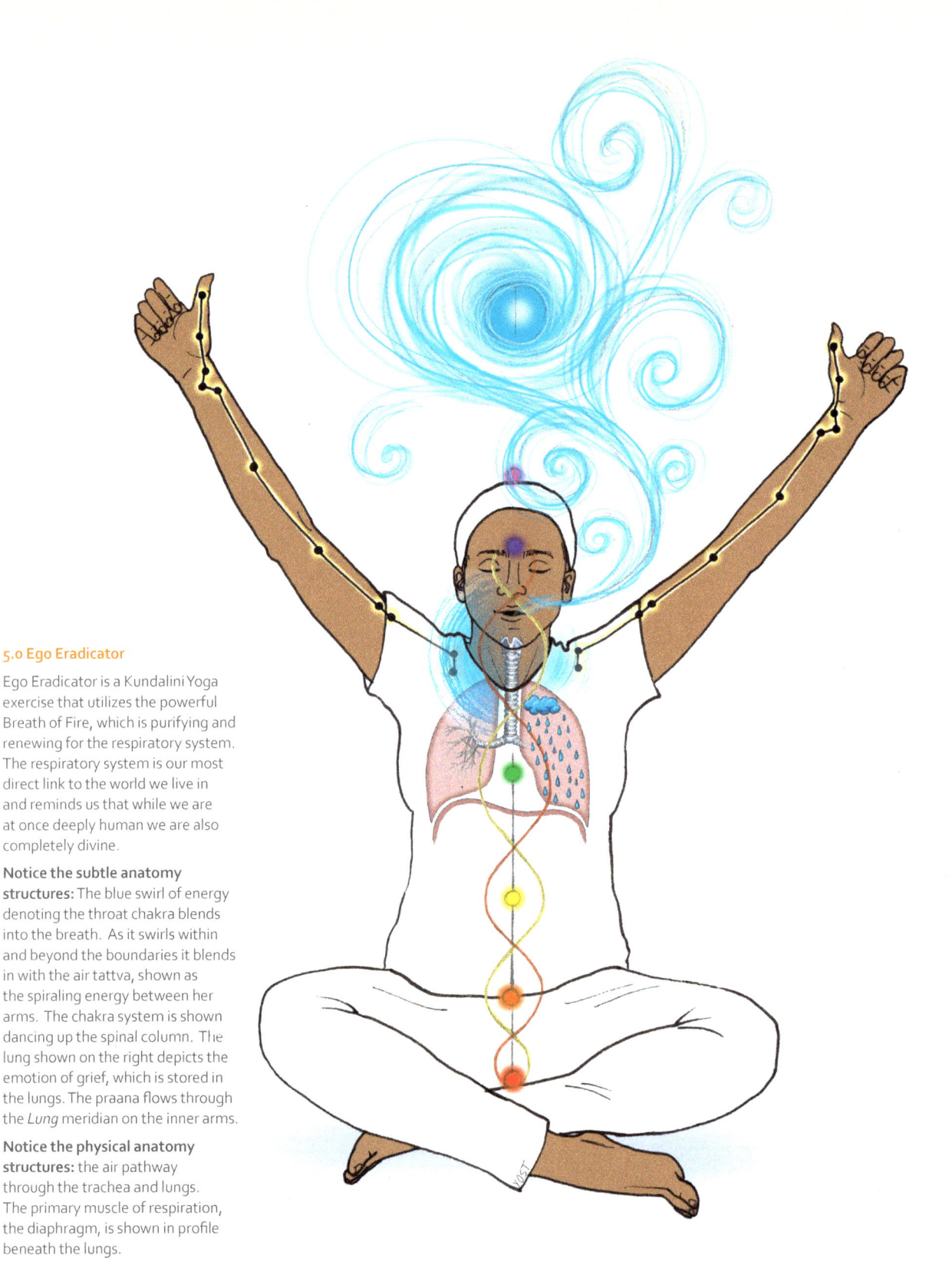

Ego Eradicator is a Kundalini Yoga exercise that utilizes the powerful Breath of Fire, which is purifying and renewing for the respiratory system. The respiratory system is our most direct link to the world we live in and reminds us that while we are at once deeply human we are also completely divine.

Notice the subtle anatomy structures: The blue swirl of energy denoting the throat chakra blends into the breath. As it swirls within and beyond the boundaries it blends in with the air tattva, shown as the spiraling energy between her arms. The chakra system is shown dancing up the spinal column. The lung shown on the right depicts the emotion of grief, which is stored in the lungs. The praana flows through the *Lung* meridian on the inner arms.

Notice the physical anatomy structures: the air pathway through the trachea and lungs. The primary muscle of respiration, the diaphragm, is shown in profile beneath the lungs.

The Respiratory System

5

The breath is the connection between the mortal experience in a human body and the vast divinity of the universe. Every time you inhale, you draw a small piece of the universe into your body. With every exhale, you give what's inside of you back to the universe. The perfect beauty of this exchange is that each party is taking what the other doesn't need, and getting exactly what it needs. Working with the breath develops an implicit trust, which builds the foundation for a relationship with the Divine.

The paradox of this exchange is that most people continue to operate under the illusion of separation. In fact, we are attached to the idea of separateness. While there is some measure of comfort in the rigidity of fierce independence, the expansion and relief that comes from leaning into the support of the Divine is immeasurably more comforting. Observe the message of the body and remind yourself that with each breath, through the respiratory system, you are constantly linked to every atom in the universe.

The respiratory system holds the messages of the human body as part of a dynamic community. It is both an independently functioning system and in critical relationships with other systems. It greatly affects and is affected by the circulatory, immune, and digestive systems. It works most directly with the circulatory system to form the dynamic process of energy and gas exchange that supports life.

The body is a balanced part of a larger community of life. You exhale carbon dioxide, exactly what plants need to complete photosynthesis. You inhale oxygen, exactly the waste product created by plants.

"When you inhale, you are taking the strength from God. When you exhale, it represents the service you are giving to the world."

—B.K.S. Iyengar,
Light on Yoga

PHYSICAL ANATOMY PERSPECTIVE

Components of the Respiratory System

- Nose
- Trachea
- Bronchi
- Lungs
- Diaphragm
- Secondary Muscles of Respiration

Benefits of a Strong Respiratory System

When the respiratory system is strong and healthy there is energy and capacity to grow in life. There is an efficient absorption of oxygen and *praana* from surrounding air and an effortless release of carbon dioxide that balances the *apaana* in the body. An appropriate blood-oxygen level is a basic marker of a healthy body.

Primary Purpose

The primary purpose of the respiratory system is to bring oxygen in and release carbon dioxide. It plays a huge role in the balance of *praana* and *apaana*.

"You live by breath, you die by breath. Make breath twenty seconds to inhale, twenty seconds you hold, and twenty seconds you exhale. …Measure by time that you breathe long and deep enough to take twenty seconds, hold it for twenty seconds, so that you can give your blood oxygen. You need it. That's better than all the vitamins in the world!"

© The Teachings of Yogi Bhajan,
September 14, 1993

Functions of Air

Oxygen is a critical component in almost all cellular functions in the body. *Praana*, which is also fed by the air, is our life-force energy. It activates everything from the ability to get out of bed in the morning to the capacity to run a marathon. Both oxygen and *praana* are delivered to the body through the breath.

The Respiratory System

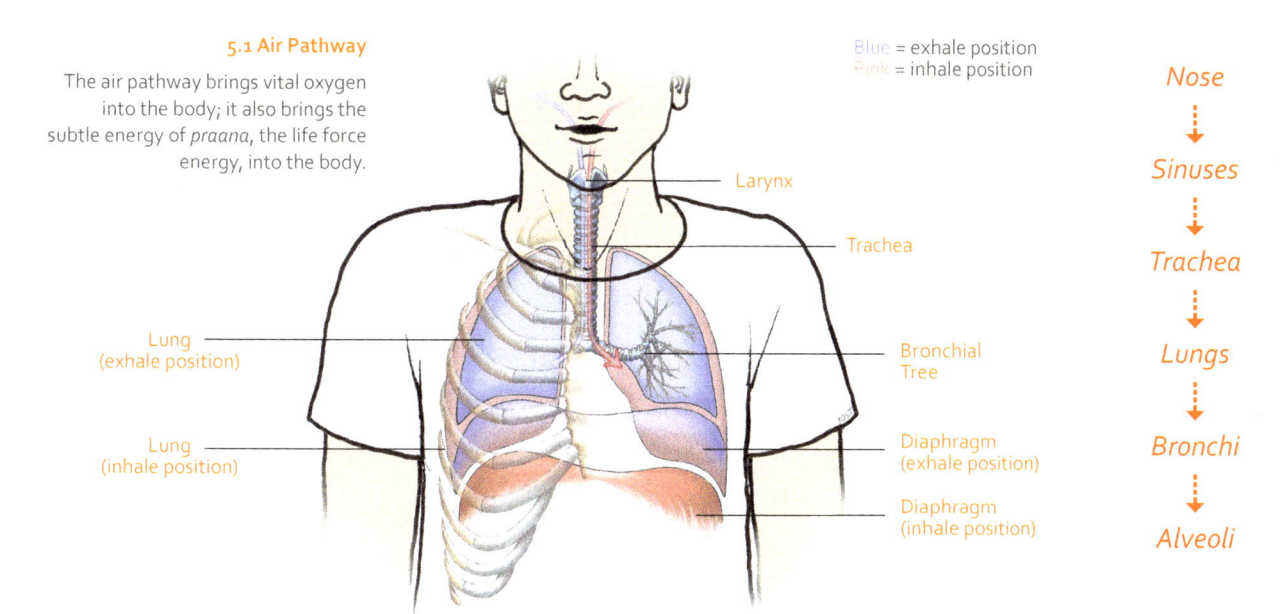

5.1 Air Pathway
The air pathway brings vital oxygen into the body; it also brings the subtle energy of *praana*, the life force energy, into the body.

Blue = exhale position
Pink = inhale position

Larynx
Trachea
Lung (exhale position)
Lung (inhale position)
Bronchial Tree
Diaphragm (exhale position)
Diaphragm (inhale position)

Nose
↓
Sinuses
↓
Trachea
↓
Lungs
↓
Bronchi
↓
Alveoli

Nose

Breathing through the nose rather than the mouth creates different effects (e.g., relaxing, energizing, cooling, warming) in the body. Understanding and applying the type of breath that will help achieve the state you want can often help.

It's ideal to breathe through the nose both in yoga and in daily life. Many people have a tendency to breathe through the mouth; it is recommended that they gently retrain themselves to breathe through the nose. There is nothing wrong with a mouth breath when it is used for a specific purpose, like detoxification or emotional release, but mouth breathing is not as gentle on the lungs or psyche as a steady breath through the nose.

"The moment you activate ida and pingala you will start feeling different."

© The Teachings of Yogi Bhajan, May 11, 1990

Ida and *Pingala*

Ida and *pingala* are energy pathways that spiral through the right and left sides of the body, ending at the nostrils. They represent and tap into different energies within the body.

The *ida* connects to the left side of the body, ending at the left nostril. It captures the energy qualities of the moon and the divine feminine; it is calm and restorative. The *pingala* is on the right side and embodies the energies of the sun and the divine masculine; it is direct and active.

The *sushmana* is the central energy channel, which runs between these two pathways. All of these energy channels are cleared and activated by the practice of Kundalini Yoga.

Exploring Physical and Subtle Human Anatomy

Nose Breath	Mouth Breath
The nostrils are smaller openings, which naturally makes the breath move slower. It's like pouring the air slowly into the lungs. This allows for more time for the gas and energy exchange.	The mouth is a large opening for air. It's like dumping the air quickly into the lungs. This can have an energizing effect. Mouth breath can be used in certain instances to quickly energize the body or quickly shift an emotional state.
Sinuses act as a natural filtration system removing dust or other particles from the air before it reaches the lungs.	Air moves directly into the lungs.
The passage to the lungs is longer, so the air has a chance to be warmed and moistened as it travels.	Air reaches the lungs with less chance for warming or moistening.
As air enters the nostrils it passes near the pituitary gland. This pathway puts a gentle stimulation into this important gland.	Less pituitary stimulation.
Connects to and activates the upper triangle of chakras.	Connects to and activates the first three chakras.
When you exhale through the nose (again because of the longer passageway and smaller openings of the nostrils) you lose less water through the breath.	Mouth breathing is detoxifying and it's important to support this process by drinking more water.
The *ida* and *pingala* are important energy pathways through the body that end at the nostrils. A nose breath stimulates and activates these channels.	

Nirmal's Mouth Breathing Story

When I started practicing yoga I became aware that I was usually breathing through my mouth. I had asthma as a child, and it's likely I created this pattern to allow more air into my body when I was struggling with an attack. I was so used to this pattern that when I did breathe through my nose, I felt like I wasn't getting enough air, and after a few breaths I would have to take a big gulp of air in through my mouth. As I moved more deeply into my yoga practice I became aware of my breath's effect on my body and realized that I no longer needed the safety mechanism of a mouth breath.

I decided I was ready to shift this pattern. I started checking in with my breath as I went about my daily life. At first it seemed like I would catch myself breathing through my mouth a hundred times a day. I would stop, take a purposeful breath or two through my nose, and then go about my business. Eventually, my habit started to shift and there were times that I would catch myself naturally breathing through my nose. Over time I found myself mouth-breathing only a few times a day. Now, I almost never catch myself breathing through my mouth unless I have a cold, am doing it purposefully, or am extremely tired. It took a long time and a lot of focused effort to make that shift, but it was worth it. Cultivating a nose breath has made it easier for me to access the peaceful feelings I get in yoga and meditation during the ordinary moments of my life.

Trachea

The trachea, also known as the windpipe, connects the nose and mouth to the lungs. There is a small structure called the epiglottis at the top of the throat that closes over the trachea when swallowing food to prevent it from ending up in the lungs. It is lined with cilia and mucus which support a clean airway. Rigid cartilaginous rings prevent it from collapsing.

Bronchi

The trachea splits near the bottom into a left and right tube called the bronchi, which carry air in and out of the lungs. The bronchi then split apart into smaller tubes and eventually tiny tubes called bronchioli. The end point of the tubes is the alveoli. The alveoli are tiny air sacs where the exchange of oxygen and carbon dioxide takes place.

Lungs

People may think of the lungs as balloons, but in reality they are more like sponges. Just like sponges, they contain small pockets of air throughout. These air pockets are called *alveoli* and are the site of exchange of oxygen and carbon dioxide.

From a physical anatomy perspective, the primary function of the respiratory system is the gas exchange of oxygen and carbon dioxide. From a subtle anatomy perspective, it is the site of absorption of *praana* and circulation of *apaana*. In both points of view the action of the lungs is to absorb what is needed, to release what is not needed, and to keep the energy flowing.

A healthy lung is bright pink and vibrant looking. Each sac in a healthy lung is a dynamic, flexible space where fluid and gas interact. Deep breaths, clean air and diet support the lungs in staying vibrant and healthy.

Shallow breathing contributes to unhealthy lung tissue. A shallow breath only utilizes the upper parts of the lungs, which can lead to stagnation in the deeper tissues. Over time when the alveoli are not stretched fully, they begin to become less elastic. Shallow breathing results in less efficient gas exchange, and can lead to general stagnation of energy and fluid in the lungs, which can lead to more serious disorders or diseases.

"Do you breathe in the lower lungs, or do you breathe in upper lungs? If you breathe in upper lungs you'll be an ordinary person with ordinary energy. If you breathe from the lower lungs you'll be an ordinary person with a stronger energy; you have to decide how you want to breathe. But your entire breathing rhythm comes from your pelvic bone, from the third vertebra."

© The Teachings of Yogi Bhajan, December 31, 1988

EACH LUNG HAS ABOUT 300–400 MILLION ALVEOLAR SACS. THE SURFACE AREA OF THE LUNGS IS ACTUALLY MUCH LARGER THAN THE ENTIRE SURFACE AREA OF YOUR SKIN.
(British Lung Foundation, n.d.).

Your Expansive Amazing Lungs

The lungs are *huge*. They reach down to the diaphragm and above the collarbones. Like a dry sponge that gets tossed into a sink full of water, the lungs expand in all directions simultaneously. This means you can breathe into your belly, chest, sides, and back. The belly expands forward as the diaphragm moves down. The sides of the body flare out as the ribs expand sideways. The back ribs bloom open as the breath moves in. The collarbones subtly lift as the breath moves up. Because of the structure of the torso, some of these movements are easier to see or experience.

With practice, there is hope for shallow breathers to restore some of the elasticity and functionality of the lungs. *Praanayam* can be effective in retraining the lungs and muscles of the ribcage to expand to their full capacity. Long deep breathing is an especially effective way to access greater lung tissue capacity, promote vitality and decrease inflammation.

Breathing

Breathing is a unique body process in that it can be automatic or voluntary. Most life-sustaining bodily processes are involuntary. The heart, for example, is not under conscious control. Breathing can happen without conscious input, or a person can purposefully take control of the breath and easily affect the body through the various breathing techniques.

Since it's often a habit to *not* expand the lungs to full capacity it can become uncomfortable (or even painful) to take a full breath. Over time this habit can lead to forgetting how to breathe deeply. Taking the time to focus on the breath and taking slow deep breaths is a meaningful tool for expanding consciousness and overall health.

With each inhalation a small piece of the universe is invited into the body. With each exhalation the body surrenders to the universe. In order to completely exhale there must be trust; trust that the universe will accept this offering and trust that the universe will continue to give the next inhalation. If there is doubt or duality in that moment it starts a cycle of shallow breathing. The shallow breath is an ill-fated attempt to gain a sense of control or

The body is asymmetrical (e.g., the right lung has three lobes, the left lung has two) which explains why a particular kriya may feature exercises that are not balanced on the right and left sides. When a kriya focuses on a particular organ it makes sense to only practice something on one side to elicit that particular effect.

Children and *Praanayam*

Zoey, a seven-year-old girl, was having trouble in school; she couldn't keep her hands to herself and kept fighting with other kids. Her parents had tried lots of things to get her to change her behavior, with no success. Then one day they decided to try a kids' yoga class. Zoey liked the class and kept coming. A few weeks later her schoolteacher called the parents. The teacher, in a shocked voice, asked the parents what they had been doing differently at home. At first the parents couldn't think of what it was, until the teacher told them what she had seen that day on the playground. Zoey had been in a situation where she was clearly getting upset and was on the verge of getting physical. Suddenly she turned around, walked away and stood behind the tree. The teacher saw Zoey bring her hand up to her nose and begin blocking off one of her nostrils. After a few moments, Zoey returned to the situation and was able to stay calm. The teacher and the parents could hardly believe it. They realized Zoey was using the left nostril breathing techniques she had learned in yoga to help calm down.

separation from the universe. Paradoxically what is needed in these moments is to surrender more deeply to the breath and the relationship with the infinite.

When you use the breath as an internal mindfulness metronome it acts as a reminder of your constant connection with the world. With every breath you are telling the world gently, "I'm here to support you, and I am accepting your support." This is the magic of conscious breathing.

Why Work with the Breath?

- Basic training in breath mechanics is the foundation of the practice of yoga.
- Breath awareness is the root of a healthy, vital life.
- Appreciation of each breath is the basis of a gratitude-filled spiritual practice.

Depth of Breath
=
Energy Available
=
Vitality

Diaphragm: The Primary Muscle of Respiration

The diaphragm is a critical component of breathing. Spanning the full breadth of the body, it attaches along the edge of the rib cage, behind the xiphoid process, all the way around and into the T12 vertebra. The diaphragm is a thin sheet of muscle, shaped like a dome, and attaches to itself by a central tendon. This muscle separates the heart and lungs from the organs of digestion and elimination. In terms of subtle anatomy it separates the lower energy centers from the upper ones. When the diaphragm is relaxed it is domed up. When it contracts, all of the muscle fibers pull toward the central tendon causing it to flatten down.

When the diaphragm contracts and flattens down, two important things happen: 1) It massages the internal organs. The diaphragm sits above the abdominal cavity, which contains the stomach, liver, intestines, and kidneys. When the diaphragm moves down there isn't enough space for those organs to move down, so they move outward instead. That's why the belly moves forward during an inhalation. 2) It increases the volume in the chest, and air rushes in to fill the space. On an inhale the air isn't pulled in, instead space is created, and air just naturally rushes in. When the diaphragm relaxes and moves up, it easily pushes the air out of the body by decreasing the available space.

The diaphragm is the primary muscle of respiration. It does most of the work to create each breath. Other primary muscles of respiration include the intercostal muscles, which move the ribcage, to create each breath.

The respiratory system delivers a message about the relationship of the individual to the Infinite: When you breathe you are not really affecting the air; you are changing your own physical body and the air is responding to whatever change you've made. There is a common saying that you create your own reality. This could be misunderstood to mean that you can manifest or attract anything by the force of your own will. If you look at the lesson in the breath it is clear that the universe cannot be molded to fit individual needs or wants. You can only change yourself. And when you do change yourself the whole universe rushes in and brings you to the exact right place. If you are constantly going out and *making* things happen you may be fighting against the divine plan. It is better to sit still, expand space in the lungs, mind, and heart and allow the infinite to fill that space with exactly what is needed.

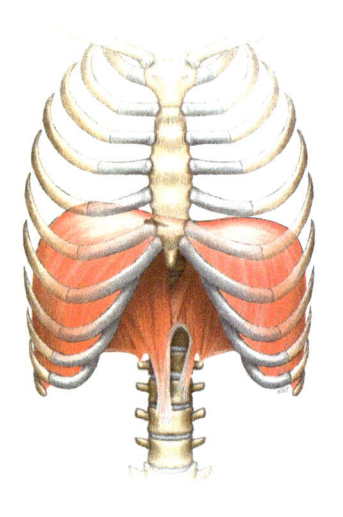

5.2 The Diaphragm
The primary muscle of respiration

A Hands-On Exploration of the Diaphragm

This is a hands-on exercise. Follow along using your hands to identify the landmarks.

Feel along the bottom edge of the ribcage. The diaphragm attaches along the inside edge of the ribcage. Let your breath be relaxed and deep. On an exhale you can start to curl your fingers around the bottom edge of the ribcage. Go slowly and gently. You may actually be able to get the fingers inside the ribcage.

Energetically, people often hold a lot of tension, fear or old trauma in this area. If you find it very difficult to access the edge of the ribcage or feel the diaphragm moving you may want to do some work on releasing tension in this area. In order to let the diaphragm completely relax and move freely you must allow yourself to feel vulnerable. In order to experience vulnerability you must feel safe and protected. It is often helpful to work on building *praana* in the body first to create this sense of safety. To build *praana*, start practicing long, deep breathing and Breath of Fire, and eating clean foods so that you can create change. When the diaphragm is easy and moving freely, we are able to trust that the breath will come, and by extension we are able trust the universe.

Diaphragm Lock

Diaphragm Lock is a technique that builds the awareness of the connection between the subtle anatomy and the physical anatomy. The diaphragm creates a physical barrier between the lower and upper triangles of chakras. The experience of Diaphragm Lock opens the subtle understanding of the energies of each of these areas.

Diaphragm Lock is performed only on the exhale. With the body completely empty of air pull the diaphragm up into the chest cavity. Imagine a parachute billowing upward. When it is correctly applied there is actually an internal suctioning feeling. It is easier to feel if the stomach is relatively empty and the diaphragm is free from excessive stress.

"Patience pays. Let the hand of God work for you."

© The Teachings of Yogi Bhajan

Chapter 5

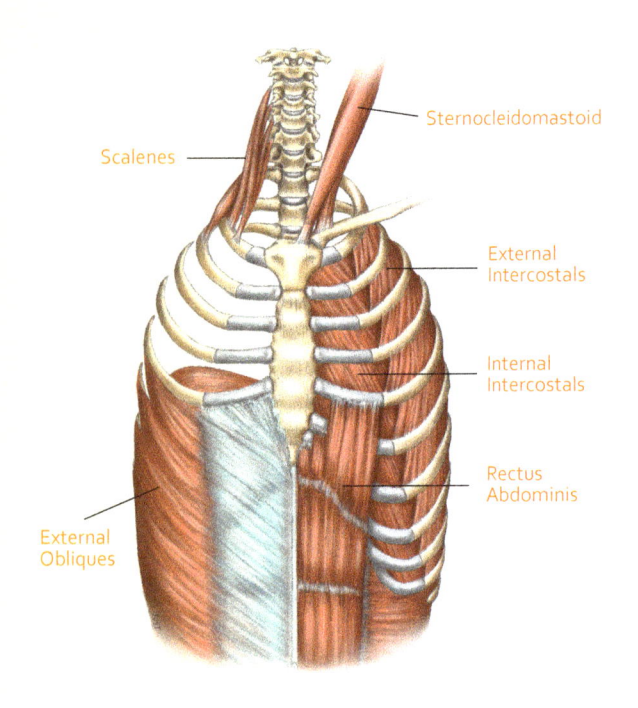

Secondary Muscles of Respiration

There is a secondary set of muscles designed to help increase the breath capacity. These respiratory muscles are designed to assist when more oxygen is needed quickly, for example, during exercise. They are the scalenes, pectorals, external intercostals and the sternocleidomastoid.

The secondary muscles of respiration help to lift the top of the ribs so that a little more air can get in with each breath. A great design in survival situations when the body needs to quickly tap into the biggest possible breath, the problem comes when you rely on these muscles for every breath on a daily basis. It is common to overuse the secondary muscles of respiration because of the fear and tension held in the diaphragm. When the diaphragm is rigid or can't move enough to draw in a satisfying breath, the secondary muscles kick in.

This pattern of breathing creates extra tension in the areas of the neck, upper shoulders, and chest. Learning to breathe with the diaphragm is an important part of avoiding the overuse and tension in those areas. The more efficient the breath is, the less tension there is in the whole system and the better the state of overall wellness. This is a relatively easy solution for a potentially complex problem.

5.3 Secondary Muscles of Respiration

SECONDARY MUSCLES OF RESPIRATION
- PECTORALS
- STERNOCLEIDOMASTOID
- SCALENES

Relationship to Other Systems

Immune/Lymph and Respiratory The respiratory system has a close relationship to our immunological response. The lungs are one possible way bacteria or other pathogens enter the body. It is important to have healthy lungs so that they function as proper barriers to such pathogens. The lungs, along with the skin and mucous membranes, function as the first line of defense in the immune response. One of the best immune system boosters is Breath of Fire (Bhajan 2010). It's a good thing to practice any time you feel like you may be getting sick. Another way to support the immune system in yoga is by breathing through the nose instead of mouth. As discussed earlier, additional filtration systems are activated by nose breathing.

The Respiratory System

Your Reason to Breathe

Breathwork has been shown to have a positive effect on the immune system, circulatory system, autonomic nervous system, and various mental or stress disorders (Novotny and Kravitz, 2007).

Digestion and Respiration Vitality comes from the amount of *praana* in the body. While *praana* comes from lots of sources, the primary ones are the nutrients from food and the oxygen in the air. In order to feel better there's a simple equation: eat better food and breathe more deeply. The process of building *praana* in the body is a bit like building a fire, you have to start small, but once the flames catch they build on each other.

Breathing techniques in Kundalini Yoga act as the kindling to start the process of building *praana*. This increase in energy can make it easier to make other healthy choices in your life, such as diet. Then the energy of the better foods can give you more energy to do other healthy things: exercise, connect with others, eat even better food, and breathe even more deeply. Your food choices and your *praanic* vitality have a very tight knit relationship! Some people might even say a better diet starts with better breathing. Air itself and the *praana* therein is like a first food to the body, allowing all other essential nourishment to occur. By practicing yoga you become a bubble of *praanic* vitality.

When you try to make dietary changes yourself, or suggest them to others, you often get a lot of resistance, often because one's *praanic* energy is too low to have the capacity to make the change. If you run into this resistance begin by adding breathwork to your regular routine. Also, focus on adding healthy foods instead of giving things up. Once the level of *praana* has increased in the body through added oxygen, more efficient detoxification, and the natural benefits of more fruits and vegetables, it becomes easier to let go of stimulants like meat, sugar, or caffeine.

Japa's Immune Boost Tip

For a quick immune booster when you think you might be getting sick or people around you are sick, sit down and do 11 minutes of Breath of Fire (see page 102 for instructions).

Food + Breath = Vitality for life

There are plenty of yogis who eat junk food. So if making a dietary change is a challenge, *praanayam* is a good place to start. Do a lot of *praanayam*; feast on oxygen, and notice the difference. Begin to pay attention to your feelings while eating. Allow junk food and, rather than dissociating from it, acknowledge your feelings as you eat and process it. Listen to your body and select choices that give you the greatest amount of *praana*!

How Much *Praana*?

Yogic texts suggest a simple test you can do to evaluate how much *praana* is stored in the body by holding your breath out for as long as you comfortably can. To begin, take a couple normal breaths, then breathe out and suspend the breath. Hold your breath out for as long as you comfortably can. A marker of good health is being able to hold the breath out for at least 30 seconds.

SUBTLE ANATOMY PERSPECTIVE

Air Tattva

The Air *tattva* represents the ability to move, shift and hold immense power. When in balance it supports creativity and the free and easy movement of life force. This *tattva* surrounds and supports every moment and each action of the body. It is the great connector between all conscious beings and the invisible provider of life. Every body type relates to the breath differently, and imbalances in this *tattva* manifest uniquely. Generally, if there is too much air, a person is flighty, forgetful or ungrounded. If there is not enough air, a person can be constipated, rigid, or unyielding.

The air *tattva* is balanced when there is trust in the unknown and unseen aspects of the divine. Meditation, stillness, and deep listening create and generate trust in the infinite. The air *tattva* also holds our ability to change and adapt to the circumstances of life. The stillness of meditation acts as a counterpoint to the constant movement of atoms in the air around us and prepares us to act and change spontaneously and consciously.

Breath and Longevity

Breath is the first and last action in life. Once it is gone, life is over. The yogis say that there are a prescribed number of breaths in life. Therefore deepening and slowing the breath lengthens life. This may or may not be true in a literal sense. But it can certainly be true in terms of the quality of life. With a more conscious breath there is greater potential to connect to the preciousness of life and to experience the gift of each moment.

Chinese Medicine Perspective

The Princess Organs The *Lungs* are called the princess organs. They get this title for a few reasons. First, the *Lungs* are very particular. They like to receive air through the nose because it is gentler. Second, they take a long time to heal when they've been ill. They need to be babied and pampered back to health. Have you ever noticed how chest colds tend to linger?

Finally, the *Lungs* embody the title of princess because of how they influence every system of the body. They are not the queen; they are not front and center, obviously running the show. They are very involved in influencing the different systems of the body. The *Lungs* are intricately connected to the immune, circulatory, and digestive systems. Their effect is very subtle but pervasive in the body.

"Deeply Listening, Recognize the ocean of virtues Within you. Deeply Listening Become In tune with Spirit, Perfectly balanced in your own humanity and nobility."

-From Guru Nanak's Japji Sahib, translated by Ek Ong Kaar Kaur Khalsa in *Song of the Soul*

"Only those who know how to breathe will survive."

—Pundit Acharya, social reformer, philosopher

> "*I believe that unarmed truth and unconditional love will have the final word in reality. This is why right, temporarily defeated, is stronger than evil triumphant.*"
>
> —Dr. Martin Luther King Jr., minister, civil rights activist, Nobel Peace Prize winner

Grief In Chinese medicine, there are special aspects of the soul that are sheltered by different organs. The *Lungs* house the emotional qualities of grief. A person may store grief in their *Lungs* and then breathe shallowly to avoid touching that grief. Grief may show up as denial or anger with the actual sadness often being suppressed for years.

When people start a yoga or breath practice they may find they cry a lot. The long, deep breathing and the movement of the lungs and muscles of respiration bring that stored grief to the surface. The practice of yoga can actually activate that stored grief. This allows the yogi to move from sadness to acceptance as the grief heals. Yoga may not make everyone cry, but crying may arise naturally as people process held or hidden grief.

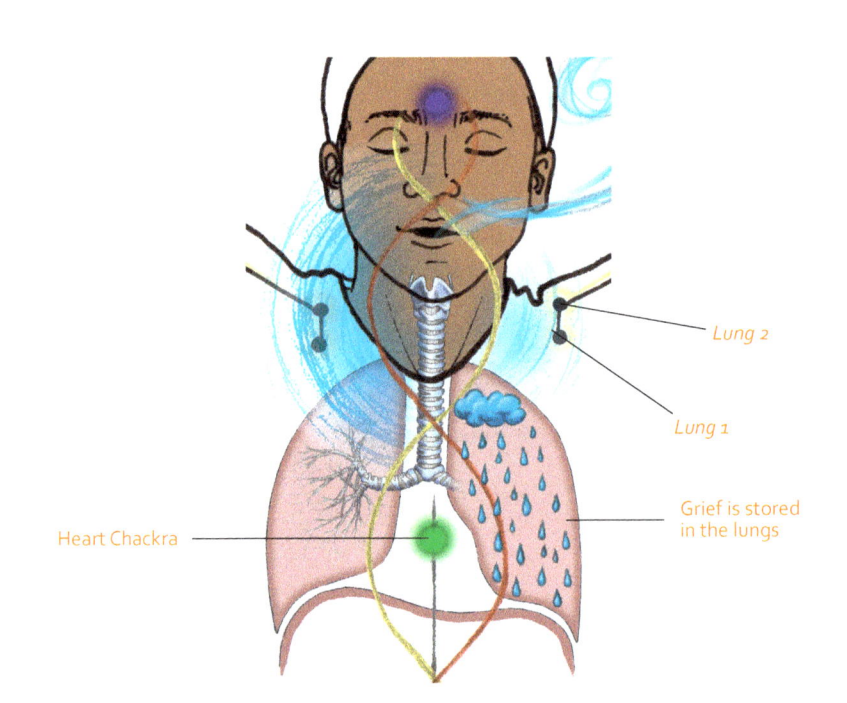

5.4 Grief & the Lungs

Our bodies can store emotions, like grief, in the lungs, which may be stirred up or released by a yoga practice like *praanayam* or other postures and exercises.

Lung 2
Lung 1
Grief is stored in the lungs
Heart Chackra

Throat Chakra, the fifth energy center, encompasses the entire throat and neck, including larynx, voice box, cervical vertebra, and the musculature of the neck. It is a relatively narrow passageway for some of the most critical tubes in our bodies. Air, food, blood, and lymph must all move through this area. Positioned right above the Heart Chakra the throat is a translation center. It supports the filtration of the subtle energies and spiritual expansion of the upper glands and chakras into a digestible form for the physical body and lower energy centers. This filtration and integration of divine and physical elements happens within the breath, which is supported by a clear, expansive Throat Chakra.

The Throat Chakra holds the energetic capacity to be authentic, truthful and to create change through the power of the word. Walking the path of truth and authenticity is a balancing act, like walking on the fine edge of a dagger. Like any balancing act though, it gets easier with repetition and practice. The conscious decision to stick to the truth, not only in terms of *not* lying, but also in terms of living in alignment with your morals and your values, your soul's purpose, leads to an ability to manifest or change situations with a powerful word. The power of the word can be potent and life changing.

On a daily basis, choosing words carefully and taking a deep breath before speaking can contribute to not only a balanced Throat Chakra but a balanced life. These techniques are especially vital to those who speak publicly. The great orators can change the destiny of an individual, a nation or the entire world simply with the power of their word.

> **Practice Suggestion**
>
> *Take three long, deep breaths every half hour (Bhajan, 1989b). Put a sticky note on your desk, steering wheel or set a reminder on your phone or computer. When the reminder comes up, stop and take three long deep breaths.*

The Respiratory System and the Pranic Body

The Pranic Body is another way to understand the subtle anatomy connection of the Physical Body to the universe. The lungs and heart bring oxygen and *praana* into the Physical Body and the Pranic Body distributes that energy to the entire system. The gentle, rhythmic movement of the heart and lungs themselves supports this distribution.

When the Pranic Body is strong and balanced, energy and courage, motivation and the ability to self-initiate on a path of truth and service to others are the hallmarks. You feel held in the energy of the universe and experience grace in facing the challenges of life. When the Pranic Body is weak we experience lethargy and a lack of motivation. Rather than feeling contained within the divine energy of the universe, we look to outside sources for energy: food, drugs, or people. The easiest way to strengthen this body is through *praanayam* or yogic breathing. Not only do these breath techniques oxygenate, energize, and release physical tension, they also act as a metronome for the Pranic Body to reset and recharge.

TIPS AND TECHNIQUES FOR A STRONG RESPIRATORY SYSTEM

The practice of yoga gives tools to quickly and easily affect the body through the lungs and the breath. The easiest way to change something that is happening in the body is to change the breath. By improving the overall health of the lungs and the depth of the breath, one can increase lung capacity, stretch the muscles around the ribs, improve the capillary bed, and increase the efficiency of the gas exchange (Bhajan, 2010).

Aasanas and Exercises

Aerobic Kriyas: Kriyas that involve lots of movement (11 minutes of dancing, for example) and get your heart beating and your breath moving more deeply increase the breath capacity by challenging it. Yogi Bhajan also taught many *PT* (Physical Training) classes and all of these PT kriyas are aerobic.

Heart Openers: Heart opening postures serve the respiratory system in the same way they serve the circulatory system. By counteracting slouching and the chronic posture of rounding the shoulders forward they create more space for the lungs to expand.

Examples: Ego Eradicator, Yoga Mudra, Camel Pose, Cobra Pose, Wheel Pose

Transformational Energy Points

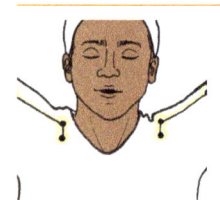

Lung 1: Central Treasury

Location: Just below the outer edge of the collarbone

Effects: Releases stored grief from the *Lung* meridian and organ, strengthens *Lung* function.

Yoga for this Point: Cobra, Spinal Flex, Plow, Yoga Mudra

Praanayam

One of the best self-care tools is breathwork. By unwinding the patterns that cause incorrect breathing you will find a quick shift in the energy balance of the whole system. That increased energy fuels growing good habits and a healthy lifestyle. When learning new breath techniques start slowly; practice for a few minutes and then rest and observe your body, mind and emotions. Be patient as it often takes time to unlearn poor breathing habits, especially when the roots of those habits go back, deep into the subconscious past.

Long Deep Breathing
- Inhale and exhale through the nose.
- Aim for a slow and steady stream of air, in and out, no big gulp or rush of air.
- Inhale and exhale are approximately the same length and intensity.
- Notice a small naturally-arising pause at the top of the inhale and the bottom of the exhale. Do not exaggerate or force the pause, allow it as you focus on the inhale and exhale.

  Note: This natural pause allows the energy and biochemicals involved in the breath time to transition after the inhale and the exhale. After the inhale, the pause allows you to absorb oxygen and *praana*. After the exhale, the pause allows the circulation of *apaana*. In both the full and empty lung there is a pause to allow the shift in *praana* and *apaana*.
- Be sure to keep the shoulder blades relaxed. The secondary muscles of respiration do not need to be activated for Long Deep Breathing, so be mindful of movements in these muscles, especially the shoulders, which may have a tendency to move up and down as you breathe.
- Finally, check for tension in your neck and face. Intentionally relax the muscles in your neck and face as you practice Long Deep Breathing.

Benefits of Long Deep Breathing
- Clear and prevent toxins from building up in the lungs (Bhajan, 2010).
- Bring about a state of deep relaxation and calmness (Cuda, 2010).
- Tap into the neutral, non-reactive mind.
- Clear the energy pathways and meridians in the body.

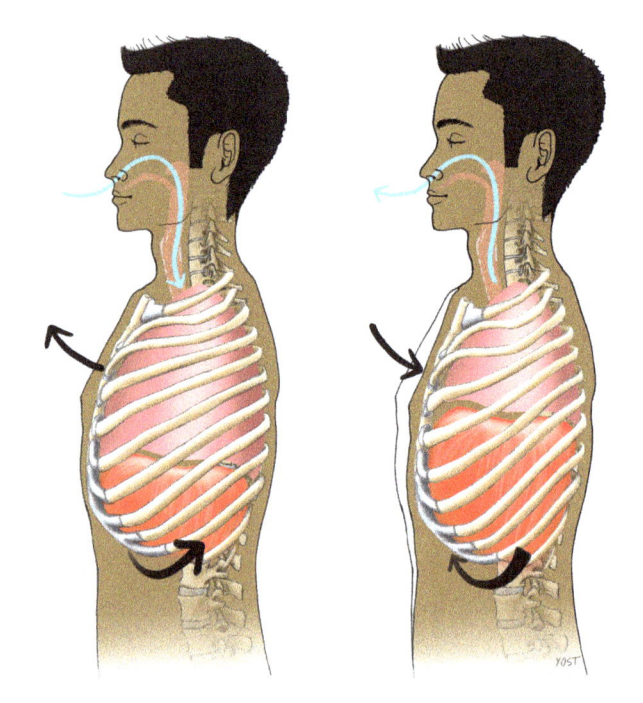

5.5 The Movement of the Ribcage
The expansion and contraction of structures in the chest cavity as they shift in relationship to the breath.

Breath of Fire

Bring one hand over the belly and begin to pant, slowly through the nose. Notice the movement of the belly and make sure the Navel Point moves *in* on the *exhale*. Now bring your awareness to the diaphragm at the bottom of the ribcage. Feel the fluttering, up and down motion of the diaphragm. As you get more comfortable you can build your pace, until you are breathing two breaths per second. Watch that you don't go too fast and that the diaphragm continues to be the driver of the breath.

- Gently pump the diaphragm. It is not a staccato or slamming motion of the navel.
- Face and neck muscles are relaxed.
- No movement of the shoulders.

Note: Women on the moon cycle or who are pregnant should not practice Breath of Fire; it places too much pressure on the abdomen.

Benefits of Breath of Fire
- Stimulates the immune system and strengthens the nervous system.
- Brings *praana* to the blood, which energizes the body.
- Breaks up stagnation and clears meridians to allow optimal energy flow through the body.
- Literally warms you up and gives you strength and courage.
(Bhajan, 2010)

Movements of the Lungs

This is a hands-on exercise. Follow along, use your hands to identify the landmarks.

Find the Forward Movement Place one hand on the belly and the other on your chest. As you inhale feel the hands moving forward away from the spine.

Find the Sideways Movement Wrap the hands around yourself, like you're giving yourself a hug, and place the hands at the bottom of the ribcage. As you inhale feel the bottom edge of the ribcage flare out into your hands. Then move your hands up into your armpits. Feel the body getting wider on the inhalation and moving back toward the center on the exhale.

Find the Backward Movement Come into Baby Pose; bring your hands to your low back. Feel the ribcage expanding into your hands with the inhale.

Find the Upward Movement Sitting in Easy PoseEasy Pose again, bring the hands to the collarbones. At the very end of your inhale feel them move out and expand up. It feels a bit like you are "puffing your feathers."

Find All Directions Sit in Easy Pose, take a few long deep breaths and see if you can move and expand the lungs in *all* directions with each breath. Think of filling the lungs from the bottom to the top. Fill every available space: belly, ribs, back and collarbone.

When you exhale everything moves back toward the center at the same time, like a balloon deflating or a flower closing its petals. Move the navel toward the spine to completely exhale.

Mantra

The mantra for the breath is the *Praan Bandh Mantra, or Pavan Guru* mantra. This mantra says that breath is the teacher and the path to ecstasy. Chant this mantra anytime you wish to feel more connected to the Breath of Life and the awe-inspiring beauty that surrounds you.

Pavan Pavan Pavan Pavan, Par Paraa Pavan Guru
Pavan Guru Wahe Guru, Wahe Guru Pavan Guru

Pavan	The Divine Breath
Par Paraa	From Beyond the Beyond
Pavan Guru	Breath is the Guru
Wahe Guru	The Experience of the Divine

Plants, Herbs, and Food

Black Pepper is a purifying substance, which Yogi Bhajan often recommended for reducing allergies and mucus. The next time you experience a lot of mucus or very moist cough, mix freshly ground black pepper with a little honey and swallow half a teaspoon a few times a day to help dry up the mucus.

Fruit In general fruits have specific properties for healing and nourishing the body that are as strong as any supplement or herbal medicine. Fruits are the potent offspring of a plant. They hold the seeds, genetic forward motion and energy of that plant. Their properties in helping to heal as plant medicine are valuable and often overlooked. They are especially useful in moistening and maintaining the health of the respiratory tissues and lungs.

The amount of Vitamin C in fruit is like a direct burst of sunlight. Vitamin C from an herbalist perspective is warming, building and strengthening, just like sunlight. That burst of fluid when biting into fruit is what allows the plant to moisten and build the *yin* or fluids of the body. Not having enough fluid is a reason people suffer from day to day complaints of constipation, cracked lips or fingers or general dryness. Yogi Bhajan often encouraged the addition of bananas or melons to the diet to restore energy and positivity.

RECIPES TO SUPPORT THE RESPIRATORY SYSTEM

BLACK PEPPER TEA

Great for lingering colds and flu with mucus and damp congestion.

- ✓ 1 tablespoon (15 ml) whole black peppercorns
- ✓ 1 quart (or liter) water

Boil down until you have one half quart (or liter) of water. Serve tea with a little honey.

©The Teachings of Yogi Bhajan, October 27, 1969

POMEGRANATE BLACK PEPPER TEA VARIATION

Make tea as directed above.
Combine with a half-quart/half-liter of pomegranate juice.

©The Teachings of Yogi Bhajan, December 28, 1998

YOGI BHAJAN'S PINEAPPLE GINGER JUICE

- ✓ One pineapple, chopped
- ✓ 1 cup (240 ml) pineapple juice
- ✓ 1 large finger (2 cm) of ginger, peeled

Blend well and serve. Good for the lungs.
(Khalsa, S.S.K., 2011)

BAKED PEARS

Pear is sweet and astringent, it balances Pitta with its sweet flavor and Kapha with its astringent nature

Chop up and core a few pears and sprinkle with cinnamon and nutmeg (optional) and a few tablespoons (30 ml) of ghee or coconut oil.
Bake them at 375° for 20 minutes until soft.
Serve as a dessert or snack.

©The Teachings of Yogi Bhajan, December 17, 1992

Fruits in general have the effect of soothing irritated tissues, building appropriate moisture in the body and calming inflammation.

Pears are especially beneficial in properly moistening the lung tissue. Try adding pears to the diet if there is a dry cough, it may help to rebalance the moisture in the body. Yogi Bhajan also extolled the virtues of the pear as the perfect way to prevent stones from forming in the body. While eating a pear, notice the gritty texture of the flesh. It is possible that components in the pear act in a preventative way to keep the body from forming cysts and stones.

Yogic Lifestyle

Neti Pot is a simple spouted pot that is filled with warm salt water and used to rinse the nostrils and keep nasal passageways clean and healthy. If you are new to this practice, or you are experiencing sinus congestion, it may take a while to feel comfortable with the water flowing through the nasal cavity. Many natural food and health product suppliers stock neti pots.

Clean Air Most of us have heard that *what goes up, must come* down. In the same way, anything that goes into the body must also come out. Elimination and detoxification are ongoing processes in the body even with the healthiest diet and lifestyle. You can avoid placing extra stress on your body by avoiding known toxins. Much as you would put the best oil and gas and other products into your car for optimal performance, putting into your body the cleanest food, water, and air possible allows your body to function optimally. Yogic techniques can often help those who want to eliminate toxins from smoking or drugs from their systems. Eating a diet of *praana*-rich foods and beverages and practicing Long Deep Breathing not only revitalizes you but can also help replace the effects of tobacco or drugs with the natural uplifting effects of *praana*.

Balance the Throat Chakra

A lump in the throat indicates that the throat in imbalanced. When the Throat Chakra is imbalanced it may be to time to tell the truth about something or set a boundary or express a need; and that takes courage. Throat Chakra imbalances are also evidenced by constant or repeated sore throats.

To Balance the Throat Chakra
- Wear blue
- Wear or meditate with a lapis or kyanite stone
- Do head rolls
- Chant
- Speak only the truth or try a period of silence
- Take a deep breath before speaking
- Gently tap or massage the throat area

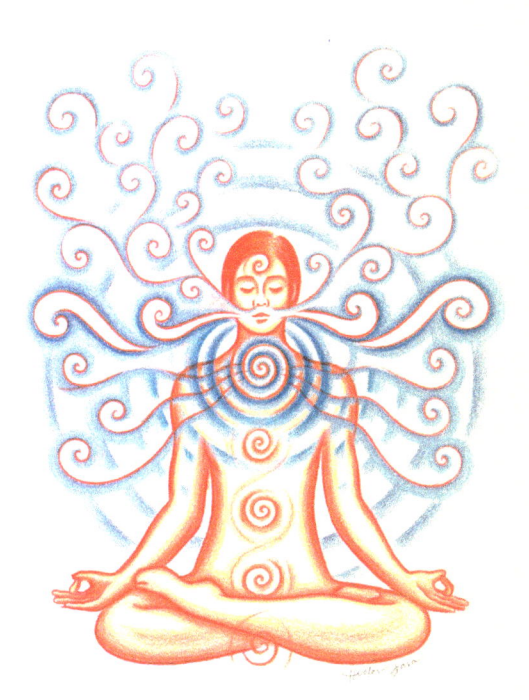

Affirmations for the Throat Chakra
I am centered in truth. My word is a treasure that uplifts me and uplifts others.

6.0 Corpse Pose

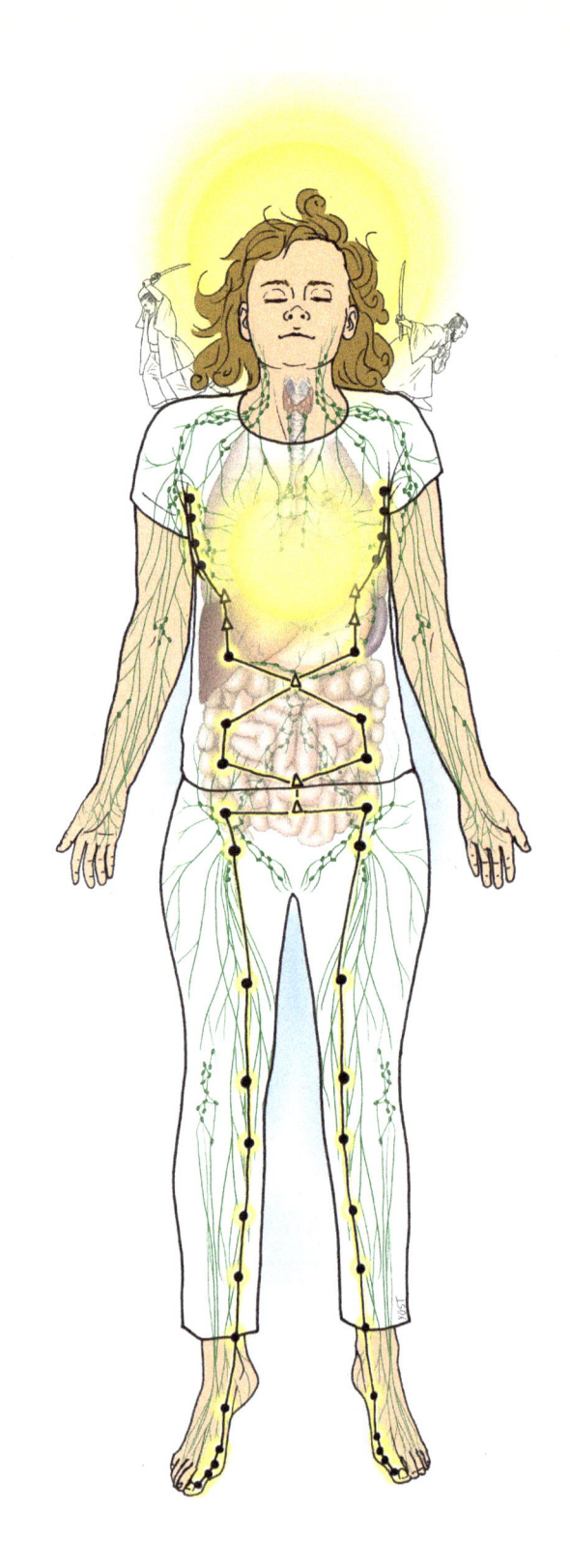

Corpse Pose is practiced at the end of every yoga class. It gives the body a chance to rest and synchronize the effects of the practice. The immune system is a delicate and important community of structures working together to keep your body healthy and vital.

Notice the subtle anatomy structures: the Arcline shown as a shimmering halo overhead and in front of her chest. The Defensive Qi warriors are ready to defend and protect. The *Spleen* meridian, is shown cycling through the inner leg and above the digestive organs.

Notice the physical anatomy structures: the vast network of lymphatic vessels, with concentration of nodes in the neck, armpit and groin, and the thyroid gland at the throat.

The Immune System

In Kundalini Yoga the practice begins with tuning in. We chant the mantra *Ong Namo Guru Dev Namo,* which creates a connection to the Golden Chain of teachers and practitioners stretching back through time and including everyone who is currently on this path. Tuning in affirms the connection to community, develops individual strength and sustains the overall caliber of a community.

Families, tribes, or communities support their members with the protection of the collective wisdom and the ease of shared work and responsibility. The immune system serves the body in a similar way through a diverse collection of cells, processes, and structures. The human body is constantly deciding what should be kept or discarded. The immune system functions as both the wise elder, guiding the body in these decisions and as the garbage collector by actually moving stuff out.

The immune system is a collective response rather than one discrete physical system; it is essentially a chain of events, a conglomeration of activities and structures that happen throughout the body. A group of organs, cells, physical barriers, and cooperative processes that protect the body from disease make up the immune response. In a healthy body the immune response is synchronous; each cell and organ communicates and responds appropriately to potential foreign particles. A functional immune response is more than just these physical parts working together; it is also interwoven with the subtle shifts in energy, mood, and perception. A positive emotional orientation to life profoundly supports an optimally functioning immune response (Cohen, 2002).

PHYSICAL ANATOMY PERSPECTIVE

Components of the Immune System

- Lymphatic Fluid
- Lymph Nodes and Vessels
- Immune Cells
- Bone Marrow
- Thymus Gland
- Spleen
- Physical Barriers

Benefits of a Strong Immune System

A strong immune response allows for vibrant health and active lives. A strong lymphatic structure protects us from short- and long-term illness and disease. From a subtle perspective, supporting the health of the immune system allows for healthy boundaries. The immune system determines what belongs to the body and what is not authentic to the body.

Primary Purpose

The primary purpose of the immune response and lymphatic structure is to keep out of the body anything that does not align with its highest potential. Its purpose is to identify and eliminate any pathogen that could cause illness, disorder, or disease. It is both an early alert system and a catalyst for relaxation and self-care.

Lymphatic Fluid

Lymph fluid is a clear, watery substance full of white blood cells that slowly pulses through your body as you breathe and move. Lymph fluid starts out as plasma (the fluid part of blood), which flows into the capillary bed through the arterial system. When the plasma leaves the capillaries it settles into the interstitial space and nourishes the cells with oxygen, hormones and nutrients. About 10 percent of this clear fluid then collects wastes and toxins and flows into the lymph vessels. The rest returns to the blood. After the lymph fluid is cleaned, it is returned to the bloodstream.

Lymph Nodes and Vessels

The primary physical structures of the immune system are the lymphatic vessels and nodes. The vessels are tubes that run parallel to the bloodstream and carry the lymph fluid, which is a critical component in arming the body with white blood cells to protect against illness.

Lymph nodes are extensions of the lymph vessels that contain specialized filters. The lymph fluid moves through the lymph nodes to be filtered. There are about 500–600 total lymph nodes in your body with heavy concentrations in the armpits, neck, and groin. Any yoga postures that apply pressure to or move those parts of the body help to move fluid through the lymph nodes.

The lymph fluid moves through the lymph vessels until it is returned to the blood, where it is again called plasma. The lymphatic drainage structure has an uneven, asymmetrical design: the right-side is responsible for clearing only the right arm and chest; the left side clears *all* of the other areas of the body; both legs, the lower torso, the upper left part of the chest, and the left arm.

Immune Cells

The immune response calls on a variety of cells with specialized jobs to carry out the work of maintaining health. Each type of specialized cell plays its part in the large, complex process of efficiently identifying and eliminating pathogens. Here are a few of the many different types of white blood cells that protect the body.

B Cells tag intruders, or pathogens. B cells float through the bloodstream when, through the intelligence that resides in their cell membranes, they recognize foreign particles, which do not have the same vibration or signal as the rest of the body. B cells recognize this item as *not-self*; they mark the *not-self* with antibodies, and the immune response begins.

Macrophages find *not-self* cells tagged with antibodies and engulf them and break them down. The lymph system then moves the debris out of the body.

T Cells are helper cells that coordinate the process of finding, tagging, and eliminating the *not-self* items.

Memory Cells are created by T and B cells so that the body remembers a specific invader. This immune memory is developed so that a stronger, quicker and more efficient response can be mounted if the same invader ever enters the body again.

Sat Nam is one of the most common mantras in Kundalini Yoga as taught by Yogi Bhajan. It means, "I am Truth," or "Truth is the Identity." The Immune response is the physical body's way of determining the truth of our bodies. The cells learn to see what is our Sat Nam and what is not-self.

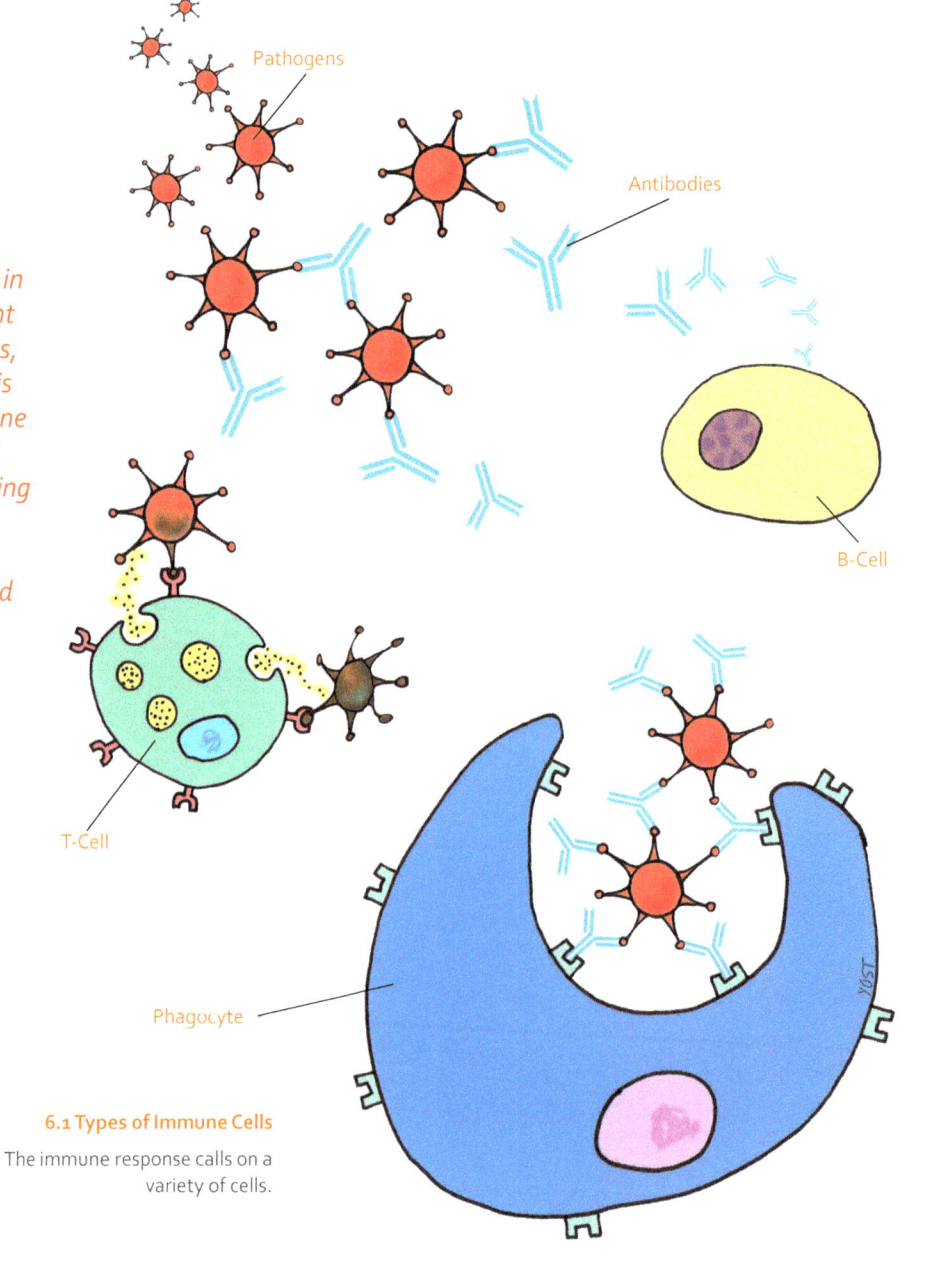

Pathogens

Antibodies

B-Cell

T-Cell

Phagocyte

6.1 Types of Immune Cells
The immune response calls on a variety of cells.

Bone Marrow

The bone marrow is located in the center of the long bones. It acts as a deep, inner reserve responsible for creating blood cells. The yellow marrow found in the humerus and femur is a soft, spongy tissue and is used to create the specialized white blood cells (WBCs) of the immune system. Some WBCs form and mature in the marrow. Others are formed in the marrow and transfer to the thymus gland to mature and specialize.

In an emergency, with a loss of blood, the body can change the yellow marrow into the red marrow that creates red blood cells.

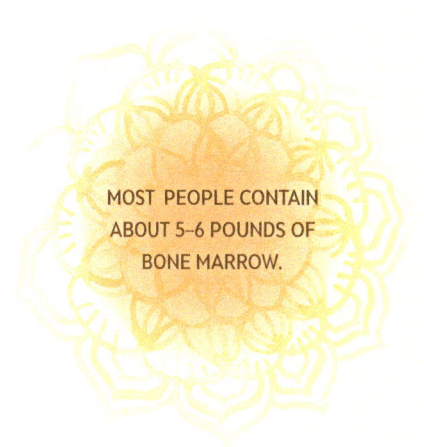

MOST PEOPLE CONTAIN ABOUT 5-6 POUNDS OF BONE MARROW.

Thymus Gland

Feeling cozy and safe allows the Heart Center to relax and the thymus to do its job of maturing white blood cells. That yummy happy feeling that comes during relaxation at the end of a yoga class is beneficial to the development of the immune response. The immune system needs stillness as a counterpoint to movement. While movement allows the cells to gather information about threats to the body, stillness and deep relaxation allows the cells of the immune system to rest next to each other and coordinate. While the body is at rest, the cells have a chance to acquire information from each other about foreign invaders and to then develop the intricate tagging systems needed to eliminate *not-self* gatecrashers.

Thymus Tapping

Try tapping your thymus gland in the center of your chest above the heart. This stimulation gives your immune system an extra boost. An especially good time for a yogi to do this is during the daily cold shower practice (see page 80).

Innate and Acquired Immunity

We build immunity and create the cellular memory involved in the immune response in two distinct ways:

Non-specific resistance (*innate*) is the body's immediate but general reaction to a wide range of pathogens. It includes swelling, running nose, and fever.

Specific immunity (*acquired*) develops slowly and is targeted at particular pathogens. When we are children and first encounter germs, the body learns to recognize *self* and *not-self*. The body then learns how to defend itself should it ever encounter that invader again.

Spleen

The spleen is an organ located toward the left side of the body. It measures about four inches (10 centimeters) long and is protected by the ribcage. The spleen filters blood and traps foreign material (pathogens). In the spleen, T cells, B cells, macrophages, red blood cells, and other cells involved in immune responses exchange information about invaders. The spleen is alerted to trouble and sends out large amounts of antibodies when needed.

Physical Barriers

Physical Barriers

- *Skin*
- *Digestive Tract Lining*
- *Stomach Acid*
- *Mucous linings of nose and lungs*

The easiest way for the body to conserve energy and prevent sickness is to stop the bacteria or viruses before they even get into the body. The body has developed a series of barriers to prevent unwanted (*not-self*) things from entering the inner circle.

Relationship to Other Systems

"We've all got both light and dark inside us. What matters is the part we choose to act on. That's who we really are."

—JK Rowling, *Harry Potter and the Order of the Phoenix*

The Circulatory System and Lymph Blood tends to be the star when thinking about fluids in the body. The lymph is the lesser-known supporting actor laboring to clean the blood and keep the flow of nutrition and waste moving in the body. The body is saturated in lymphatic fluid. The lymph, unlike the blood, is a no pressure system and does not have a pump to move it. The lymph fluid relies completely on the physical movements of the body in order to spread through the cellular spaces and vessels.

The Metaphor of the Lymph

The lymph, as the supporting actor of the body, slowly absorbs toxins and facilitates healthy circulation, all without fanfare or much acknowledgement. It is easy to ignore the shadows and the emotional depth the lymphatic system embodies but it plays a crucial role in both physical health and subtle radiance. There is much talk about connecting to the inner light and letting it shine brighter. But just like a candle flame cannot be seen if the glass around it is dark and dirty, the inner light of the yogi cannot shine without the tireless effort of the lymph.

SUBTLE ANATOMY PERSPECTIVE

Challenges to the Immune System

Often the immune response is compared to a military action in the body. There are lots of parallels drawn to identifying invaders, killing, and defense. While these comparisons can be helpful, there is a gentler, more expansive reframing of this system available. Instead of thinking about the fight of the immune system, think of it more as a community project. Everything in the body is working together to move along the path. Sometimes that path involves getting sick. All sickness, from the flu to something dire, creates a time of realigning with what *is* possible and important in life. Often the immune response is the body's way of asking for some downtime, self-reflection or lifestyle changes.

Japa's Story: Sickness Adds to the Sweetness of Life

A friend of mine recently contracted amyotrophic lateral sclerosis, also known as Lou Gehrig's disease or ALS. He is the last person on earth one would associate with serious illness. He is a jock and a fun-loving guy who at the age of 41 with two young children suddenly became ill. Not one to be daunted, he wrote online about his desire to drive a Krispy Kreme truck and give out donuts. Krispy Kreme contacted him right away and gave him a vintage delivery truck with the words, "One Sweet Ride," on a banner across the top. Now he drives this truck around delivering donuts to cancer patients, high school students, and people in need. He gives inspirational speeches as he hands out the treats, reminding folks to appreciate life, worry less, and savor the sweetness of every moment. His acceptance of his sickness as a blessing is an inspiration; it allowed him to reveal even more of his energetic and giving presence. He is a lighthouse to all. (Breitling, 2014)

Why We Still Get Sick

The amazing thing about the body is that *most* of the time it is able to keep us healthy. Most of the *not-self* stuff in the world never even makes it inside. If it does, it is usually handled before it results in illness. There is a general belief that a germ gets into the body and automatically causes sickness. The reality is that bacteria and viruses are everywhere. It is not guaranteed that sickness will occur just because they make it inside the body. Sometimes viruses sneak

> THE IMMUNE SYSTEM TEACHES US THIS: THERE IS NO NEED TO REACT TO EVERYTHING AROUND YOU; JUST STAY STEADY AND ALLOW FOR CHALLENGES TO PASS WITHOUT DISTURBANCE.

past the barriers, or the bacteria outwit the immune cells. But *most* of the time the body keeps them out or destroys them before they have a chance to become a full-blown illness.

In one study at the University of Michigan, researchers found that when subjects were purposefully infected with the flu virus, only half actually became sick. That is because the immune system is really good at finding and eliminating pathogens before sickness occurs. Illness arises when the immune system is overwhelmed by other factors and fails to respond. Holistic medical practitioners are more concerned with strengthening the vital force and increasing the health of the immune system than fending off pathogens. The principle is to support the environments in the body with a clean diet, regular movement, and consistent rest, which allows the immune system to respond appropriately and consistently (Hunag et al., 2011).

Allergies Exposure to environmental irritants is an important factor in developing a strong immune system. A study of Amish children in *The Journal of Allergy and Clinical Immunology* found a lower rate of allergies and asthma among Amish children who grow up on farms, drink raw milk, and play and work outside in the fresh air and dirt. It is possible that immune systems are not challenged enough in environments that are too sterile or that control environmental factors with air conditioning and air purifiers. In fact, there is even research that has shown babies are healthier later in life if they grew up around furry pets. (Journalism of Courage, 2014; Holbeich et al, 2012; and Bergoth et al, 2012). It is also interesting to consider that as babies naturally test and try everything they can touch or put in their mouths they are building their immunity through constant exposure to different germs and pathogens.

While products like cleaning wipes and hand cleaners that tout killing 99.9% of germs have value in not spreading germs, the reality is that germs will always exist and are necessary in helping us build strong immune systems. So, when children eat dirt or share lollipops with the dog, it may actually be good for them! They are building a stronger immune system through exposure to pathogens.

The Immune System and the Arcline

The Arcline is the energetic structure of the Sixth Light Body. It can be visualized as a halo around a person's head, running from temple to temple. Women have an additional Arcline that runs from nipple to nipple. The Arcline is our connection with the divine and also holds an imprint of our karmic record. When there is clarity of intention and projection, the Arcline is bright, and the universe delivers. To reach that state of clarity and brightness requires steadiness in your practice and a commitment to connecting to the higher self.

The immune system is intertwined with the Arcline because of the relationship between illness and our karmas. Sickness trains the immune system to respond appropriately to challenges in the same way that the universe pushes us to face challenges. When a person is able to see sickness as a blessing or gift in his or her life, no matter how challenging the illness, the Arcline is cleared of those karmic debts. The Arcline becomes brighter and clearer when there is a conscious surrender or trust in the Infinite. Any yoga or meditation that strengthens the Arcline also protects the body and helps to transform sickness.

> THE ARCLINE IS STRENGTHENED PRIMARILY WITH THE POWER OF PRAYER, STEADINESS IN YOUR PRACTICE, AND BY BEING IN COMMUNITY WITH OTHERS.

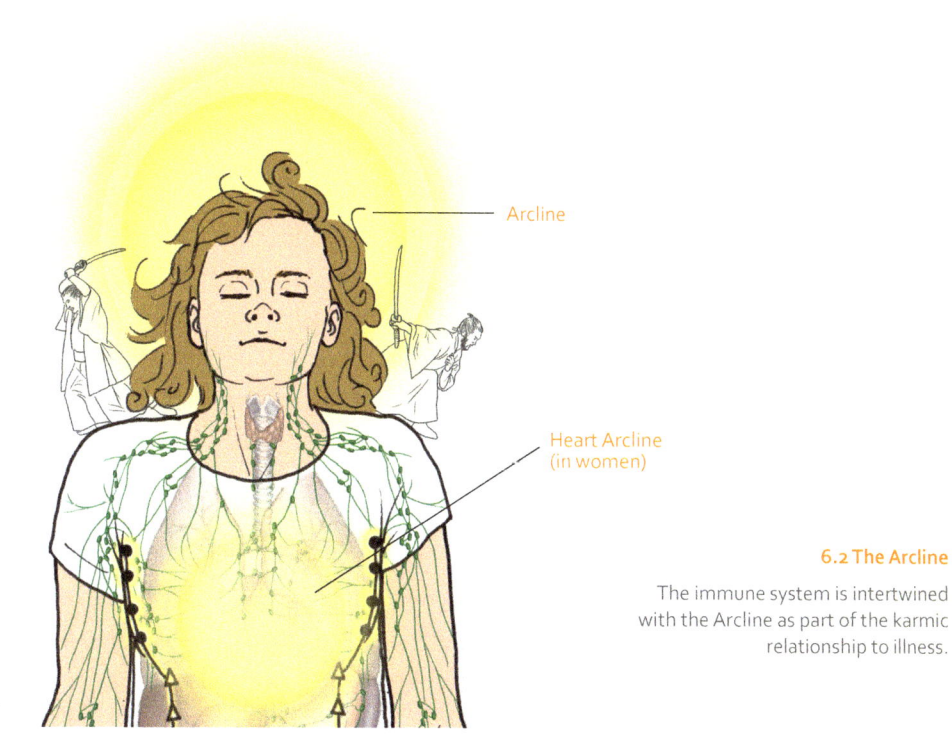

6.2 The Arcline

The immune system is intertwined with the Arcline as part of the karmic relationship to illness.

Exploring Physical and Subtle Human Anatomy

Another way to strengthen the Arcline is through the power of community. Arclines of different people link up with each other and create change that spans beyond time and space. Yogis believe that even smiling at someone else generates a spark of energy and creates a link in the Arclines. The power of linked Arclines creates a sense of connection and expansion which can be tapped into for deep healing. In a spiritual community, family or tribe people often gather together when someone is sick. The combined link of their Arclines creates the power to uplift and shift the illness.

Japa's Secret Family Healing

When I was about eight years old, my Great Aunt Lucy pulled my mother aside and whispered a healing secret to her that had been passed down among the women in my family for generations. My mother now holds the family secret to wart removal. To tap into this secret healing a person with a wart must do two things: one, send my mother a picture of the wart, and, two, believe that it will be healed. Family lore says that her secret process works as well as any chemical on the market. My own theory about why this family secret works is that the subtle linking of Arclines combined with the recipient's belief in the process helps the immune system get rid of the wart.

Sangat, or Spiritual Community

Community is about connecting with people in real life; sitting down with them face-to-face, talking together, eating together and meditating together. Community means creating and nurturing bonds with people. The spiritual practice of living in community, or *Sangat*, is a powerful metaphor for the immune system; and serves to strengthen it as well.

As human beings when we're in community, we're much stronger than when we are on our own. There is a magical, whole-is-greater-than-the-sum-of-its-parts thing that happens. This does not mean that being in community is always blissful and challenge-free. A community of people around you acts like the immune system in the body. When sickness happens it presents a growth opportunity for the body, just as challenges in families and communities are an opportunity for growth and trust. Through challenging situations both the immune system and communities of people learn, heal, and grow toward more expansive versions of themselves.

The Immune System

Just like a healthy community filters out troubles and collectively shares in the highs and lows of the human experience, the discrete physical structures of the immune response work together to keep *not-self,* or pathogens, out of the body and collectively move toward health and vibrancy. Being in the world is messy. Even though there are germs everywhere, *most* of the time the body gets rid of pathogens without a lot of visible effort. Occasionally something makes its way in that causes sickness, but as the body heals itself, it is also learns and prepares to better handle that problem in the future.

Being around people is messy. Even when we're trying our best we're occasionally going to hurt someone's feelings, have our own feelings hurt, or in some other way experience the drama of being human. When we're intentionally connecting to other people, and these challenges arise, we have the opportunity to experience the pain and learn how to move past it. As our minds and souls heal we learn and prepare to handle ourselves better should a similar situation arise again.

On the other hand being around people on a similar spiritual path of growth is inspiring. When we feel crazy for wanting to get up at 4 a.m., or sit for two and a half hours in meditation, or give up sugar, having people around us on the same path helps to normalize our behavior and keep us going. And we can do the same for others. There are studies that show that having a "gym-buddy" makes people significantly more likely to stick to a fitness routine and get better results during their workouts. Having a *sangat* around you makes you more likely to stick to your spiritual fitness routine. When we connect with like-minded souls, we see the light of our souls mirrored back to us. That mirroring allows our own light to shine brighter (Irwin, 2012).

There is no germ-free; there is only the ability to respond to the environment.
There is no problem-free community; there is only the ability to respond and grow.

Collective Wellbeing

There is a practice in some indigenous cultures where one member of a tribe will offer thanks when they see another member doing something to improve his or her own health. This supportive belief is that when any one member gets healthier, it improves the collective energy of the whole tribe. The next time you're driving in your car and you see someone out for a run, consider offering them a silent thank you for their contribution to the collective wellbeing!

Chinese Medicine and the Immune System

The tickle in the throat or chills at the back of your neck when a cold is approaching are the Wei Qi warriors at work.

Immunity in Chinese medicine is viewed as a wave of energy, called *Wei Qi,* which rises up to protect your body at the first sign of illness. This defensive force field rises up to fight off sickness like a line of warriors defending a fortress. The strength of *Wei Qi* is developed through truthful and healthy living.

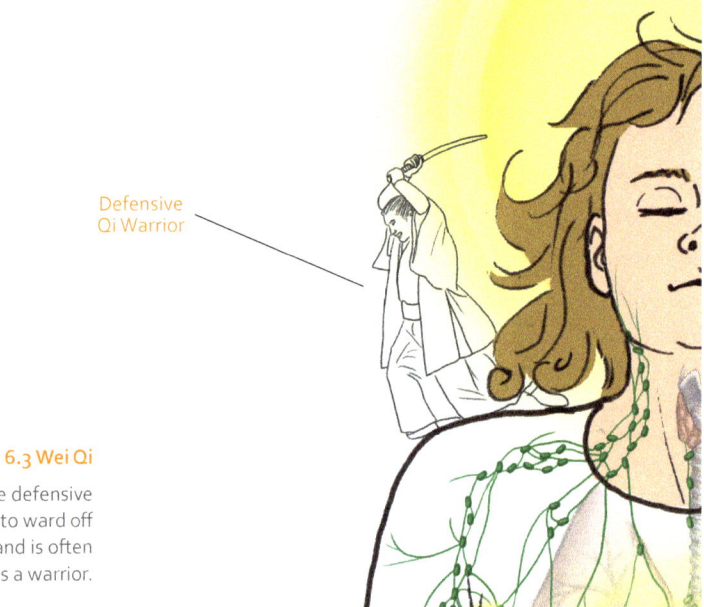

Defensive Qi Warrior

6.3 Wei Qi

In Chinese medicine, the defensive energy that rises up to ward off sickness is called Wei Qi and is often depicted as a warrior.

When this specific type of *Qi* is depleted it is easier for colds, flu, or other pathogens to penetrate the body. *Wei Qi* is spread throughout the body in different organs (just like the physical immune system). The lungs are the first line of defense and stimulating them is an easy way to turn on the *Wei Qi* and establish a barrier against colds.

In Chinese medicine the *Spleen* is considered a part of the immune system. It works in harmony with the pancreas and adrenal glands to process all information, events, and food. Students who stay up late studying and reading are described as taxing their *Spleen*. Everything from the food you eat to what you watch on television to how your spouse speaks to you is processed by the *Spleen* and the Physical Body.

The Immune System

The *Spleen* is also a major component of detoxification for the whole body. Eating "clean" is one of the best things to support its health. If you are filling up your body with loads of junk the *Spleen* has to work twice as hard to keep up. Have you ever noticed that you feel exhausted after a fight or stressful interaction with another person? This is because worry and mental stress can also tax the *Spleen*. The *Spleen* responds well to rhythm, good food, and a steady schedule. It is like a sweet baby inside of you that needs to be warm and dry. It is the part of you that must be nurtured, so that you can deal with everything that life throws at you.

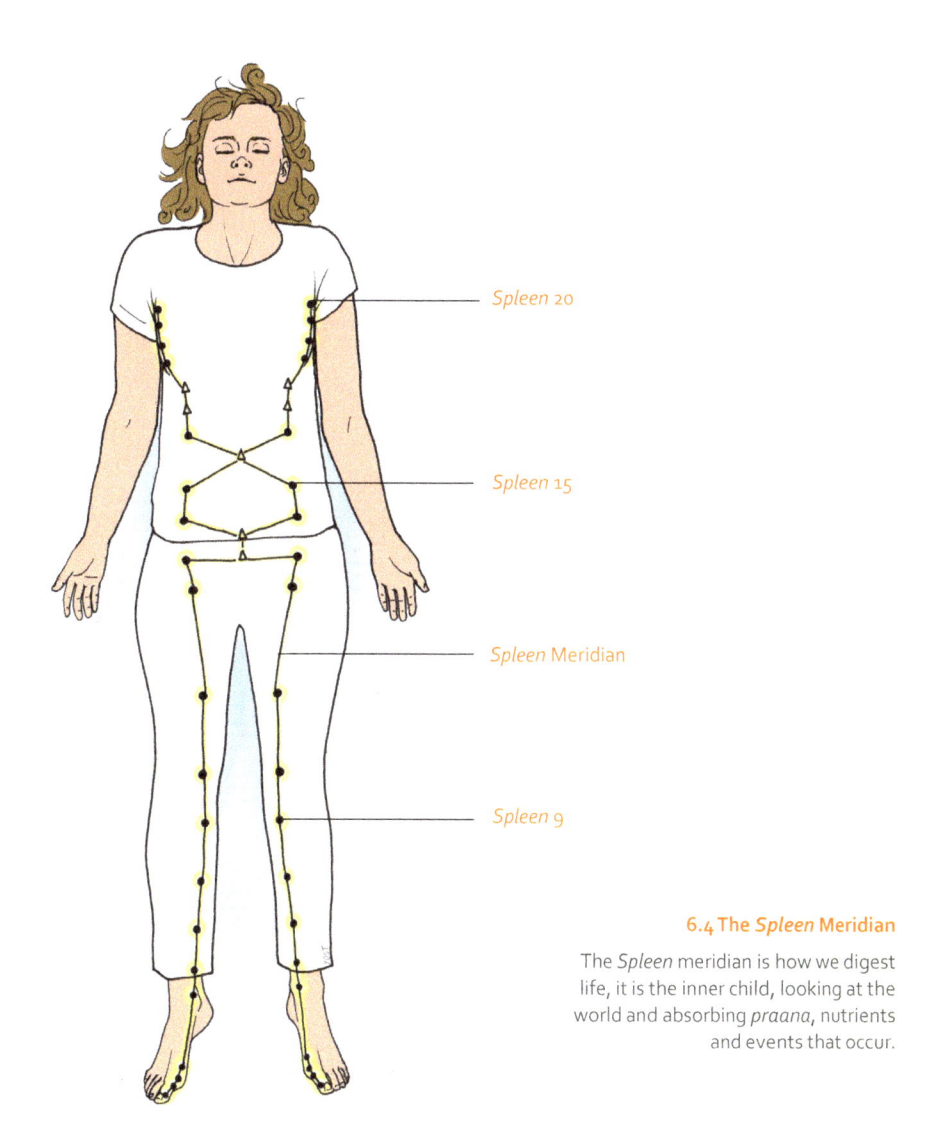

Spleen 20

Spleen 15

Spleen Meridian

Spleen 9

6.4 The *Spleen* Meridian

The *Spleen* meridian is how we digest life, it is the inner child, looking at the world and absorbing *praana*, nutrients and events that occur.

Exploring Physical and Subtle Human Anatomy

TIPS AND TECHNIQUES FOR A STRONG IMMUNE SYSTEM

Aasanas and Exercises

Moving Lymph: Any posture that moves or applies pressure to the neck, armpit or groin will help push lymph fluid through the nodes.
Examples: Head Rolls, Leg Lifts, Shoulder Shrugs, Sat Kriya, Arm Swings, Shoulder Stand
Twisting Postures: Twisting postures are detoxifying. Wrings the body tissues out like a dish rag. Moves the lymphatic fluid that surrounds every body cell.
Examples: Seated Twists, Static Twist, Moving Twists, Windmill
Thymus Pressurizing Postures: Anything that creates pressure across the chest or the spleen will activate the thymus.
Examples: Bear Grip, Heart Center Kriyas, Cobra, Camel, Shoulder Stand

"The deep relaxation at the end of a Kundalini Yoga kriya is the single most impactful aspect for stabilizing the immune system. It is in this still point that immune response function is balanced and restored."

—Shanti Shanti Kaur, PhD
Director and founder of the Guru Ram Das Center for Medicine and Humanology

Transformational Energy Points

Spleen 21: Great Embracement

Location: On the side of the ribcage at about elbow level

Effects: Alleviate physical pain, brings harmony to the entire being

Yoga for this Point: Meditations where the elbows strike the ribcage

Mantra

Mantras work on the mind to slowly create feelings of contentment and peace. These feelings support the immune system and our ability to relax and be happy and healthy.

Ra Ma Da Sa
Sa Se So Hang

This mantra helps to build healing energy by calling on the power of the sun, moon, Earth, and the infinite. It is used to send healing to individuals near or far.

Ek Ong Kaar Sat Nam
Karta Purkh Nirbhao Nirvair
Akal Moorat
Ajoonee, Saibhang
Gur Prasaad
Jap
Aad Sach, Jugaad Sach, Haibhee Sach, Nanak Hosee Bhee Sach

This mantra is called the Mool (root) Mantra. It awakens the ability to heal oneself and soothes depression. It creates a safe, firm, and energetic foundation for life. It is said to be a fate-killer that can remove karmic illness.

Ek Ong Kaar Sat Gur Prasaad
Sat Gur Prasaad Ek Ong Kaar

This mantra is about the internal sweetness of life. The forward and backward nature of the words create a turnaround. It is good to use when feeling stuck in negative thoughts or experiences. It can be chanted over water or food to bring sweet healing energy into the substance.

Exercise Your Smile Muscles: *Be Happy!*

Happiness and immune function go hand in hand. The happier you are, the easier it is to stay healthy. The brain does not know whether a smile is from happiness or whether happiness leads to a smile. A very glum mood can change just from forcing a smile or a laugh. After a few minutes one may simply start to feel better. There are practices in Kundalini Yoga that tap into this phenomenon with big belly laughs, chanting *Haree*, whistling, or even forcing a goofy smile. These are simple ways to impact the nervous system and shift from a downward cycle to focusing on the positive (Khalsa, S.S.K, 2010).

Traditional Healing

In some indigenous or traditional healing methods, when a tribal member goes to the medicine man for healing, the medicine man will determine the root of the illness by asking three questions: When did you stop singing? When did you stop dancing? When did you stop telling your story? (McKay, 2014)

Plants, Herbs, and Food

Cloves Clove tea is typically used in the springtime in the first warm days of the season. Clove tea has anecdotally been successful as a cold and flu preventative. Cloves are a spice known for reducing parasitic activity in the body. According to Yogi Bhajan, viruses breed in the springtime and drinking clove tea every morning for the month of May will increase protection. The nose, ears, throat, and bronchial tissues will absorb the protective capacity of the clove (Bhajan, 1995b).

Fruit All fruits are powerful immune boosters due to their high vitamin and mineral content.

Astragalus Next time you feel a cold or flu approaching pick up some astragalus root. This herb, shaped like a tongue depressor, shows up in clinical trials along with echinacea and ginseng as immune system enhancing. It is known for its ability to increase the effectiveness of the immune system. To use astragalus root, cook it at a low boil until the water becomes a pleasant gold color. If you're feeling adventurous you can also add a stick or two when cooking soup or gravy for added flavor (Block et al, 202; Clement-Kruzel et al, 2008).

Many spiritual traditions encourage the blessing of food before eating a meal. In the Kundalini Yoga as taught by Yogi Bhajan© community the words Sat Naam are repeated three times before a meal with the hands in prayer mudra at the heart center.

Yogic Lifestyle

Community (*Sangat*)

A study of the world's longest-living and happiest centenarians examined 260 people. Those who were part of healthy communities, including people belonging to faith communities, and those living in multigenerational households lived the longest and measured highest on happiness factors (Buettner, 2012). Community, or *sangat*, is an important aspect of Kundalini Yoga. Kundalini Yoga is not just taking a class, it's a lifestyle. Sharing meals after class, doing service projects together, and coming together twice a year for the large solstice sadhana gatherings are all important community-building activities for Kundalini Yogis. Building healthy relationships with a community of people helps contribute to the possibility of a long healthy life. As people come together to support each other, community is created and immunity is enhanced.

Abhyanga

Abhyanga (self-massage with oil) is an Ayurvedic self-care technique that is both calming and stimulates the immune system through the skin. Daily massage of the skin releases beneficial chemicals, helps to strengthen immunity, and circulates the lymph fluid. People with a dominant *Vata* dosha especially benefit from oil massage and can use sesame or almond oil. To support *Pitta* dosha try coconut or olive oil. *Kapha* dosha can do a dry massage with mustard or safflower oil. Also, some Ayurvedic product retailers sell oils specifically blended for each body type.

RECIPES TO SUPPORT THE IMMUNE SYSTEM

MAY CLOVE TEA RECIPE

Soak a handful of cloves in a porcelain or ceramic bowl overnight. Take two to three teaspoons (15ml) in the morning before breakfast. Don't overdo it; just two to three teaspoons (15 ml) are enough..

(Bhajan, 1995b)

YOGI BHAJAN'S IMMUNE-BOOSTING SHAKE

Balances *Vata* and *Pitta* doshas. Increases *Kapha* dosha.

- ✓ 2 apples, cored and chopped
- ✓ 2 bananas, scrape and include white strings from the skin
- ✓ 1 red bell pepper
- ✓ 8 blanched almonds
- ✓ 3 tablespoons (45 ml) of sesame seeds

Blend ingredients together with one cup of water until a smooth shake is made. This recipe will give you energy and immune-boosting power.

Ayurvedic Self-Massage

- Stimulate the skin with a dry brush or rough towel. Rub every limb toward the heart.
- Warm a small amount of oil by running it under hot water.
- Rub oil into scalp in circular motion.
- Using more oil as needed massage the upper body with small circular motions; cover as much of the arms, neck, chest, and back as you can reach.
- For women, spend some time on each breast and over the breastbone.
- Continue to massage in circular motion the hips, low back and legs. Pay special attention to each joint. Direct the pressure of strokes *toward* the heart.
- Give each foot a good squeeze, soothing the nerve endings on the soles of each foot.

The whole process can be done in about 3 to 5 minutes. You can then take a light shower to remove excess oil, or you can choose to leave a thin film of oil on the body for the whole day (Chopra, n.d.) .

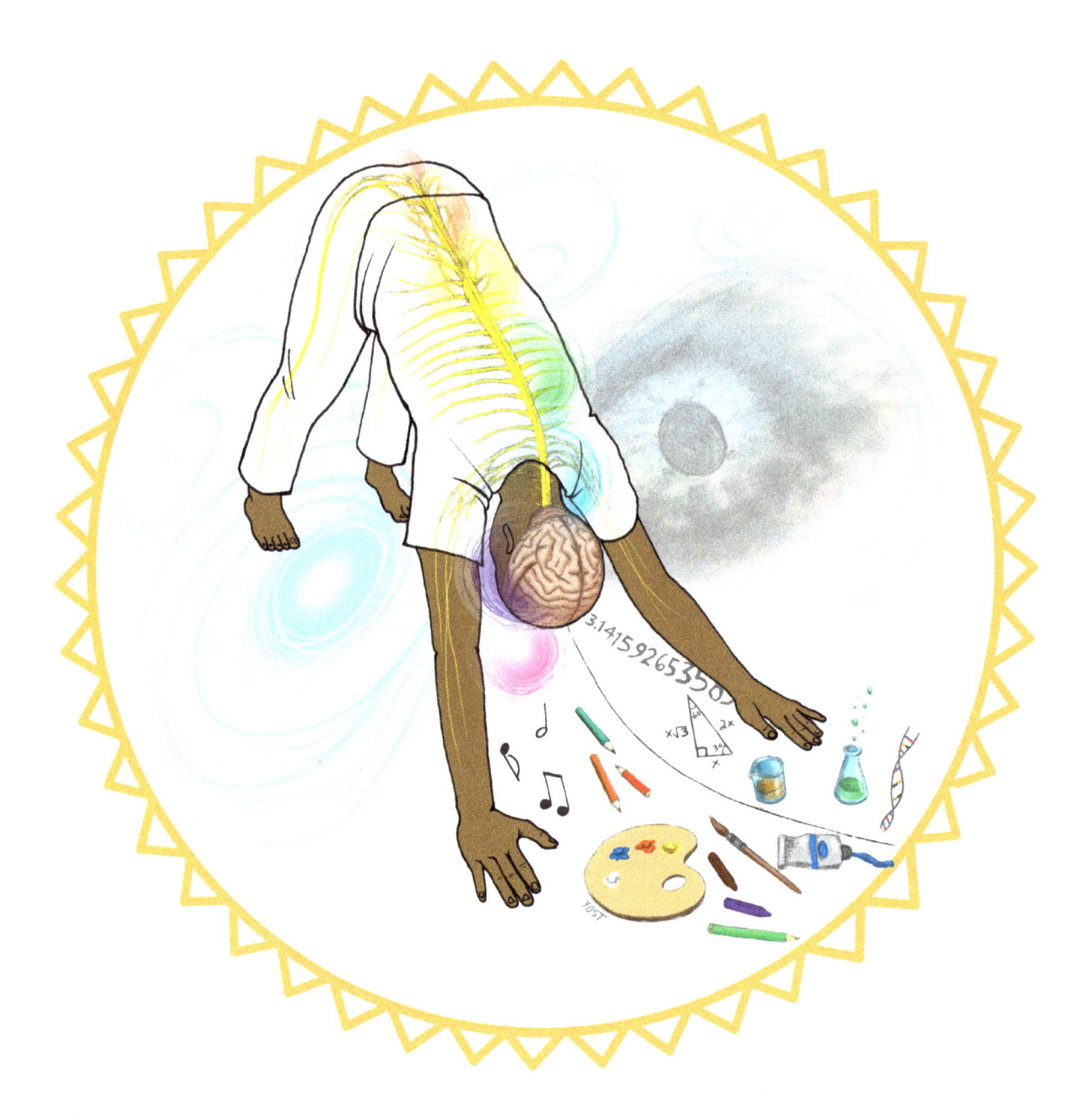

7.0 Triangle Pose

Triangle Pose builds upper body strength and lower body flexibility. It is a gentle inversion that is healing and supportive to the nervous system. As one seeks to find the balance point between the hands and feet, so we recognize the importance of balance in the nervous system.

Notice the subtle anatomy elements: the swirling energy of the air and ether tattva, the left and right brain functions represented by the items between his hands and the Radiant Body represented by the pointed golden circle.

Notice the physical anatomy structures: the network of the brain, spinal cord and nerves as they exit from the spinal column.

The Nervous System

The nervous system is involved in every function of the body and is the fulcrum of life. A complex system of interconnected signals, which monitor and manage most major physical actions and processes, the nerves relay information, directions, and input about the environment and maintain homeostasis in an ever-shifting world. The nervous and endocrine systems work together as managers of the body. When they are balanced, the body is balanced.

Balance is a foundational concept in the practice of yoga, meditation and mindfulness. Individuals on a spiritual path are constantly asked to find the balance between fanatical devotion and the elements of everyday human existence. Kundalini Yoga is the yoga of a householder who lives in the world but is not of the world. There is no escape to a cave or monastery; the yogi must find the balance between spiritual practice and the demands of family life. The efficiency of this technology opens up the possibility for an ever more graceful life. With regular practice, there is more *praana* available for maintaining a home, having meaningful work, and the blessings of serving society in creative ways.

Kundalini yogis must have a sense of the spiritual ideal: chanting for two and a half hours before the sun rises every day, eating the perfect diet, giving money to charity, and perfecting every yoga posture. They must also accept the real: sleeping through your alarm, eating on the go, weighing your need for new tires with your monthly commitments to gifting, and recognizing that bound lotus just may not be in your future. One yogi can rarely do everything perfectly. Each individual must find balance between the spiritual life and a home life. This is why we gather as a spiritual community. Some yogis are better at *sadhana*, some are generous with philanthropy, and some are warriors about eating the perfect diet. With each individual contributing in their own balanced way, the greater collective energy is uplifted for all. Finding this balance is essential to maintaining the health and vitality in the nervous system, because even well-intentioned actions can tax the system when they are taken to the extreme.

The nervous system is involved in everything from enjoying a sunset or understanding the sensation of hunger to picking up a pencil. Maintaining the health of the nervous system is critical to the enjoyment of life.

PHYSICAL ANATOMY PERSPECTIVE

Components of the Nervous System

- Brain
- Spinal Cord
- Nerves

Benefits of a Strong Nervous System

The nervous system is the command center of the body. When it is strong the body experiences effectiveness and ease in both purposeful movement and automatic body processes.

A strong nervous system gives us the ability to quickly adapt and respond to stimuli. Life happens at an increasingly quick pace; being able to respond quickly and efficiently allows us to keep up. If the nervous system becomes overtaxed or overstretched, we become susceptible to overwhelm, depression, and even illness.

Primary Purpose

The primary purpose of the nervous system is to receive input from the environment, both external and internal, and to send signals through the body when action is needed.

"One of the most beautiful actions we can take in our life, with a lot of courage and wisdom, is to relax."

© The Teachings of Yogi Bhajan, February 22, 1990

Central Nervous System

The central nervous system consists of the brain and the spinal cord. It processes all sensations—from the physical feeling of cold or hot to the sensation of imbalance in an internal organ. The central nervous system is also where conscious bodily movement begins by directing the action of the skeletal muscles. Because they are crucial to continuing life, the brain and spinal cord are well protected. The body's design features protective boney cases for the brain, spinal column, and cerebral spinal fluid to keep them safe.

The Brain

Different sections of the brain have very specific functions.

The Frontal Lobe is situated directly behind the forehead. This is where decisions and conscious thought processes happen. Accidents involving traumatic brain injuries to this area can have catastrophic results because of the loss of conscious decision-making and higher-level thinking abilities.

Limbic System Deep in the center of the brain is the limbic system, often referred to as the reptilian brain. This part of the brain is primarily concerned with survival. The reptilian brain *can't* think frontal lobe thoughts. The frontal lobe can contemplate how to meaningfully contribute to community or choose salad over French fries; but when the reptilian brain has needs, they must be met *now*. The reptilian brain will push others away to make sure its needs are met. Unlike the frontal lobe decisions, which take into account consequences, the reptilian brain is designed to take over during times of extreme stress or fear and dictate a reaction to keep us alive. Problems arise when it emerges at moments that are stressful but not necessarily life threatening. This can lead to decisions or actions based on fear instead of higher-level cognition.

The frontal lobe can be activated and strengthened through meditation to allow for more evolved decision making to emerge. The yogic lifestyle supports making decisions from the frontal lobe instead of the reptilian brain. Eating healthy foods, cleaning out the mind with *sadhana,* and being mindful in our actions support making these front-lobe decisions, especially when feelings of stress arise. Sometimes you are only able to identify that you *are* acting from your reptilian brain rather than from your higher self but you are unable to stop the actions. Continuing on the path of contemplation and mindfulness reveals these old survival behaviors and helps to develop the ability to act from a more conscious frontal lobe place instead.

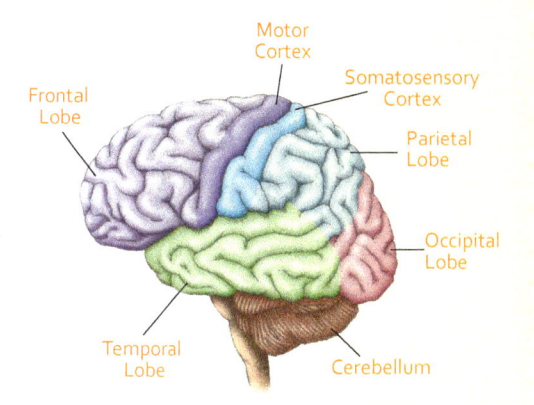

7.1 Sections of the Brain

"To live off each other or to live at each other is not human. To live for each other is human."

© The Teachings of Yogi Bhajan,
April 8, 1990

Nirmal's Story of Sharpness

Throughout my life I've found myself in roles where I am organizing people, coordinating activities, lists, or needs. And even though I had good organizational skills before I started practicing yoga, I lacked the skills to handle my stress. Everything felt like a big deal, and when we would get close to the big event, I would find myself snapping at people. Due to the stress of the event I felt I was justified in lashing out. Even though I would feel bad later, when I was in the moment I just couldn't seem to help myself.

As I began practicing yoga and meditation, I noticed that sometimes even as I was saying the words, snapping was not really the interaction I wanted to have. This helped me to apologize right away and repair the damage of my sharp tongue. Lately, I've noticed that even when I have the thought of sharp words, I am at times able to catch them before they come out of my mouth. I can take a moment to reflect on why I'm feeling stressed or angry and communicate with my friend or coworker in a way that reflects my frontal-lobe thinking or higher self. This allows me more time to relax or work instead of spending so much energy repairing the damage done by my sharpness. I am by no stretch of the imagination perfect. I still make mistakes and say things I shouldn't. But it happens less now, a lot less. This is the benefit of a regular contemplative practice. It gives you the ability to zoom out in times of stress and act in accordance with your values rather than innate survival strategies.

Impact of Meditation on the Health of the Brain

Time-tested yogic meditations are now being put through the rigors of scientific study. Often these ancient techniques are proving to be powerful tools for improved health and wellness. In the realm of brain health specifically there have been studies showing significant effects of meditation on Alzheimer's prevention. Medical studies have analyzed the results of 12 minutes a day of Kirtan Kriya, a meditation involving chanting and specific hand positions, see page 254. The caregivers who did the meditation showed less stress and inflammation. The patients who practiced the meditation showed a significant reduction in memory loss. Even changes at the DNA level were discovered which indicate meditation may be part of helping someone ward off genetic predispositions to particular diseases.

(Khalsa, 2014).

The Nervous System

Hemispheres of the Brain

The two sides of the brain have different capabilities and strengths.
- **Right Brain:** Processes feelings and emotions; sees the big picture.
- **Left Brain:** Processes facts, language, and details; sees the logistics.

Most people tend to be either more right-brained or left-brained. However, for optimum function, both sides of the brain should work more or less equally well and communicate back and forth with ease. When the pattern of either left or right brain dominance is identified, yoga and meditation can be used to cultivate balance between the hemispheres (Bhajan, 2010). It is important that both sides of the brain are strong, healthy, balanced and communicating with each other.

Third Ventricle

The third ventricle is a fluid-filled space deep in the center of the brain that contains cerebrospinal fluid and is known in many yogic paths as the "cave of Brahma" (Khalsa, 2013). From a mystical perspective, it acts as a connecting point between the rational upper parts of the brain and the deeper survival-based functions of the lower brain. The third ventricle is the space that connects the workings of the pineal and pituitary glands and the thalamus. It is possible that these structures work together in subtle ways to create the nectar of a spiritual practice. The third ventricle, like the center of a flower, is a space for many unique elements to come together and create sweetness.

Deep meditation stimulates change in this area. During meditation pearls of wisdom arise in this vestibule of *ojas* and cerebrospinal fluid. Physical and subtle anatomy merge in this space as the glands create the biochemical experience which correlates to the subtle experience of meditation. It is that sweet spot when the efforts of the dedicated yogi result in a pure glandular secretion. These *Aha!* moments of bliss happen amid the subconscious murmurings of the mind. The entire nervous system is soothed and rejuvenated as the newly invigorated cerebrospinal fluid circulates and bathes the nerves.

Our feelings of deep bliss, peace, and oneness that develop over many years of practice originate in this portal to universal knowledge, the third ventricle. It is the foundation of the body-mind-spirit connection. This cavern in the brain is the common space that allows for the transformation of consciousness (Khalsa, 2013).

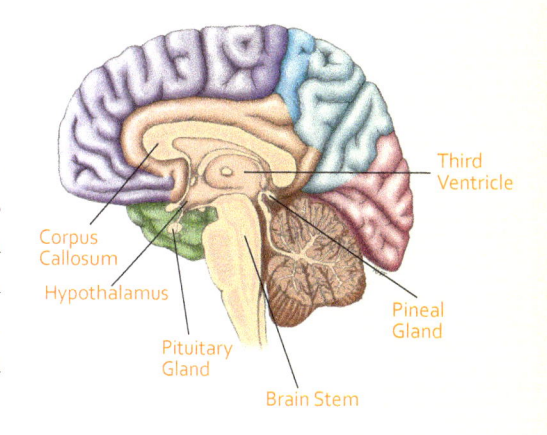

7.2 Cross Section of the Brain

"By its design, our right mind is spontaneous, carefree, and imaginative. It allows artistic juices to flow free without inhibition or judgment. In contrast, our left hemisphere is completely different in the way it processes information. It takes each of those rich and complex moments created by the right hemisphere and strings them together in timely succession."

—Jill Bolte Taylor, Neuroanatomist and author of *My Stroke of Insight*

Exploring Physical and Subtle Human Anatomy

> "We are going to arouse the energy, through the spinal column to change the serum to affect the gray matter in the brain, and to affect the patterns of the neurons."
>
> © The Teachings of Yogi Bhajan, January 23, 1991

The Spinal Cord

The spinal cord is the information highway connecting the brain with the rest of the body. It is about 1.5 centimeters in diameter and runs down the center of the vertebral column. Like the brain it is made of both gray matter and white matter. Most often the spinal cord is just the middle step between the brain and the body. However, in certain situations a reaction is needed far more quickly than a signal could make it to the brain. In those cases the spinal cord acts as a reflex arc. If someone were to touch a hot stove, the intensity of the heat signals would prompt the withdrawal even before the brain has time to cognitively feel the pain, much less send a signal to retract the hand.

The spinal cord is surrounded in three layers of connective tissue, which protect and separate it from surrounding structures. These thin, filmy layers are called the dura, and they overlay the brain and spinal cord.

Cerebrospinal Fluid If you were going to pack up your fine china, you would find a nice, sturdy box to pack it in. But you would first secure each dish in bubble wrap to create padding and protection. The body has packed the brain and the spinal cord in a similar way. They are safely in the hard boxes of the spine and skull, and they are surrounded by the anatomical equivalent of bubble wrap—the Cerebrospinal Fluid (CSF), which pads the brain and spinal cord. It is also responsible for nourishing tissues of the central nervous system. It flows around the structures delivering nutrients and removing wastes.

Peripheral Nervous System

> "Put your hand on a hot stove for a minute, and it seems like an hour. Sit with a pretty girl for an hour, and it seems like a minute. That's relativity."
>
> —Albert Einstein, theoretical physicist, Nobel Prize winner

The nerves that branch out from the central nervous system are called the peripheral nervous system. They travel to the muscles, glands, and organs to monitor and affect the processes of the body. One of the miracles of the body is the huge volume of information that is passed through the nervous system each day. For every single conscious action and many unconscious activities (hormone secretion and heart rate, for example) there are electrical impulses being sent to, around and from the brain.

A Snapshot of the Nervous System

Right now your nervous system is sending thousands of messages:
- The temperature of the room and whether to start sweating or shivering to maintain internal body temperature;
- The amount of light in the room and whether it is time for the pineal gland to start secreting melatonin; and
- The sensations in your digestive tract and whether it is time to eat or go to the bathroom.

The peripheral nerves carry information about the state of the body to the brain, and they carry directions from the brain to the structures of the body. The nerves don't interpret information or make decisions; they are simply the messengers.

Neurons and Nerves

Neurons are the individual cells that make up a nerve. Nerves are the networks on which messages travel around the body. Messages travel along the nerves in waves of electrical currents. It's a beautiful complicated dance of chemicals moving across the membranes of the neuron. As electrical impulses travel down the length of the neuron, information is passed along. At the end of the neuron there is a small gap, which the message must jump across before it goes on to the next neuron. It jumps across this gap via another special set of chemical agents called neurotransmitters. Like the members of a relay team, the message is seamlessly handed off from neuron to neurotransmitters to neuron until it reaches its destination.

> **MOST NERVES ARE COVERED IN A PROTECTIVE LAYER CALLED A MYELIN SHEATH, WHICH HELPS SIGNALS TO PASS MORE QUICKLY DOWN THE LENGTH OF A NEURON.**

1,000 Thoughts

Yogi Bhajan said you have 1,000 thoughts per wink of the eye (Bhajan, 1994b). Only a small percentage of those thoughts register on your conscious level. The other thoughts must go somewhere. They feed into the unconscious and subconscious minds. When practicing yoga and meditation you can start to identify those deep, subconsciously held thoughts that create your unconscious habits and patterns of being. Once they come into conscious awareness you can start processing and healing those thoughts in order to make better choices.

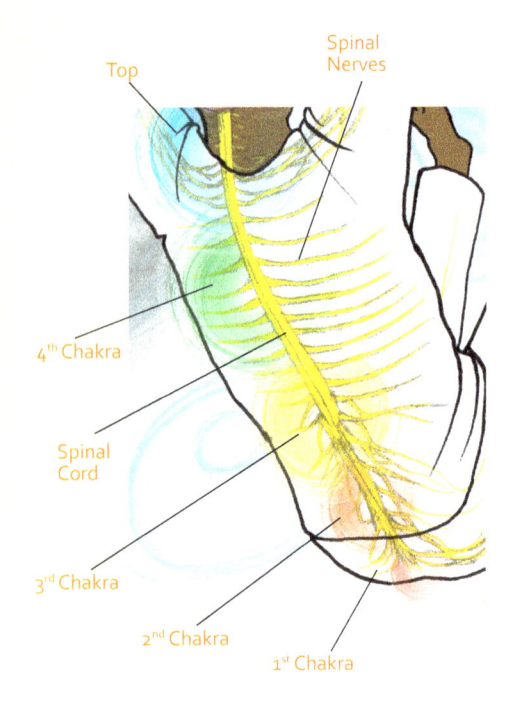

7.3 Spinal Cord and the Chakras

Spinal nerves exit between vertebra of the spinal column and correlate to principal chakra energies.

Sensory Nerves There is a huge amount of sensory information available at any given moment. In a split second, multiple sensations are simultaneously captured: the color of the walls of the room, your rumbling stomach, and the realization that a truck is headed toward you. The brain has to take all of this information in and make sense of it. The complete overload of sensory information is one of the reasons most of this happens on an unconscious level. Consider for a moment all of the sensory input you are not *actively* aware of, like the feeling of your clothes against the skin or the amount of light in the room.

Motor Nerves carry action instructions to the body. The impulses of the motor nerves trigger all actions of the skeletal muscles.

Spinal Nerves branch off from the cord and exit between the vertebrae of the spine as they head out to whatever organ, gland, or muscle they work with. The level at which the nerves exit relate to the different chakras.

Connecting Concepts chart, on page 137, describes where each nerve exits, what chakra it relates to, and what Chinese organs it innervates.

Cranial Nerves support smell, vision and eye movement, facial sensation and movement, hearing, tongue movement, and shoulder shrugging. By exiting directly from the brain, they remain protected even in the event of lower level spinal cord damage.

The vagus nerve is one of twelve cranial nerves and is the only cranial nerve that leaves the cranium. It has the widest ranging influence of any nerve in the body. It takes a long and wandering path. The vagus nerve

Vagus Nerve Activity

Try this the next time you are feeling entitled or bent out of shape in some way. Imagine there is a gold chain connecting your chin and the little hollow in the center of the base of your neck and shorten the chain by pulling the chin down into an exaggerated Neck Lock (Khalsa, 2011). Take a few long deep breaths or try sitting in this posture for 11 minutes a day and see what changes arise in your attitudes. This posture is said to energize the vagus nerve, activating feelings of compassion, altruism, and perspective (Disalvo, 2009).

Connecting Concepts

The Spine, Chinese Medicine Organs, and Chakras

Crown and Third Eye	Cranial Nerves
Throat Chakra	C1–7
	Influences parasympathetic response
	Stimulates general relaxation
Heart Chakra	T3: *Lungs*
	T5: *Heart*
Navel Chakra	T9: *Liver*
	T10: *Gallbladder*
	T11: *Spleen*
	T12: *Stomach*
Second Chakra	L2: *Kidneys*
Root Chakra	L4: *Large Intestine*
	S1: *Small Intestine*
	S2: *Urinary Bladder*
	S3-S5: Parasympathetic nervous system

innervates multiple organs and crucial life systems, such as the heart, lungs, and digestive tract. It is part of the parasympathetic nervous system, which slows heart rate, controls blood pressure, and regulates breathing.

Research on the vagus nerve has revealed that it is also involved in our feelings of compassion, empathy, and goodness. Research participants with higher vagal nerve activity expressed higher feelings of altruism, love, and happiness. This is because of the vagus nerve's influence on communication, heart rate, and its ability to trigger the release of oxytocin—a hormone responsible for feelings of bonding and connection. Research on children shows more cooperation and helpfulness when a child's vagus nerve is more active (DiSalvo, 2009).

This unique nerve holds the key to the ability to be present, aware, and compassionate. It is also one of the nerves most profoundly affected by the practice of yoga and meditation. Kundalini Yoga activates the vagus nerve

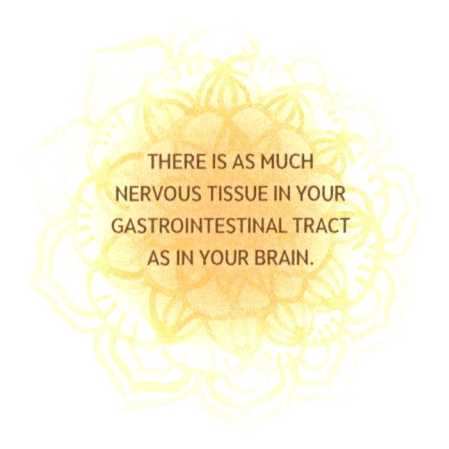

> THERE IS AS MUCH NERVOUS TISSUE IN YOUR GASTROINTESTINAL TRACT AS IN YOUR BRAIN.

with chanting, singing, whistling, pulling neck lock, eye focus (drishti), and practicing postures such as shoulder stand, plow pose, and cobra pose (Bhajan, 1982, 1989c, 1993d).

Enteric Nervous Plexus There are independently operating neurons in the digestive tract that are part of the autonomic nervous system. The mind is not limited to the brain. These neurons control things like the fluid balance and movement of food through the digestive tract. They also play a role in the experience of the "gut" feelings—like butterflies in the stomach or warm happy feelings when seeing a good friend.

The digestive system contains more neurons than the spinal cord, and like the brain, it plays a role in processing memories and generating gut feelings. Neurotransmitters like serotonin and dopamine are present in the gut, and it is becoming evident that the health of the digestive function greatly impacts mental mood and clarity by influencing brain chemistry.

Functional Categories of the Nervous System

Beyond the main components of the central and peripheral nervous systems, the nervous system is further classified by its predominant activity: autonomic, sympathetic, parasympathetic, and somatic.

Japa's First Teacher

A caution to readers: Many people have been helped with health issues from a regular yoga practice. But this is one person's story and is not meant to be taken as medical advice.

My first yoga teacher, Shiva Singh Khalsa, suffered from profound grand mal seizures as a teenager. He explained that during his youth in the 1960s he was prescribed heavy medications with lots of negative side effects. When he started doing Kundalini Yoga he asked Yogi Bhajan if he had any suggestions that would help. He was told to practice the Seven Wave Sat Nam Meditation for 31 minutes a day. This began a slow process of changing the course of his illness. Within a year he was able to stop taking the medication. Over time he was able to repair the damage to his nervous system, and he has been able to manage his seizures without medication for more than 35 years. He continues to meditate and maintain a healthy diet in order to prevent the return of symptoms.

Autonomic Nervous System

The autonomic nervous system controls the automatic functions of the body. It allows the body to keep running without having to remember to breathe, digest, or keep the heart beating. This frees up space for higher-level cognition.

The autonomic nervous system is further divided into the parasympathetic and sympathetic systems. These two divisions are the most impacted by a regular practice of yoga and meditation.

Sympathetic Nervous System

The sympathetic nervous system is the crisis management team of the body. It's what the body calls on in a fight, flight or freeze situation when responding to stress. The sympathetic nervous system coordinates a wide range of reactions in preparation for stressful or dangerous situations, including:
- Dilating pupils;
- Making the heart beat faster;
- Deepening the breath; and
- Releasing glucose for quick energy.

The sympathetic nervous system is also the danger alert system. It responds the same to *actual* danger as to *perceived* danger. In our modern society there are stressful situations, like a toxic boss or a challenging relative, which the body interprets as danger. This causes an overly activated sympathetic nervous system, which means that food cannot be digested effectively. Perhaps the chronic digestive problems of modern society stem from this chronically overstressed state? To get the most out of food it is important to be able to move easily and quickly into the safe, relaxed state of the parasympathetic state.

Parasympathetic Nervous System

The parasympathetic system is the nourishing and relaxing system. It coordinates a host of changes in the body, which support relaxation. Including:
- Slowing and softening the breath;
- Stimulating digestion;
- Cell rejuvenation; and
- Sexual arousal.

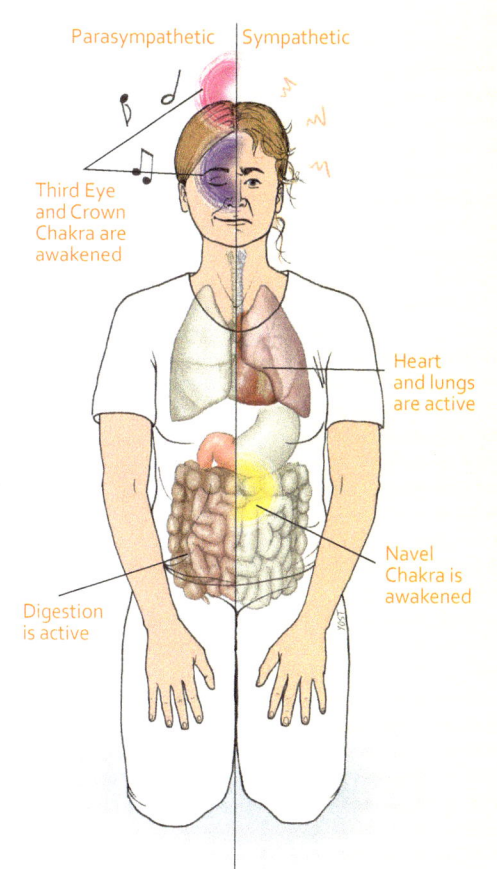

7.4 Parasympathetic and Sympathetic Nervous Systems

For comparison purposes, the left half of the body is shown in a peaceful and relaxed state characteristic of the parasympathetic nervous system: smooth digestion, restful or meditative brain activity, activation of higher intuitive energies of the Third Eye and Crown Chakras; while the right half of the body demonstrates stress responses characteristic of the sympathetic nervous system: increased heart rate, more rapid breathing, roused brain activity, increased alertness, Navel Chakra activation.

Sympathetic

- *Stress and Sweat*
- *Gas Pedal*
- *Fight, Flight, or Freeze*

Parasympathetic

- *Paradise*
- *Brake Pedal*
- *Rest and Digest*
- *Feed and Breed*

The parasympathetic nervous system and the vagus nerve are given a lot of emphasis in the yoga world. Many postures directly impact these systems to restore the ability to relax, deeply and completely. It's good to remember that the sympathetic system is also toned by yoga. Difficult or irritating postures that challenge nerves are a way of provoking and then relaxing the sympathetic nervous system. In order to be a responsive and compassionate yogi, both systems must be toned and nurtured so that all of the nerves are conditioned. A healthy nervous system can easily and efficiently switch into either an activated (sympathetic) or relaxed (parasympathetic) state. This is one of the strengths of Kundalini Yoga. It trains the nervous system to switch quickly and smoothly between these two states.

Many forms of yoga or meditation primarily focus on developing the parasympathetic response because of the amount of stress in modern life. Yet just as important as a strong parasympathetic response is the ability to switch back and forth quickly and easily. This is where Kundalini Yoga really shines. It has exercises that are irritating or challenging, like Breath of Fire or flapping of the arms, that stimulate the sympathetic system. After each exercise is a small rest to calm down, observe the mind, breathe, and stimulate the parasympathetic. The next exercise repeats that same cycle.

Somatic Nervous System

The somatic nervous system works with skeletal muscles to move and respond to stimuli in the environment. This system coordinates the voluntary actions of the body. Remember that to create even a simple body movement, a whole symphony of precise muscular activation and relaxation is required. Any time you dance, walk, raise your hand, or give a hug you are tapping the wisdom of the somatic nervous system.

Relationship to Other Systems

Nervous System and Endocrine System The nervous and endocrine systems work together to control and monitor *every* action, process and reaction in the body. The nervous impulses and the glandular or hormonal signals influence every function; from smelling dinner cooking to stimulating the desire to eat to finally eating. The nervous system creates change in the body through electric charges, while the endocrine cells communicate through the interlocking of target cells and hormones. They work together in many cases to create feelings of sexual arousal, rage, love or wonderment. The main connection point between the nervous and endocrine systems is the hypothalamus gland. This gland communicates between nervous and endocrine systems to facilitate smooth functioning of all body systems. The hypothalamus has both nervous and endocrine functions. By improving the health of either one of these systems the health of the other is automatically improved.

These are also the two systems that Kundalini Yoga impacts most effectively. The strength and health of the nervous and endocrine systems are directly related to the capacity to withstand stress, both good and bad. Everyone has stress in their lives; it is a natural part of the human experience. Often good things are just as stressful as bad ones. Getting married and having kids can be as stress-producing as having a family member die or losing a job.

Because it isn't possible to live a life without stress it is better to be prepared to handle life's stresses. Imagine stress as a liquid filling up a teacup. Once the stress level overflows the teacup stressed-out behaviors begin: becoming short-tempered and snapping at people, or having an increased risk of heart diseases or digestive problems (Mayo Clinic, 2014).

Yoga and meditation train the nervous system to better handle stress. Instead of a teacup's worth of stress sending someone off the deep end, it's more like a bathtub's worth of space to hold and process that stress. Deepening the practice allows for the creation of more space so that there is room to process all of the stress. A strong nervous system changes the capacity to handle stress. Like a tub with a good clear drain, a strong nervous system provides a clear channel for processing millions of stimuli and impulses—keeping your bathtub from backing-up or overflowing!

Both the endocrine and nervous system rely on rhythm. The cycles of the day and the rhythms of life are what keep them working and balanced. If there is a sense that these systems are not working at their top level, then resetting the rhythm can be helpful.

SUBTLE ANATOMY PERSPECTIVE

Challenges to the Nervous System

Air, Ether, and the Nervous System

In Ayurvedic medicine the nervous system is affected through the *tattvas* of air and ether. The air *tattva*, like a windy day, represents movement and the ability to set other objects into motion. The air *tattva* manages the nerves that speak to each other and the subsequent changes that occur. Air is the quality and flow of movement and information in our bodies.

The ether *tattva* manages the gap between nerves. Ether is the space or gaps between matter, and is connected to the realms of manifestation and possibility. It is the subtlest of all the elemental *tattvas* and the most closely connected to the vibration of sound or the 'sound current'. What we perceive of as sound (music, mantra, talking) is actually a unique combination of sound and silence. These silences, or gaps, are where the impact of the sound is felt and how the sound current creates its impact.

These two *tattvas* are the least dense of the elements, which is how they support the frequency and speed of the messages from the nerves. The subtle quality of the nervous system and the interplay of the two least grounded *tattvas* leave it vulnerable to stress and feeling overwhelmed. These two tattvas are especially vulnerable to the effects of screen devices. The physical presence of computers and cell phones can create a subtle heat or electric pressure on the body. Combined with the demands of rapid communication and expectations of constant electronic availability, screen devices apply maximum pressure to the nerves. Excessive stress or demanding expectations requires too much movement (air) over the specific nerves and gaps between the nerves (ether) which creates an accumulation of electricity in the body and leads to feeling fried.

In modern society there is an expectation to be connected and informed at all times. This creates a constant pressure to be busy and to perform. It can be difficult to unplug but making a few simple choices can create a calm and balanced life that protects the nervous system and balances the *tattvas* of air and ether. When these *tattvas* are balanced we experience security in a state of relaxation and a meaningful connection to our soul, other people and the divine. Balancing the air and ether *tattvas* is an ongoing process of clearing and strengthening the pathways of the nerves, the spaces between nerves, and the spaces in our lives.

Cold Depression

What happens when the nervous system is overwhelmed with day-to-day stress? A feeling of pressure, frustration, and overload arises. Cold Depression is a term Yogi Bhajan used to describe a specific type of depression that is unique to the time we live in and that manifests itself under those feelings

Living in an Electronic World

Simple choices to reduce the impact of electronic device
Sit down for meals and turn off the television, computers, radios, etc.
Turn off all electronic lights and screens at least one hour before bedtime.
Sleep in a completely dark room (no electric lights).

Simple reset if you're feel overexposed to electronics
Stand barefoot on the ground outside for five minutes.
Wash your hands, face, and feet in cold water.
If working on a computer, set a timer to take 3 Long Deep Breaths every 30 minutes. (Bhajan, 1989b) (see page 99 for how-to).

---

of being overloaded (Bhajan, 1998). Cold Depression is incubated in the challenges and pressures of the Aquarian Age. For many, gone are the days when you had to go home to listen to your answering machine or get an important phone call. Now communication devices travel with us, so we are virtually never disconnected. Many people living in this hyper-connected way do not consider the extra stimulation a problem. Yet something as seemingly simple as carrying a phone with you everywhere you go brings so much added stimulation into our lives; having so much so readily available can launch a cycle of wanting, striving and accumulating more and more without ever feeling truly satisfied. If unchecked, a mindset can develop from this cycle where we may feel that we can never get enough success, money, food, or wealth, leaving us feeling empty, sad or unfulfilled. The speed of communication and information exchange can exacerbate this outward striving, keeping us from checking inward to slow down and connect with the reality and truth of our being.

A person with Cold Depression may not even appear to be depressed in the typical way we imagine depression. In fact they may be very active or even considered an overachiever. Cold Depression can sometimes be a state of almost manic overdoing that leads the body to burnout and numbness. Cold Depression is exacerbated by our tendency to be disconnected from the frequency of our own soul and can be "a very sizzling hot anger in the personality (Bhajan, 1988a)". Often people experiencing this condition

Men, Women, and Brains

Anatomically and physiologically men and women are, in fact, quite different. One of the biggest areas of difference between the genders is in the brain. This is still an active area of research and the findings so far are mixed. Some studies suggest that men have significantly more grey matter in the brain (Holmes, 2008). This is the type of brain tissue responsible for holding facts and processing information. Women have significantly more white matter, which is the type of tissue responsible for making connections between pieces of information (Holmes, 2008). This makes women well-suited to see relationships between people or concepts. It makes men well-suited to follow through on tasks and solve problems.

Another major difference between male and female brains is the corpus callosum—the structure that connects and shares information across the two hemispheres of the brain. Studies show that women tend to have a significantly larger structure than men (Ardekani et al, 2012).

There are some interesting new areas of brain study with individuals who identify as transgendered. Initial findings show that often these individuals may have brains more similar in structure to the gender identity they express rather than that of their anatomical sex (Hamzelou, 2011).

will engage in risk-seeking behavior to try to counteract the experience of feeling numb in life. They may consume excessive amounts of caffeine, food, or alcohol; they may engage in random, unprotected sexual experiences, or risky sports or activities just to recapture some sense of being alive.

Kundalini Yoga and Meditation can be an effective remedy for Cold Depression because it is *both* stimulating and relaxing. It connects the body to the soul through mudras, mantras, and the elevated frequencies it produces in the body. It quickly creates an alternative way to cope with stress and be present in the moment. Connecting to spirit can help to create a sustained relationship with the self and alleviate the emptiness of Cold Depression (Khalsa, S.S.K).

The Nervous System, the Organs and the Chakras

The *Shu*, or acupuncture points of the back, are contained in the paraspinal muscles, the large muscle group that runs parallel to the spine. These points have a powerful influence over the body; by stimulating the pathways that branch off of the spine and circle around the body they activate the internal organs.

While some of the physical body systems correlate to a particular chakra, the nervous system has a broader relationship with the whole chakra system. The goal of the chakra system is not to have one strong center; it is for all of the chakras to be in balance and communicate easily and frequently. Similarly, the nervous system works as a cooperative of energy centers to effectively direct all life's processes.

The entire spine works in harmony to influence the state of mind and consciousness. Any posture, such as rolling up and down on the spine or Plow Pose, massages these points and is like giving an acupressure treatment to the organs. Postures that extend or compress the spinal column also affect these energy pathways and the corresponding internal organs.

7.5 Shu Points Along the Spine

The Nervous System and the Radiant Body

The Radiant Body is the Tenth Light Body. It contains all of the other bodies and can appear as a gold lining around the aura. When it is strong it boosts the power of all other nine Light Bodies. Someone with a strong Radiant Body will be confident, calm, and magnetic, with the ability to easily attract good things. She or he may appear to be someone who is lucky or has it all in life. The nervous system, like the Radiant Body, acts as a protective shield *and* informs all body functions.

Have you ever seen a person walk into a room and easily draw attention and control of the room? This is the type of leadership of someone with a strong Radiant Body. It is common in yoga circles to hear this capacity referred to as "holding the space." Although ubiquitous, this phrase is still often confusing or misunderstood. A person who can gain control over the physical space of the nervous system and tap into a strong Radiant Body creates a sense of steadiness for those around them. *This* is holding the space.

> "*We are just an advanced breed of monkeys on a minor planet of a very average star. But we can understand the universe. That makes us something very special.*"
>
> —Stephen Hawking (1988), theoretical physicist, cosmologist

In the yogic perspective this type of person is a warrior saint, someone who protects and serves others and is generous to all. The warrior saint must have strong armor in place and that armor is a strong nervous system with the capacity to handle immense loads of stress and still maintain balance. A warrior saint must be able to drop into a space of deep humility, vulnerability and tenderness in order to uplift and serve others, but maintaining this depth of sensitivity is only possible because of their strong nervous system.

Meditation and a yogic lifestyle can help you build a strong nervous system. When thoughts and sensations are filtered through a steady contemplative practice your capacity to handle what comes your way improves. Meditation is a little like taking out the garbage. When practiced regularly, you have the space and capacity to take in and let go of whatever comes your way!

TIPS AND TECHNIQUES FOR A STRONG NERVOUS SYSTEM

Aasanas and Exercises

Armpit Postures can help adjust and balance your nervous system. Yogi Bhajan said that the armpit is the center of all of the nervous systems. And they can all be adjusted by applying pressure, massaging, or moving the armpit area (Bhajan, 1994a).

Examples: Ego Eradicator, Arm Swings, and massaging the armpits.

Forward Bending helps nourish and bring circulation to the brain. Any time the brain is below the hips it creates an antigravity effect. The bowing motion promotes the flow of cerebrospinal fluid and blood to the brain, enhancing memory. Forward-bending postures bring fresh oxygen to the face.

Examples: Baby Pose, Bowing, Guru Pranam, and Life Nerve Stretch

Unusual Movements develop and prune pathways in the brain. The new actions are stimulating for the brain, which is forced to learn something new.

Examples: Fish Fry, Bundle Rolls, rhythmic clapping, contra-lateral movements, or any mudra.

Pumping the Navel Point stimulates the brain in the gut. Pumping the Navel Point clears the subconscious mind and makes space in the nervous system; it helps to reset the functional rhythm of the nerves.

Examples: Sodarshan Chakra Kriya, Sat Kriya, and any navel pumping

> *"Stretch the armpit so that...your nervous system ...is stimulated. Stretch out your universe. It will set the pattern in the neurons of the brain."*
>
> © The Teachings of Yogi Bhajan, June 25, 1990

> WHISTLE AND SING EVERY DAY TO KEEP YOUR SENSE OF INTERNAL HAPPINESS ALIVE.

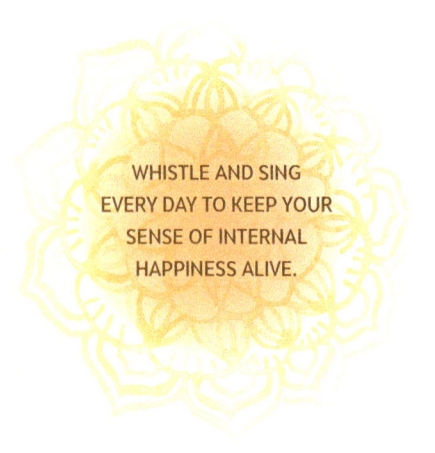

Mantra

Chanting serves the nervous system by creating a specific rhythm in the body. The vibration of sound travels through the bones of the skull and massages the brain. There are also specific meridian points on the roof of the mouth that are stimulated by the movement of the tongue in chanting, which in turn tonify the entire nervous system.

Sa Ta Na Ma

This is a mantra that balances all of the *tattvas* and soothes the mind. It invokes the simplicity of the original sounds of the universe.

Using Mantra to Focus on Work

Nirmal's dad works in specialty antique clock and watch repair. He spends his days repairing delicate, ancient, and tiny machines. One day he decided to play some mantra music in his shop. Very quickly he noticed that when he played this elevated music, he made fewer mistakes, lost fewer parts, and was generally more successful in this detailed work. The effects of the vibration of the mantras on the nervous system allow him to be more focused and relaxed in his work.

Plants, Herbs, and Food

Trinity Roots: Garlic, Ginger, and Onion These three roots are used to strengthen the body and to maintain order in the consciousness. Many teachings state that those wishing to maintain a celibate lifestyle should not eat garlic or onions. These roots are thought to be too stimulating to the mind, which could result in sexual thoughts and feelings. In the Kundalini Yoga tradition, the householder lifestyle, including family and marriage, is advocated over celibacy. The use of garlic, ginger, and onion is encouraged for its ability to build the nervous system and reduce parasites and bad bacteria in the gut. Eating the trinity roots together is a strengthening tonic that fortifies and purifies the body.

The Nervous System

According to the Teachings of Yogi Bhajan, ginger is for the nerves, onion is for the eyes and ears, and garlic is for semen and reconstructive energy. The spicy heat of these plants helps to cleanse and strengthen the immune system, clear toxins from the body at a fast rate, boost the immune system, and strengthen the nerves. Traditionally they are combined into a masala, which is then added to cooked beans to provide flavor. Adding them to the diet in creative ways is beneficial (Bhajan, 1992, June 30).

RECIPES TO SUPPORT THE NERVOUS SYSTEM

JAPA'S BASIC MASALA RECIPE

- ✓ 2 onions, chopped
- ✓ 2 fingers ginger, minced
- ✓ 2–3 garlic cloves, minced
- ✓ Ghee or olive oil
- ✓ 1 teaspoon (5 ml) cumin
- ✓ 1 teaspoon (5 ml) coriander
- ✓ 1 teaspoon (5 ml) turmeric
- ✓ 1 teaspoon (5 ml) fennel
- ✓ Salt and pepper to taste

Combine onions, ginger, and garlic cloves. Sauté with ghee or olive oil until onions are translucent. Toward the middle of cooking time, add spices and add more ghee or a little water if necessary to keep the trinity roots from sticking. Add this mixture to any prepared rice and beans dish to add flavor and healing properties.

DASHMULA

Dashmula is a famous Ayurvedic formula made of ten roots that are especially soothing for the nervous system. It is amazing for those times of overwhelm, anxiety, and fatigue from insomnia. It is known for balancing *all* body types and *tattvas* and especially supports the nervous system. Mix it in hot water for tea or if feeling adventurous, sauté it in ghee, and add it to soup stock for an interesting flavor.

(Khalsa, K. P. S., n.d.)

Exploring Physical and Subtle Human Anatomy

8.0 Sat Kriya

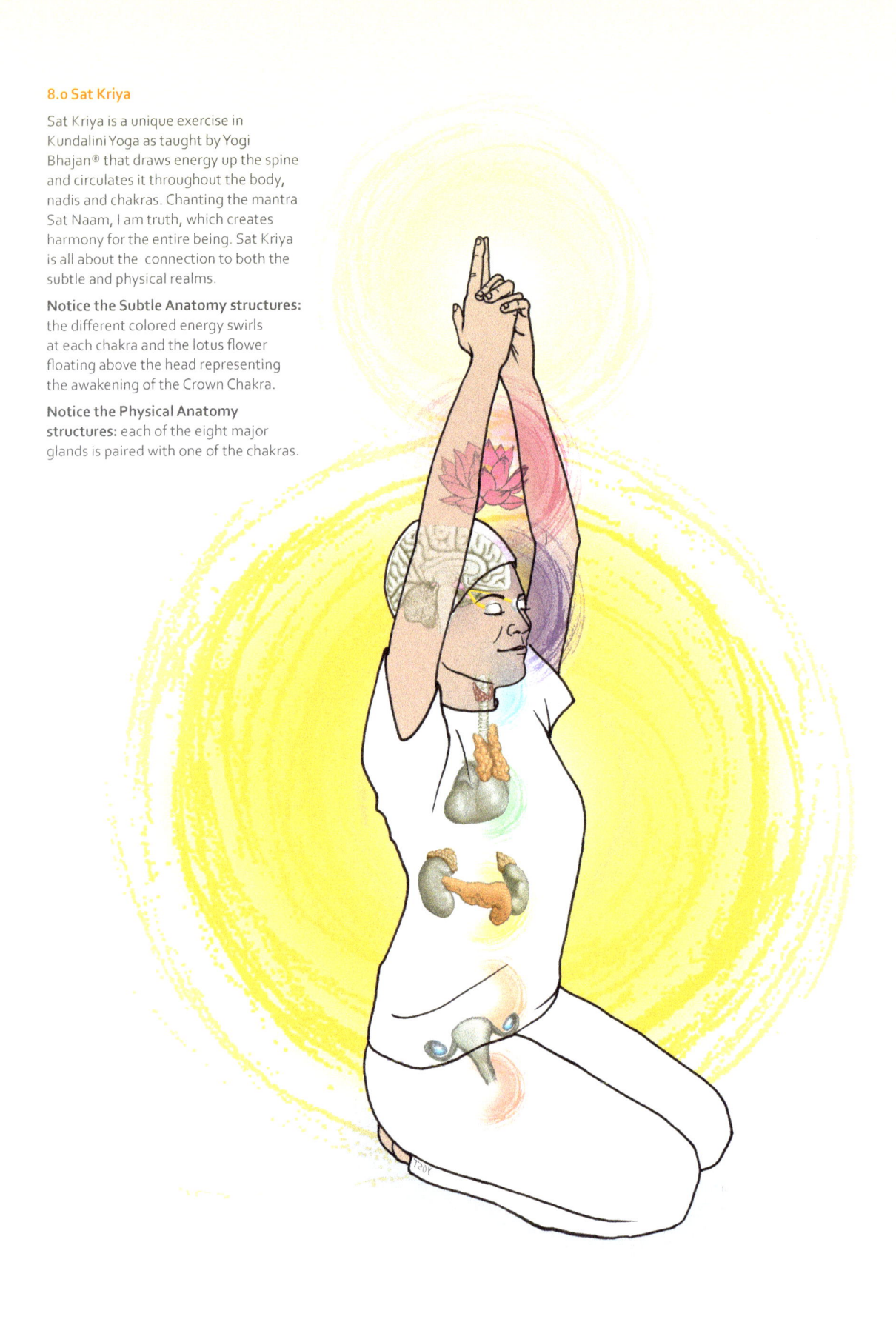

Sat Kriya is a unique exercise in Kundalini Yoga as taught by Yogi Bhajan® that draws energy up the spine and circulates it throughout the body, nadis and chakras. Chanting the mantra Sat Naam, I am truth, which creates harmony for the entire being. Sat Kriya is all about the connection to both the subtle and physical realms.

Notice the Subtle Anatomy structures: the different colored energy swirls at each chakra and the lotus flower floating above the head representing the awakening of the Crown Chakra.

Notice the Physical Anatomy structures: each of the eight major glands is paired with one of the chakras.

The Endocrine System

Group *sadhana* is a daily spiritual practice, such as yoga, meditation, or prayer, done in a community of people. This type of practice creates a subtle but powerful force in the lives of the participants. It connects them to a frequency that is greater than the sum of its parts. Similarly the endocrine system is a subtle but powerful force in the community of the body. Each of the endocrine glands can exert an incredible influence on the physical body, yet without each other they are powerless. Glands cannot work in isolation; they must exist in harmony with each other.

The endocrine glands are nurtured by the repetition of a daily practice; sadhana and its steady rhythm mirror the glands' pulsations. The glands manage the entire body's homeostasis the same way that group sadhana underlies the balance in a healthy spiritual community. Healthy discipline creates healthy communities that are connected and supportive of one another.

The endocrine (glandular) system along with the nervous system, controls almost all functions in the human body. Each endocrine gland has a discrete location without a dedicated connection system; instead the glands rely on parts of the blood, lymph, and nerve networks to communicate with each other.

> "*Our biological rhythm is the symphony of the cosmos—music embedded deep within us to which we dance, even when we can't name the tune.*"
>
> —Deepak Chopra, physician, author, alternative medicine advocate

> "*Glands are the guardians of the health.*"
>
> © The Teachings of Yogi Bhajan, Dec. 17, 1992

Lymph Glands or Nodes?

People often confuse the glandular system and the lymphatic system. While these three are closely related and work together, they are distinct systems and structures. This confusion is sometimes perpetuated by variations in language. In European schools lymph nodes are called lymph glands. Sometimes Yogi Bhajan referred to glands, meaning lymph nodes. At other times when Yogi Bhajan said "glands" he was actually referring to endocrine glands, so it is necessary to look at the larger context of a particular lecture if there is any doubt in the meaning intended.

PHYSICAL ANATOMY PERSPECTIVE

Components of the Endocrine System

- Hormones
- Glands

Benefits of a Strong Endocrine System
When the endocrine system is strong, the body is able to maintain homeostasis. A healthy endocrine system supports correct rhythms and processes in the body and impacts a person's state of well-being in a profound way. Hormones affect everything from mood to energy level to stamina.

Primary Purpose
The primary purpose of the endocrine system is to monitor the status of the body and secrete hormones to either bring the body back into homeostasis or to perpetuate the cycles and rhythms of life.

Hormones

> THE BLOODSTREAM, LIKE A TRAIN SYSTEM, PLAYS AN IMPORTANT ROLE IN THE ENDOCRINE SYSTEM TRANSPORTING HORMONES THROUGHOUT THE BODY SO THEY CAN DO THEIR JOBS.

Hormones are chemical substances that glands release into the bloodstream to have a particular effect on the body. Hormones are crucial to the communication network in the body. They play a role in regulating bodily processes including sexual arousal, hunger, and sleep cycles. There are even hormones that create the emotional state of bliss and connectivity. Hormones are triggered by all kinds of actions: changes in blood chemistry, seeing an attractive person, changes in light. The connectivity hormone (oxytocin) can even be stimulated by the subtle work of meditation. The feeling of bliss and connection to the universe that happens in deep meditation is partly a hormonal experience.

Hormones have a much more complex and delicate effect on our bodies than obvious at first glance. Because hormones circulate in the bloodstream they have the potential to affect a wide range of structures. As an example, estrogen is most commonly thought of in terms of female reproduction yet plays a major role in emotional stability, protection of the cardiovascular system and bone health.

The Endocrine System

Sex Hormones develop characteristics that differentiate females and males. In males, this means deeper voices and more muscle mass; in females, breasts, rounder hips and regulation of the menstrual cycle. They also play specific, crucial roles in sexual reproduction.

However, the sex hormones also have more subtle effects on the energies, projection, and consciousness of women and men that extend beyond our typical ideas of sex or sexual characteristics. Testosterone is a significant part of the male psyche. It allows men to penetrate and achieve in a linear way. Estrogen, which regulates the menstrual cycle, creates a certain sparkly expansiveness in the consciousness that is unique to being a woman (Duncan, 1994).

"We are not human beings having a spiritual experience; we are spiritual beings having a human experience."

—Pierre Teilhard de Chardin, *The Phenomenon of Man*

Multitasking Female Sex Hormones

While parallel in many ways, the endocrine systems of men and women do have some differences. Women have a more complex series of hormonal loops related to the menstrual cycle and pregnancy involving three different hormones: estrogen, progesterone, *and* a little testosterone. Men have one main sex hormone, testosterone, and it has a relatively straightforward function in the body.

Glands

Endocrine glands are a grouping of tissues which monitor particular activities or states of the body. They secrete a hormone to bring the body back toward balance, or facilitate a particular process when necessary.

How Glands Work

Each gland creates a specific set of hormones. The gland is then stimulated when that hormone is needed in the body. Glands can be stimulated to release their hormones in a variety of ways. A change in blood chemistry or a nervous system impulse might tell a gland that the body needs more calcium or that it is time to go to sleep. The gland then releases the hormone into the bloodstream, where it travels to the entire body. The hormone eventually finds its target tissue where it elicits a particular response, like sleepiness, hunger or activating osteoclast cells.

We are spiritual beings having a hormonal experience.

Exploring Physical and Subtle Human Anatomy

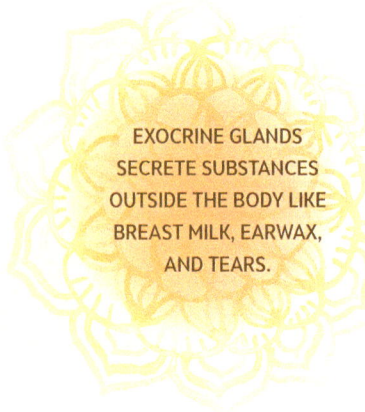

> EXOCRINE GLANDS SECRETE SUBSTANCES OUTSIDE THE BODY LIKE BREAST MILK, EARWAX, AND TEARS.

This is generally how glands monitor the states of the body and elicit responses. Let's look at a specific example in more detail. The pineal gland is responsible for regulating the sleep-wake cycle. We know that the presence of light helps our bodies to know when it is time to be awake and when it is time to sleep. But how exactly does that happen? Light hits the retina in the back of the eye, this is perceived by the brain in a nervous system signal. As the impulse passes along the optic nerve it stimulates the pineal gland. The pineal gland interprets the data about the amount of light and decides when/how much melatonin to release into the body. When the light gets lower the pineal secretes more melatonin, which makes us feel sleepy.

Hormone Pathway

Gland detects something needs to change in the body

↓

Secretes hormone

↓

Hormone travels through bloodstream

↓

Hormone reaches target tissue

↓

Change occurs

The Endocrine System

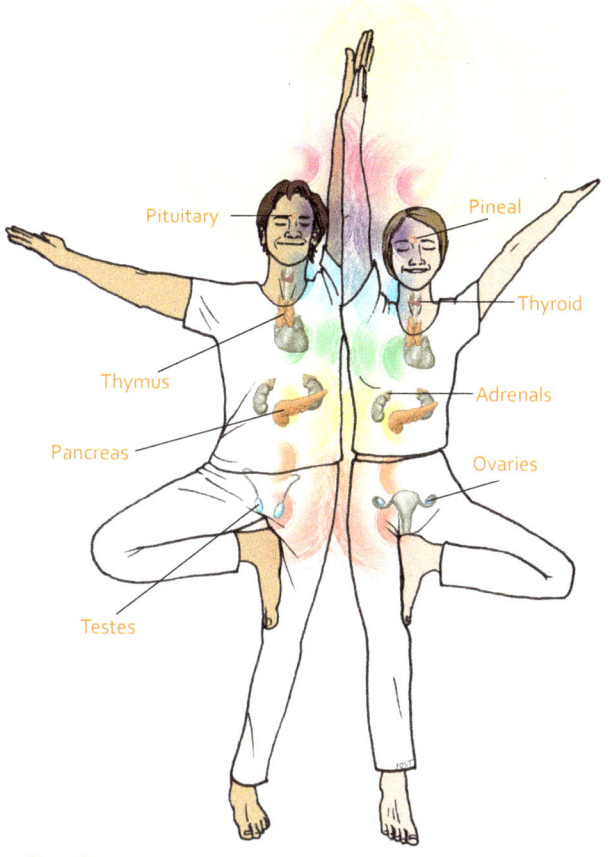

8.1 The Major Endocrine Glands

The Major Endocrine Glands

8.2 Pineal Gland

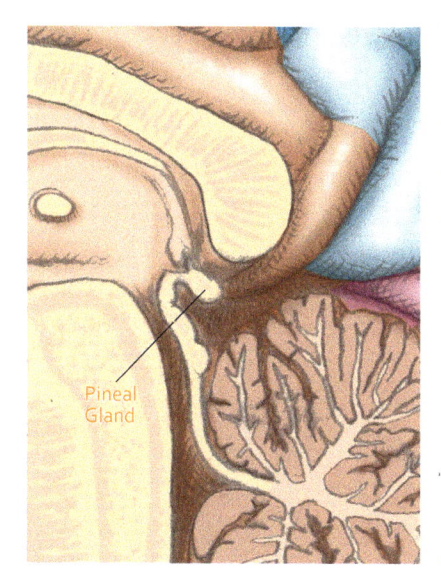

Location	Center of the head
Chakra	Crown, Seat of the Soul, Thousand-Petaled Lotus
Hormones	Melatonin
Main Action	Regulates sleeping and waking cycle
Other Fun Facts	• Scientist used to think it was a "dead" gland after a certain age.
• The pineal gland is shaped like a pinecone. There are several spiritual traditions that use pinecone imagery as a representation of spiritual enlightenment. The pineal gland is activated during spiritual experiences.
• Using a strong Neck Lock during meditation allows the pineal gland to be stimulated.

Exploring Physical and Subtle Human Anatomy

8.3 Pituitary Gland

Location	About the size of a pea (0.5 grams), protruding off the bottom of the hypothalamus at the base of the brain, consisting of three distinct lobes (Anterior, Intermediate and Posterior).
Chakra	Sixth Chakra, Ajna, Third Eye
Hormones	**Anterior Lobe:** Human Growth Hormone, Thyroid-stimulating Hormone, Adrenocoticotropic Hormone, Prolactin, Luteinizing Hormone, Follicle-stimulating Hormone **Intermediate Lobe:** Melanocyte-stimulating Hormone **Posterior Lobe**: Antidiuretic Hormone, Oxytocin
Main Action	• Growth • Blood pressure • Pregnancy and childbirth • Breast milk production • Sex organ functions in both males and females • Thyroid gland function • Metabolism • Water balance • Temperature regulation • Pain relief
Other Fun Facts	• Often referred to as the Master Gland because it directs the activity of so many other glands. • Rolling the eyes to the Third Eye Point during yoga and meditation stimulates the pituitary gland via the optic nerve. • The pituitary gland arises from two different embryonic tissues. In the budding fetus precursor tissues of the upper palate and the nervous system develop into the pituitary gland (Moore, 2013). So when we chant and strike the tongue against the roof of the mouth, we are influencing the pituitary gland at its birthplace. (Gresham, L.S.K., 2015)

8.4 Hypothalamus

Location	Center of the brain
Chakra	Third Eye
Hormones	Produces hormones responsible for homeostasis and manages the release of hormones by the pituitary
Main Action	• Stimulates or inhibits pituitary gland • Maintain homeostasis • Metabolism • Body temperature • Hunger/thirst • Circadian cycles (the rhythms of our days, eating, sleeping, etc.) • Attachment behaviors (See page 163)
Other Fun Facts	• Acts as the main connecting point between the nervous and endocrine systems • The optic nerve crosses the space between the pituitary and hypothalamus. This is why eye focuses have such a powerful effect on these glands.

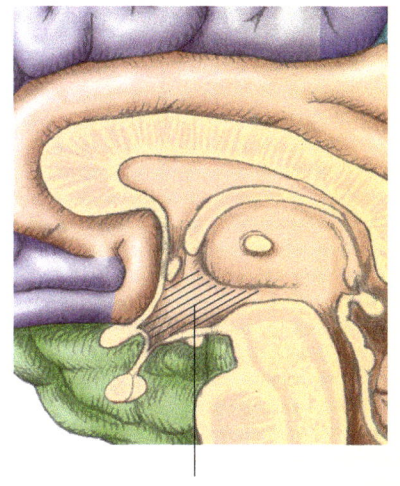

Hypothalamus

Hypothalamus and Pituitary Relationship

The pituitary gland is referred to as the master gland, and it is heavily influenced by the hypothalamus. The two together are the link between the nervous and endocrine systems. The hypothalamus is hard wired into the nervous system and then translates the nerve impulses to the pituitary, which regulates the hormonal processes for all the other glands. Think of the pituitary as the CEO—the one that gets all the glory. The hypothalamus is the secretary—the one behind the scenes, who is tending to all of the details and filtering information to the CEO.

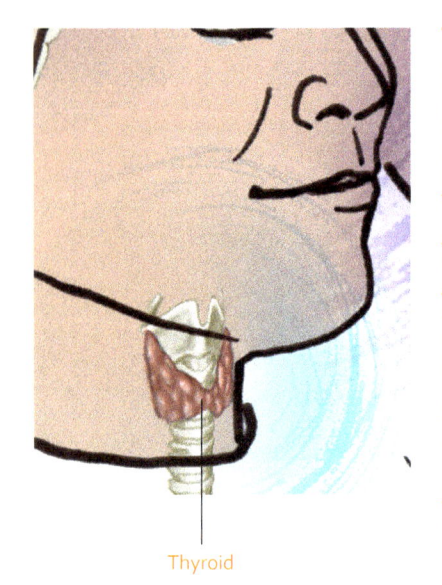

8.5 Thyroid

Location	Consists of two lobes on either side of the windpipe (trachea)
	Just behind the thyroid are the parathyroid glands. Anything that affects one will also affect the other.
Chakra	Throat
Hormones	Thyroxine and triiodothyronine
Main Action	• Regulates weight (metabolism*)
	• Iodine uptake
	• Calcium balance
	• Maintains youth*
	• Stability*
Other Fun Facts	• This area can often hold psychological fears. It is one of the reasons the throat constricts when we're scared.
	• With its location on the front on the throat, the thyroid gland often gets compressed with a standard self-protective fear response posture (dropping the head, rounding shoulders forward)
	• Goiters, a pathological enlargement of the thyroid gland, in holistic medicine are sometimes linked to a fear of the future and the unknown.
	• Working on the thyroid gland helps balance the energy of the Heart Chakra and Navel Point.

* Bhajan, 1992

Thyroid

The Endocrine System

8.6 Adrenals

Location	Above the kidneys
Chakra	**Navel:** The adrenal glands are located in the physical area of the Navel Chakra. They also have a function in regulating your stress response. For this reason they are often associated with the fire energy of the Navel Point. **Root:** The adrenals also play a huge role in the fight-or-flight response, which is one of our most basic, fundamental survival mechanisms. For this reason they can also be associated with the Root Chakra.
Hormones	Adrenaline, cortisol
Main Action	Fight or flight response, muscle growth, stress response
Other Fun Facts	• The body responds in the same way to actual danger as to perceived danger and the same to actual emergencies as to imagined emergencies. This is why the heart races when watching a scary movie. In modern society there are lots of things that the body reacts to as if it were a life-or-death situation, even something as banal as a never-ending stream of emails. The problem here is that the adrenals are being called on constantly to perform a task they are meant to perform occasionally or rarely. This can lead to adrenal fatigue. When the adrenals become less and less able to respond to the actual stresses in life, it can lead to feelings of exhaustion, numbness and apathy. • Adrenal fatigue often goes hand in hand with cold depression (see the Nervous System chapter for more information about cold depression).

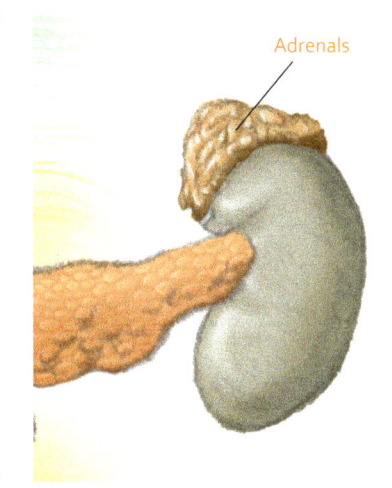

Exploring Physical and Subtle Human Anatomy

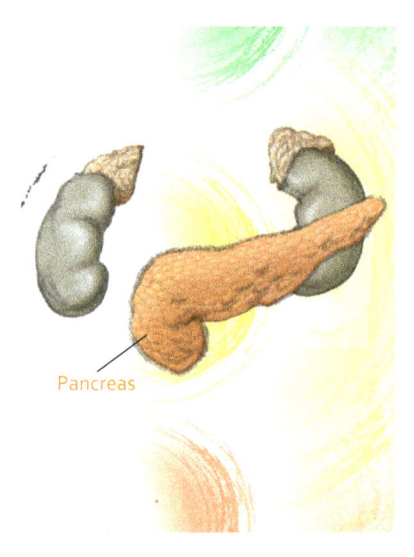

8.7 Pancreas

Location	Behind the stomach
Chakra	Navel
Hormones	Insulin and glucagon
Main Action	Regulate blood glucose levels The pancreas regulates blood glucose levels by stimulating the muscles to absorb glucose.
Other Fun Facts	• If the pancreas isn't working properly blood glucose levels will be unstable which leads to feelings of anger, frustration, short temper and lethargy. It creates an unstable environment, which is challenging for the other glands and internal organs. • Diet and exercise are the best ways to affect the health of the pancreas. While it is particular to each individual, generally the pancreas performs best with a low sugar diet and regular exercise.

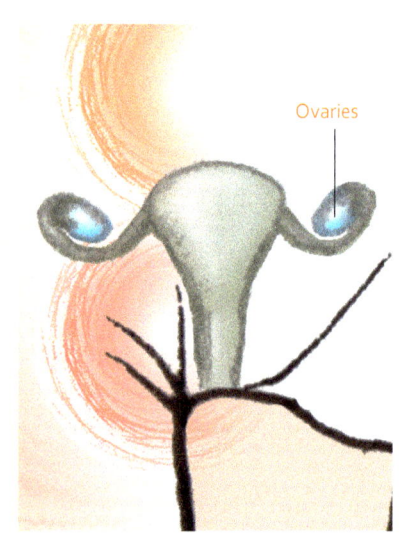

8.8 Ovaries

Location	In the pelvic cavity
Chakra	Second
Hormones	Estrogen, progesterone, and some testosterone
Main Action	• Reproduction • Secondary female sex characteristics
Other Fun Facts	• At birth each ovary already contains all of the egg cells it ever will.

8.9 Testes

Location	Testicles
Chakra	Second
Hormones	Testosterone
Main Action	• Reproduction • Secondary male sex characteristics
Other Fun Facts	• The testes are the only glands that only secrete one hormone.

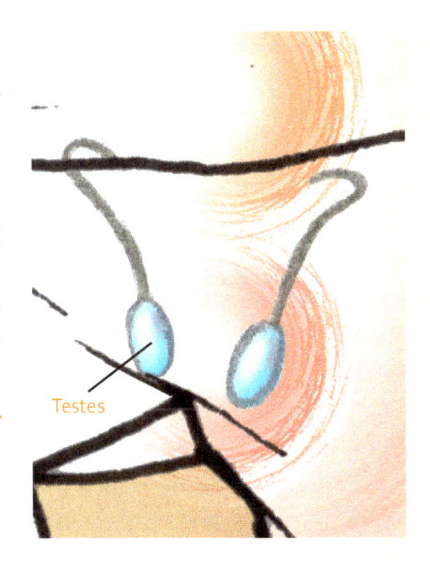

Relationship of Endocrine and Other Systems

It is important to remember that when a gland secretes a hormone it travels through the bloodstream to the *whole body*. Its most obvious effect will be on its target tissue, where it elicits the response we most commonly associate with that hormone. The glands, however, are able to exert a subtle effect on all parts of the body. The hormones profoundly impact every organ and body system regardless of its primary function.

Liver

Sometimes there are excess levels of hormone in the bloodstream: residual hormones in the system once they have completed their function or too many hormones are secreted from a gland in the first place. The liver metabolizes these excess hormones, during sleep, by breaking them down and either directing the elements to be recycled or excreted. If the liver is overloaded with toxins or hormones, the excess will continue to circulate in the blood stream until the liver has the capacity to clean them all up. Often "hormonal feelings" are a result of an overloaded liver that is unable to remove the excess hormone from the bloodstream.

Yoga can help with the removal of excess hormones from the bloodstream by supporting the health of the liver. Every posture that massages or compresses the liver moves blood through the organ. It then fills with fresh blood as the posture is released like a sponge that is squeezed, releases fluid, and then refills with fresh fluid. All yoga, but specifically any pose that compresses the right side of the body, has a cleansing effect on the liver, which leads to healthier blood and more optimally functioning glands.

The liver also plays a role in our response to stress. During stress the liver keeps the level of blood glucose high by regulating the hormone levels and interacting with the pancreas and adrenal glands. This helps the body to have the energy to respond to the stressful situation and is an example of dynamic interplay of the body with the glands. After the stress has passed the liver allows for the reabsorption of glucose from the bloodstream.

Endocrine System and Nervous System

Strengthening the nervous system supports the health of the endocrine system. The nervous system connects directly to the glandular system and often starts the chain of events that lead to the release of hormones, the interlock of target cells, and the resultant shifts in the body. This connection happens at the hypothalamus. With a consistent practice of Kundalini Yoga and Meditation the communication lines between the nervous system, hypothalamus, and endocrine system are streamlined and improved.

Yogis and Glands

The yogi taps the thymus gland in the shower and activates it. During meditation, the yogi engages neck lock, which stretches the vagus nerve and activates each chakra and gland. It is the interplay of these two systems through daily practice that results in the calm, peaceful steadiness of the yogi. The cross communication between nervous and endocrine allows for the development of new neural pathways and the gradual strengthening of glands through a consistent practice. Over time there is a deeper experience of personal balance and steadiness of mind.

SUBTLE ANATOMY PERSPECTIVE

Challenges to the Endocrine System

Permanent Habits Attachment behaviors fall into the category of what Yogi Bhajan called "permanent habits," which create the foundation of your potential. First you create your habits, often laid down early in life, and then the habits create you. A wide range of behaviors and patterns from favorite foods, to addiction to alcohol or sugar, to how introverted or extroverted you are around strangers can all be traced to the habits laid down early in life (Bhajan, 1993c).

Habits often get created to serve a particular function when we're children but are no longer helpful as adults. Because habits are regulated through the endocrine system, they can be affected by eye focus, chanting, and breathwork. When we are ready for a new way of being, we must first shift the unhelpful permanent habits from our childhood. That shift must begin with an adjustment of the hypothalamus, which in turn can shift deep, hard-wired patterns in both the nervous and glandular systems.

One example of a permanent habit is weight. Losing weight is hard to do unless a permanent change is made in lifestyle around food and exercise. It is one thing to change habits for six months, but to keep weight off, the change has to be permanent. This type of permanent change requires a complete adjustment of the consciousness and projection. Those looking to maintain weight loss would be well served to add a supportive practice for the endocrine system to their diet and exercise routines, such as chanting, long deep breathing or a meditation with drishti (eye focus).

Trauma and Hormones Certain traumatic life events cause significant shifts in hormonal patterns. Some examples would be a car accident, loss of a loved one, and even the normal stresses of adolescence or pregnancy. Trauma disrupts the firing process of the brain and glands by sending the body into either a shutdown or hyper-aroused mode as a means of self-protection.

Once the rhythm of the glandular system is changed, new and unexpected metabolic processes, such as weight gain or heart palpitations, can lock into the body under the new, survival-based glandular rhythm. In order to unravel the trauma-induced pattern, an integrative approach is often successful. Working with a primary care doctor or specialist for diagnosis, modifying behavior, practicing yoga and meditation, and getting massage and bodywork are all part of supporting the renewal of the endocrine system.

Meditation works in a way that allows the brain and glands to relax and recharge. Repetition and rhythm are the soothing balms that repair the glands, which allow for a core-level shift in the body and consciousness. Over time, the applied discipline of meditation can unweave the traumas embedded in the physical and subtle anatomy to allow for a renewed sense of health, radiance, and balance.

Chinese Medicine and the Glandular System

Chinese medicine doesn't directly reference the glandular system; the connection instead is to the concept of moisture and longevity. As we get older the moisture and fluids in the body (*Kidney Yin, ojas*, sperm, menstruation) begin to dry up as the glands secrete less hormones. This shows up in the body's decrease in sexual function, lack of menstruation, grey hair, and a general drying up of essential bodily fluids. A tangible example of this would be the hot flashes of menopause. In a hot flash the body's *Yin* is stressed from aging, which causes it to overheat and dry the body even more.

To maintain optimal functioning and youthfulness we want to keep the glands secreting properly. To keep the glands secreting properly we must maintain the moisture and fluids of the body. Techniques like Tai Qi, yoga, and herbal remedies can strengthen the glands, which create a better quality of life through a gradual slowing of the aging process.

Third Eye and Crown Chakra The Third Eye is located between and just above the eyebrows. It contains the capacity for intuition and insight. When the Third Eye opens, the unseen becomes seen and a greater mental capacity is revealed. The Crown Chakra is located at the very top of the head. It is the Seat of the Soul and embodies the capacity to be authentic, blissful and to live with raised consciousness. It is the sweet spot that is activated as the Kundalini energy rises.

Both of these energy centers are intricately linked in with the glands, especially the glands deep in the brain. Often in meditation, the eyes are focused at the Third Eye or the crown of the head, which energetically charges up these centers. It also creates a pressure, via the optic nerve, which stimulates the pituitary, pineal, and hypothalamus glands. The interplay of the pituitary, hypothalamus, pineal, and the ventricles of the brain contribute to the sense of deepening intuition that comes with a regular spiritual practice and the opening of the Third Eye. The expanded functioning of these glands also contributes to the regal acceptance of self and natural state of bliss that comes into play with a balanced Crown Chakra.

Yogi Bhajan taught that the glands operate in a rhythmic energetic frequency (Bhajan, 1993e). The vibration (through the upper palate) of chanting and the pressure from the eye focus in meditation influence the glands to change, heal, and expand. These experiences can lead to a new level of sensitivity to environments, energies, and personalities.

Head Coverings

Kundalini Yogis suggest covering the head during meditation. This helps to protect individuals experiencing increased sensitivity and keep the energy contained within the body. When the Kundalini energy rises to the Crown Chakra it can be contained and recirculated within the body.

The Endocrine System and the Aura Talking about the Aura can get a bit tricky because the Aura is a part of both the chakra and the Ten Light Bodies systems. And even within the Ten Bodies system, the Aura encompasses the energetic realms that exist outside of the physical boundaries of the body. The Aura is simultaneously its own palpable entity and the unique combination of these other subtle anatomical structures.

The Aura is like a lucky charm, drawing in what is needed in the moment and repelling things that aren't in your best interest. When it is strong it can extend out nine feet (three meters) in every direction. When the Aura is weak, it's as if a layer of protection is stripped from the body. You might put yourself into compromised situations or give in to peer pressure, or be attracted to addictive behaviors as a way to feel expanded or uplifted. Unsheltered by the safe cocoon of your own electromagnetic field, you may seek the sensation of expansion in false circumstances.

The proper functioning of the endocrine glands allows for a strong Aura. This leads to a radiant glow, both physically and subtly. When the glands are at peak function, and the Aura is radiantly strong, others start to notice and respond.

> *"There is an electromagnetic energy field that surrounds the body which includes the Arc Line the Radiant Body and the Subtle Body. When people talk about Aura they're talking about this energy field."*
>
> —Nirvair Singh Khalsa, *The Ten Light Bodies of Consciousness*

Japa's Aura Story

My son is adopted. He has brown skin, eyes, and hair. My husband and I are both fair skinned with blue eyes. People often comment that we look alike even though we don't share a genetic connection. I believe that people see something in the subtle anatomy in those moments. They are seeing a shared destiny, a common Aura, and a family connection that is beyond physical. My child, his smile, and his spirit are deeply connected to us and it shows in his Aura.

THE AURA IS ALSO REFERRED TO AS THE *DIVINE SHIELD* OR THE *ELECTROMAGNETIC FIELD*.

The Endocrine System

TIPS AND TECHNIQUES FOR A STRONG ENDOCRINE SYSTEM

The endocrine system is healthy when the hormone levels in the body are balanced. We can support the glands in secreting the *just-right* level of hormones through physical pressure or movements that energize the glands. Certain kriyas compress a part of the body that contains a specific gland and then continues in a synchronized order, giving each gland a chance to be massaged by the angles of the postures. Certain postures will press a nerve directly on a gland. This pressure acts as a way for the nerve to provoke the best performance out of the glandular tissue.

Aasanas and Exercises

Any posture or movement that stimulates the location of a gland can be healing for that gland. Movements may compress a gland, vibrate it, or even stretch it. Almost every yoga aasana affects at least one gland.

- Bowing — Brain Glands (Pituitary, Hypothalamus, etc.)
- Bow Pose — Pancreas
- Camel — Thyroid
- Cat-Cow — Adrenals
- Frogs — Ovaries/Testes
- Shoulder Shrugs — Thymus and Thyroid

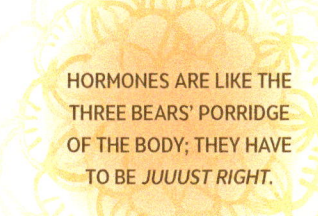

HORMONES ARE LIKE THE THREE BEARS' PORRIDGE OF THE BODY; THEY HAVE TO BE *JUUUST RIGHT*.

Transformational Energy Points

Governing Vessel Meridian: Hall of Impression

Location: At the forehead, in the gap between the eyebrows

Effects: Soothes the mind-spirit connection

Yoga for this Point: *Drishti* (eye focus)

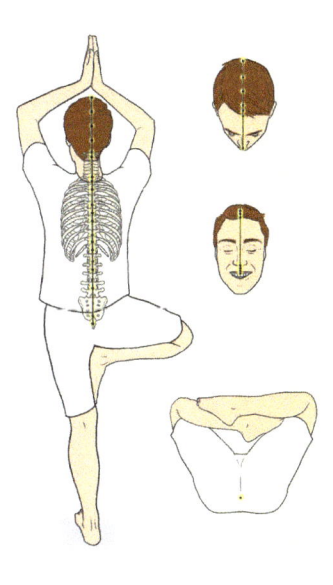

Exploring Physical and Subtle Human Anatomy

Eye Focus (Drishti)

Drishti is the practice of putting the eyes in a particular focus while holding a posture or meditation. This practice impacts the glands deep in the brain because of the physical closeness of the optical nerve to the pineal, pituitary, and hypothalamus glands.

Gazing at the tip or the root of the nose are the most common eye focuses in Kundalini Yoga, and they are both means of activating the "blue pearl gateway," stimulating the pituitary and pineal glands and creating a general ease in the mind. The blue pearl is a specific place in meditation that is simultaneously created and seen when you are in deep meditation. The pressure you feel in holding these eye postures are from the optic nerve, which applies pressure to the pituitary gland and hypothalamus. (Bhajan, 1992c).

> "*That God in you is the power in you. And when you balance that power you are God... Balance yourself and see what happens, just watch it.*"
> © The Teachings of Yogi Bhajan, April 18, 2001

EYE FOCUS ON THE THIRD EYE POINT AFFECTS THE PITUITARY GLAND AND EYE FOCUS ON THE TIP OF THE NOSE OR THE CROWN CHAKRA AFFECTS THE PINEAL GLAND.

8.9 Kirtan Kriya L-Shape

Eye focus (*drishti*) is practiced in Kundalini Yoga as taught by Yogi Bhajan® and is a way to benefit the glandular system. Some common eye focuses are the tip of the nose, the Third Eye point, the chin. These may be practiced with eyes closed, 9/10ths closed, or open depending on the specific desired effect.

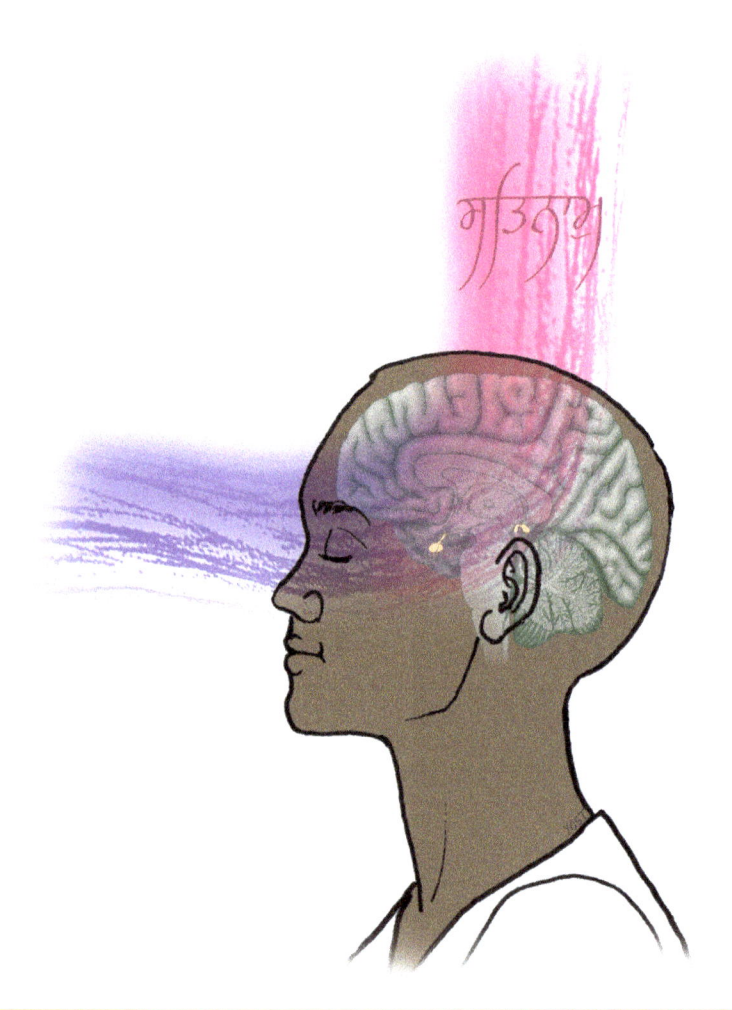

The Endocrine System

The practice of using a *drishti* during meditation is believed to loan a person control over his or her entire glandular system. It is important to recognize that it is just a loan, because day-to-day life can easily turn control of the nervous and glandular system control back over to stress. A regular practice of staring at the tip of the nose for even just 11 minutes can give 24 hours of stability and stress relief to the endocrine system. This specific eye focus is a key part of many Kundalini Yoga meditations for elevating consciousness and bringing prosperity (Bhajan, 1993a, 1991a).

Mantra

Chanting creates an elevation of consciousness through its impact on the glands. There are 84 meridian points inside the mouth that are activated as the tongue strikes them with the sounds of sacred music. The impact of chanting in a rhythmic way also indirectly stimulates the glands in the brain via the vibrations of the skull bones. Yogi Bhajan called this stimulation an "actionary revolution," where the brain stem, nervous system, and body can change the consciousness and become more connected to infinity in thought, word and deed. Chanting generates *tapas* on a subtle level which purifies and protects the Physical Body as it changes the frequencies of the *tattvas* and produces greater health (Bhajan, 1993a).

Har Haray Haree Wahe Guru

Translation: Bliss is experienced through all aspects of Creation
More Information: This mantra reveals the three qualities of the word Har: seed, flow and completion. It is a Shakti/Bhakti mantra that uses the primal force of creativity to rid one of obnoxious situations in life and can bring you through any block and opens up your creative energy.

Yogic Lifestyle

Sleep In our electronic world, there are so many items that create light in our bedrooms while we sleep. The small light from the clock radio, the bright outdoor lights shining in through the windows, and the tiny light from the fire alarm that stays on constantly. All of these sources of illumination result in a chaotic impact on the endocrine system. Eliminate sources of artificial

> *"The science of chanting is, there are two things in your life you have to control: one is your hypothalamus and second is your frontal lobe of the brain. Frontal lobe of the brain is controlled by meditation. And hypothalamus is controlled by chanting. Is that clear? Now you can chant or not, it is up to you."*
>
> © Teachings of Yogi Bhajan, December 28, 1993

Yogic Tips for the Best Night of Sleep

- Wash your feet in cold water; this helps to break energetic connections to the day and brings the blood down to the feet and out of the head
- Avoid eating a big meal 2–3 hours before bed
- Turn off all electronic screens at least 1 hour before bed
- Set a schedule. Go to bed and wake up at the same time each day
- Massage the feet with lavender scented oil
- Brush hair with a wooden comb or brush

(Khalsa, 2010)

light while sleeping in order to support the proper secretion of melatonin. The body's sleep and wake cycles are best protected by a dark bedroom during sleep (Ratzburg, n.d.).

The entire glandular system benefits from a healthy sleep routine. Yogis developed a few tips for getting a good night's sleep. The hour before you actually close your eyes sets the stage for the length, depth, and quality of your rest.

Deep Relaxation At the end of every yoga practice, there is a period of deep relaxation. This time of stillness allows you to integrate the effort and the effects of the yoga (Bhajan, 2010). The body can adjust and create a new homeostasis. The energizing or healing impact of the kriya can be fully integrated as the nervous system goes into parasympathetic mode, and the endocrine system responds to the pressures of the poses with renewed hormonal balance. As the muscles relax and soften, they absorb the changes on a cellular level. The entire experience quietly builds a better functioning body.

The Deep Relaxation Difference

Practice a kriya and take a nice long relaxation at the end. Notice how you feel at that moment *and* for the rest of the day. The next day, practice the same kriya without relaxation. Notice how you feel, how the rest of your day goes, and your thoughts. Don't just *believe* the difference deep relaxation makes—*experience* it!

Plants, Herbs, and Food

Adaptogenic herbs are a particular type of herb that supports the body in maintaining or regaining homeostasis. They are especially helpful to tone and improve the function of the endocrine system. Adaptogens like ginseng or licorice are known for their ability to improve the function of a particular gland, regardless of whether the gland is over- or under-performing.

Licorice is an herb that specifically helps the adrenals by giving them a break from producing too much cortisol. It is known in herbal realms as a harmonizing agent in that it generally supports and helps any other herbs taken with it because of its action on the adrenal glands. Without sacrificing effectiveness, its chemical components break down and help extend the half-life of cortisol so that the adrenals do not have to produce as much cortisol. As an interesting side note, it seems that licorice supplementation is best in liquid or chewable form; there is actually something about the body tasting the licorice that begins this harmonizing action.

Cruciferous Vegetables On a chemical level, specific vegetables, like broccoli and cabbage, have elements that are able to link up with excess hormones in the body. They create a compound that can exit the body more easily. When the bloodstream is cleared of these excess hormones, people automatically get that healthy glow and feel more balanced.

Balance the Third Eye Chakra

Your Third Eye may be out of balance if you feel confusion, indecisiveness, foggy thoughts, or experience headaches.

To Balance the Third Eye Chakra
- Practice using intuition on small decisions.
- Wear indigo.
- Wear or meditate with a sapphire or azurite.
- Meditate in silence.
- Chant.
- Roll the closed eyes up as if looking out through the Third Eye point.
- Gently tap the Third Eye point.

Affirmations for the Third Eye

I trust that the unknown is known to me. I am awake in my spirit and my sight, I am fully connected.

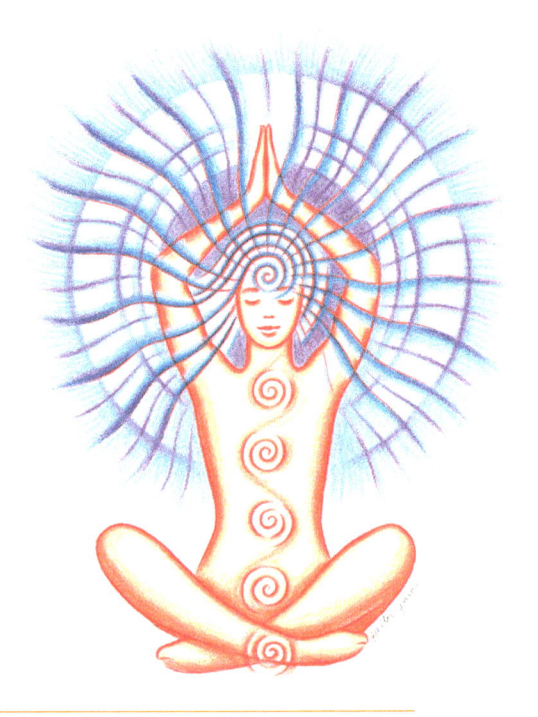

Balance the Crown Chakra

If the Crown Chakra is out of balance you feel disconnected from soul or the divine, and generally feel uninspired about life. This imbalance may manifest as headaches, restlessness or trouble sleeping.

To Balance the Crown Chakra
- Wear light purple or violet.
- Wear or meditate with a diamond or cubic zirconia.
- Roll the eyes up, as if looking out through the top of the head.
- Chant.
- Deeply listen and reflect on spiritual writings.
- Tap or massage the top of the head.

Affirmations for the Third Eye

I am part of all that is. My divinity and grace flow through me and surround me, uplifting all that I am and all that I will be.

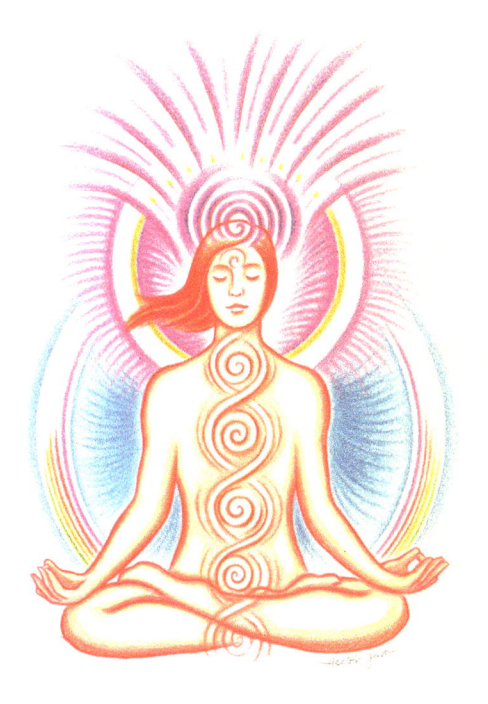

9.0 Crow Pose

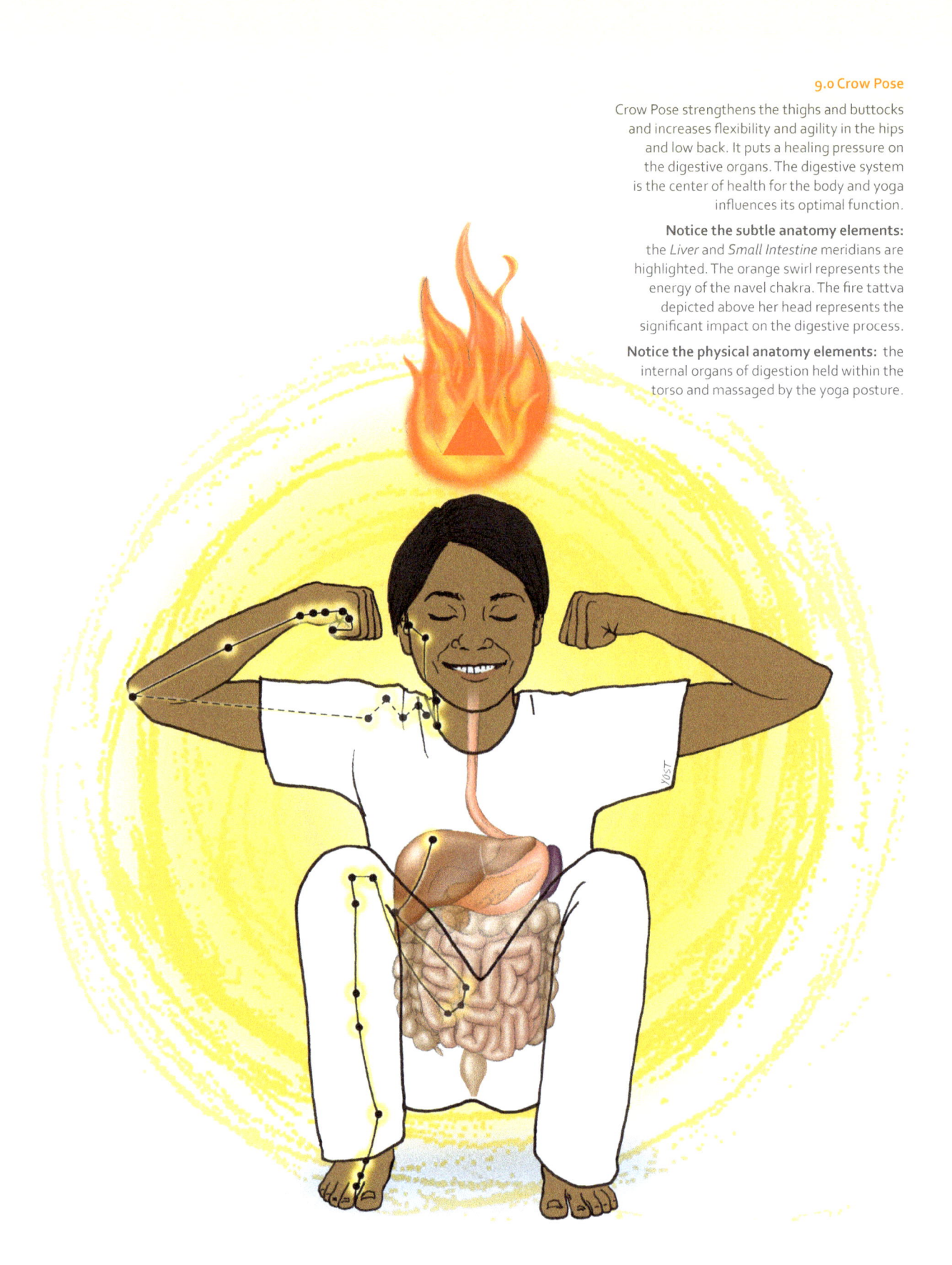

Crow Pose strengthens the thighs and buttocks and increases flexibility and agility in the hips and low back. It puts a healing pressure on the digestive organs. The digestive system is the center of health for the body and yoga influences its optimal function.

Notice the subtle anatomy elements: the *Liver* and *Small Intestine* meridians are highlighted. The orange swirl represents the energy of the navel chakra. The fire tattva depicted above her head represents the significant impact on the digestive process.

Notice the physical anatomy elements: the internal organs of digestion held within the torso and massaged by the yoga posture.

The Digestive System

The digestive system is the churning, metabolic factory that transforms food into energy. It is at the core of the human being, both literally and figuratively. The process begins at the mouth and continues through the length of the torso, passing by and interacting with a vast array of other systems, organs, and structures as it moves to the organs of elimination and rectum. Digestion is an all-consuming process that absorbs the body in virtually every moment. The health and vitality of both the physical and subtle anatomy hinge on the quality of our digestion.

The impact created by the digestive process affects a wide range of bodily functions: from moods, feelings, and sensations to complete systems. Healthy digestion reduces inflammation and stress on the body, which frees up resources and energy for all systems to function at their peak.

A healthy digestive process models a balanced relationship with the surrounding world; taking in exactly what is needed, without over consuming, and easily letting go of what is not needed. Embodying this quality contributes to the community of life. It's like uncluttering a home. By letting go of the sweater that is two sizes too big, giving away that unread book, and dropping the attachment to *stuff*, the person who receives these things will be kept warm or entertained by them, and you will feel lighter and more energized. Letting go of stuff and digesting food establishes you and your role in the community of humanity.

"It is not what you eat and how much you eat, it is how much you digest and how much your body accepts out of it...and how much it distributes to yourself."
© The Teachings of Yogi Bhajan, August 27, 1994

One man's trash is another man's treasure.
—Proverb

Chapter 9

PHYSICAL ANATOMY PERSPECTIVE

Components of the Digestive System

- Mouth
- Esophagus
- Stomach
- Small Intestine
- Large Intestine (Colon)
- Rectum

Accessory Structures

- Liver
- Gallbladder
- Pancreas
- Mucus

Benefits of a Strong Digestive System

A strong digestive system is the foundation for a healthy organism. Easily absorbing nutrients and energy from food is like putting high-quality gas in the car: everything just runs better. And just as important as absorbing energy from the food is allowing what is not absorbed to efficiently pass through the system.

Primary Purpose

The primary purpose of the digestive system is to turn food into *you*.

Strong digestion
⋮
Healthy Body
⋮
Capacity for Elevated Consciousness

The digestive process is a series of mechanical and chemical steps to break food down into its component parts, followed by the absorption of nutrients and the elimination of food components the body does not want or cannot use. The digestive tract is a tube—open on both ends—anything within it is actually considered *outside* the body. This understanding shifts our relationship with food. Food is still *outside* as it passes through and is broken down by the body. The elements that make up food must gain entry through the walls of the digestive tract. Once they have crossed that barrier they cease to be food and become a part of the body.

ENLIGHTENED BODIES

The Digestive System

Another important role of the digestive system is to protect the body from the outside world. The digestive tract plays an important role in the immune response by breaking down and kicking out foreign invaders.

Mouth

Mechanical and chemical breakdown begins in the mouth. Chewing food breaks it up into smaller physical parts, and the saliva begins to chemically break down the food.

Esophagus and Stomach

Food and saliva travel down the muscular tube of the esophagus to the stomach. The powerful stomach acid continues the chemical breakdown of food into its nutrient parts and begins dividing out the proteins, fats, and fiber.

Small Intestine

While food passes through the small intestine, the process shifts from breaking down the structure of food to absorbing nutrients. The walls of the small intestines allow proteins, vitamins and other nutrients to cross from the digestive tract and into the bloodstream. Those nutrients are now a part of the body's energy and metabolism.

The walls of the intestines are delicate. They are covered in hair-like projections (called villi), which increase surface area to allow for more absorption of nutrients. Certain chemicals, often found in processed foods, in excess amounts can damage the intestinal villi, which makes it harder to absorb nutrients and can lead to the modern-day phenomenon of being over-fed but under-nourished.

Large Intestine (Colon)

Once the food moves into the large intestines, also called the colon, most of the nutrients that *can* be absorbed *have* been. In the colon water is removed from the waste product and reabsorbed into the body. The colon relies on a proper balance of bacteria to complete the digestion and to efficiently process waste for elimination.

> THE PURPOSE OF THE DIGESTIVE SYSTEM IS TO BREAK DOWN THE FOOD THAT PASSES THROUGH THE BODY AND TO EXTRACT FROM IT THE THINGS THAT CREATE THE BODY CELLS, TISSUES AND ORGANS. YOU LITERALLY ARE WHAT YOU EAT.

> *"That's why the Yogic way is to sit down, do the prayer, calm down… and thank God for the food and food as a gift, as a nurturing and nursing. It's a total science of self-healing. How you do it? . . . How can you heal yourself? You can't. You can heal through the nourishment, you have to concentrate on it, you can put your praana into your nourishment, to get it in."*
>
> © The Teachings of Yogi Bhajan, Feb. 26, 1991

Exploring Physical and Subtle Human Anatomy

Rectum

After the digestive process is completed, the remaining substance (not really food anymore) moves to the rectum. The final step is to eliminate the things that are not needed. The rectum compacts and prepares the waste for excretion.

Accessory Structures

There are many other organs that contribute to the process of digestion without being part of the tube that food actually passes through.

The Liver plays roles in many different bodily systems. In digestion the liver is responsible for secreting bile, which helps break down fats.

The Gallbladder plays a supporting role in storing bile.

The Pancreas is both an endocrine gland and an exocrine gland. As an endocrine gland it produces and delivers insulin to the bloodstream to regulate blood sugar. As an exocrine gland, it secretes enzymes which support the digestive process.

Mucus While not an organ, mucus is considered an accessory structure in digestion. It is a crucial element to the entire process. Mucus lines the digestive tract from the mouth all the way to the rectum. Mucus moistens the entire tract and allows food to move through the digestive process smoothly, like the coating of the throat that lets food slide down. Mucus is also a chemical barrier, like in the stomach, protecting the delicate lining of the organ from harsh stomach acid.

"You have to chew your food. You need twenty-five percent saliva per bite of food."

© The Teachings of Yogi Bhajan, June 22, 1992

The Digestive System

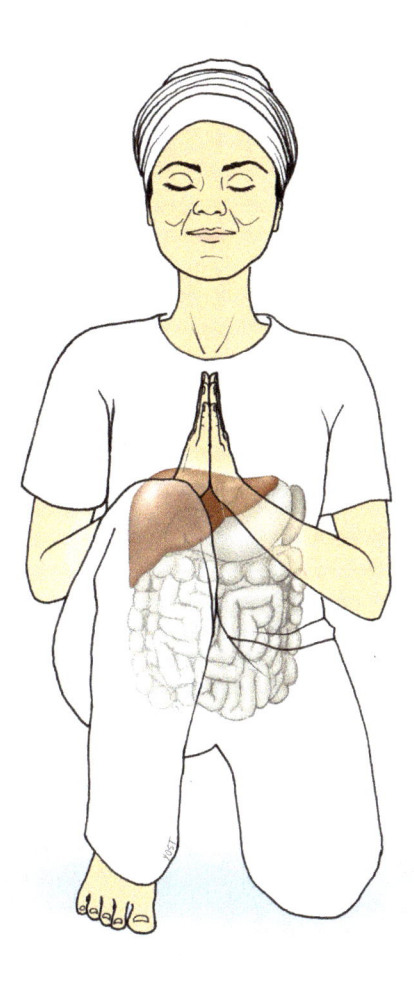

9.1 Asymmetrical Postures

Hero or Warrior Pose (Viraasan) is an example of a posture that takes advantage of the asymmetrical design of the body. It puts pressure on the liver, to release fear and build courage. It is a posture of the spiritual warrior, ready to defend the innocent and defenseless, but also surrendered in the peaceful mudra of Prayer Pose.

The Asymmetrical Body

These organs are an example of a general observation about the structure of the body. Our bodies are *not* symmetrical. The liver is on the right side, the spleen is toward the left, and the large intestine has a completely different flow on the left and the right side of the body. Sometimes we do things asymmetrically in the practice of Kundalini Yoga to create a particular effect within our asymmetrical design.

For example, in the Aquarian *sadhana* practice, we sit in *Viraasana* for 22 minutes. This posture is always done sitting on the left heel with the right knee up toward the chest. Sometimes people ask, "If we're doing it for 22 minutes *every* day, wouldn't you want to do it on the other side sometimes?" The answer to that question is "no" because of the asymmetrical design of our bodies. Having the right knee up creates pressure on the liver and *Liver* meridian. The *Liver* plays a huge role in the digestive process, keeping the blood clean and the hormones balanced. The *Liver* also energetically stores anger. Always doing this posture with the right knee raised compresses this vital organ and creates a gentle and healthy way for people to clear out their anger.

Relationship to Other Systems

Digestive System and Nervous System There is a large amount of nervous tissue within the lining of the digestive tract that acts as brain-like cells in the gut. This explains expressions like, "trust your gut" or the feeling of butterflies when nervous. There is cognitive function in the belly.

The process of digesting food is regulated by the parasympathetic nervous system, which puts the body into a relaxed state. Therefore, digestion works best when relaxed. This explains the tradition of blessing food: taking a few moments before eating to slow the mind and body primes the nervous and digestive system to prepare for the incoming meal. In fact, the very sight and smell of food begins the process of digestion.

Digestion and Joint Health Joint pain can point to a larger issue in the core of the body or digestive system. As food is absorbed, the digestive tract constantly discerns which substances to keep and which ones to throw away. If the digestive lining is irritated or unhealthy, it is harder for the digestive process to prevent inappropriate substances from getting into the blood stream. The weaker the digestion, the more likely it is to allow in substances that create inflammation in the joints. This can lead to chronic inflammation, weakening of connective tissues, or other injuries. A simple way to remedy this is to take large quantities of turmeric, which repairs the lining of the gut by eliminating viruses and bacteria. Turmeric acts as a joint-repair tonic, primarily by reducing inflammation in the intestines. See page 57 for easy recipes using turmeric.

The Digestive System

SUBTLE ANATOMY PERSPECTIVE

Fire *Tattva*

The fire *tattva* is the energetic fuel of life. It creates the energy to get out of bed in the morning and the capacity to processes and transform food. The fire *tattva* in digestion relies on the balance of the other *tattvas* for support. If there is too much air, for instance, the fire can burn too hot or blow out. Or, if the air is too weak, the fire can burn too cool and be unsustainable. Fire must also contain some of the water *tattva*, otherwise it is too drying for living systems to tolerate.

From the subtle perspective, fire is the root of anger, both misplaced indignant anger *and* righteous anger that ignites the desire for change in society or oneself. If left unchecked the fire *tattva* can burn out of control, like a forest fire, causing damage to the body or to relationships. When nurtured and balanced the fire *tattva* is like the flame of a candle at a vigil, passed from person to person slowly creating a gentle healing light.

Emotions and Digestion

Digestion is also intricately linked to and affected by your emotions. When a person is depressed the nervous system operates below optimal capacity, including the mesenteric nervous system in the gut. Food will not move through the gut optimally, and the process of absorbing nutrients will not be as effective.

This can start a downward cycle. When the digestion is not working well, sugar cravings are a natural way to try to increase energy. Eating too much sugar negatively affects the intestinal flora, which means there is less absorption of nutrients from food. Absorbing fewer nutrients leads to lower energy and lack of ambition to take initiative to change. And the downward cycle continues.

We can see how emotions impact the ability to digest and process food, which is why it is important to create a relaxing, safe, and uplifting environment when eating so that we initiate the switch to the parasympathetic nervous system and promote optimum digestion. Traditionally in Kundalini Yoga communities, meals are shared. The process of eating with other people makes your belly happy. It is easier and more efficient to digest your food and process the ups and downs of life in a calm, supportive environment.

> *The fire tattva is at its best when tended to and fed steadily over time and kept in balance with the other tattvas.*

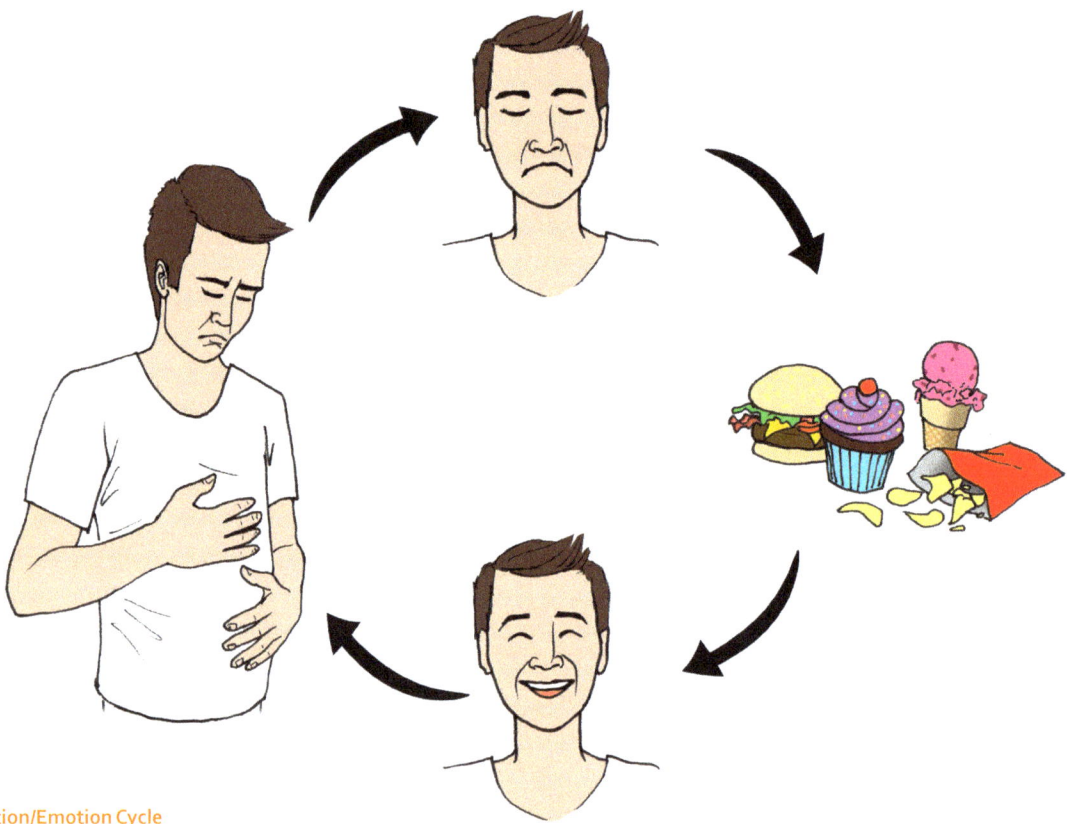

9.2 Digestion/Emotion Cycle

Your food choices, digestion and emotions are directly connected. The cycle of addiction plays out and is healed through direct experience of our feelings and body awareness.

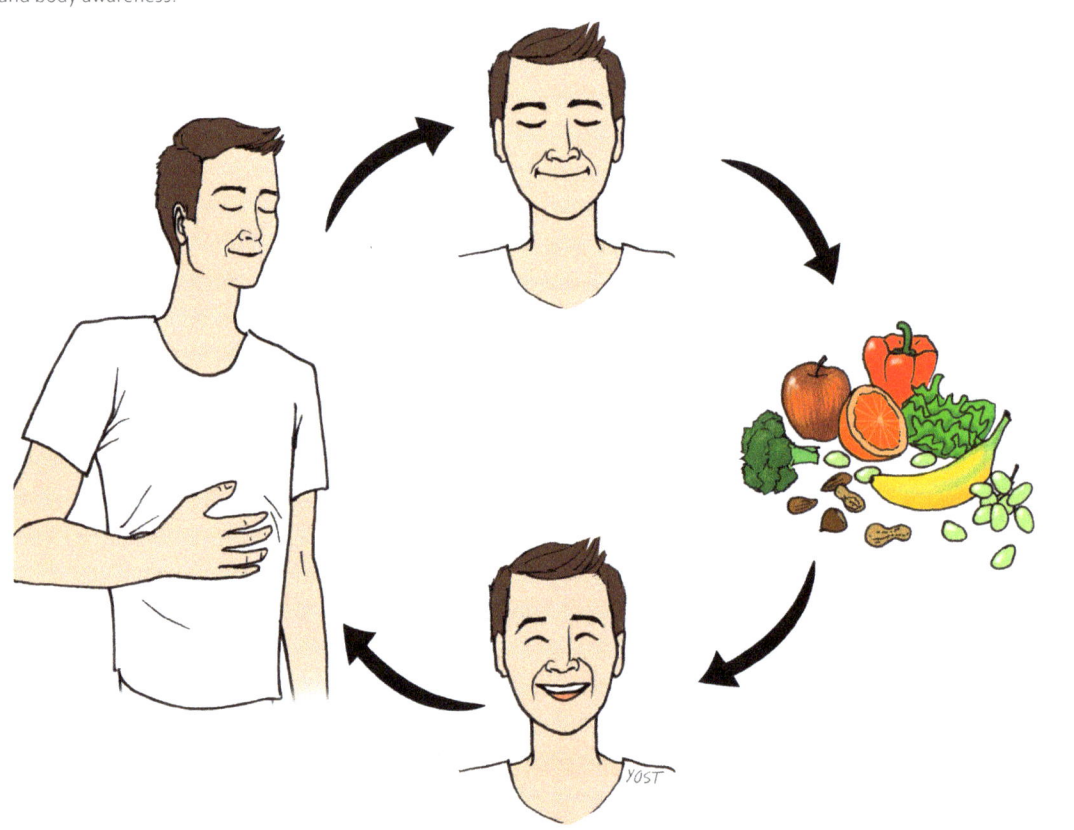

Some studies show that families who share meals together have statistically lower rates of substance abuse and depression, the children have larger vocabularies, family members have stronger immune systems, and all are less likely to be overweight. By sitting together, sharing stories, and connecting with others a sense of safety and relaxation permeates the experience and helps you digest your food (Cook and Dunifon, 2012). On the flip-side, picture a chaotic family meal where children may be screaming, parents yelling, or, perhaps even worse, a completely cold and silent family meal. These kinds of environments lead to poor digestion and leave your stomach and intestines in knots. Who we share our meals with and *how* have a direct effect on good digestion and healthy digestive processes in our bodies. Share your meals with people you feel relaxed and happy to be around. If you find yourself in a tense situation at meal time, it may actually be healthier for you to wait until you are calm to eat.

Digestion and Whole Foods

Picture celery for a moment; the cellulose provides celery with structure, but it is the micronutrients within the celery that nourish you, not the cellulose. The body takes in the micronutrients and discards the cellulose.

Challenges to the Digestive System

A healthy digestive system is the cornerstone of a healthy body. There are several indicators to become aware of as you evaluate the health of your digestive tract.
- Transit Time
- Food Quantity
- Intestinal Flora
- Acid-Alkaline Balance

Digestion Defined

Digestion is defined as the breakdown and separation of food into an absorbable state. What happens in the GI tract is more than just digestion, which includes absorption and elimination. People often refer to bad digestion when they really mean bad elimination or bad absorption.

Food Remedy for Diarrhea

Grate an apple finely and leave it out for a few hours until it turns brown, then eat it.

Transit Time

Transit time is how long it takes a particular food to make it through the digestive process. In *Foods for Health & Healing*, which contains recipes and remedies based on the Teachings of Yogi Bhajan, the directive is clear: "Eat only what you can eliminate within twenty-four hours" (KRI, 1983). Meats, cheese and eggs are common foods that take beyond twenty-four hours to digest. If your time is longer than twenty-four hours and you're not eating any of the culprit slow-digesting foods, it may be time to consider a cleanse for your digestive system. *Foods for Health & Healing* recommends giving your digestive system a day off once a week to allow digestive organs time to rest and do a little preventative "housekeeping". When you discover your body's digestion is slow, it is also a good time to check in and ensure you are drinking enough water to support your body's digestive processes. Beyond the physical factors, psychological factors such as anxiety and stress can also play a role in slow or stagnant digestion.

Test Your Transit Time

Eat a meal with lots of beets and record the time you eat this meal.

The beets will dye your stool bright red, when this happens, record that time and the difference between the two times should show you the approximate transit time through your digestive system.

If your transit time is not within a 24-hour window there may be an imbalance in your digestive system. If your transit time is too rapid, your body does not have enough time to absorb nutrients. The more common problem is digestion that is too slow. Transit time that is too long generally indicates that food is staying in the body and blocking up the system.

Tips to speed up your transit time include drinking more water, include more whole foods and plants in your diet, move more, try a probiotic, practice *praanayam* techniques.

Tips to slow down your transit time include eating fiber-rich foods like bananas, rice, apples, and toast, rest, take a nap, put on calming music and generally reduce stressors.

Food Quantity

It is important to avoid overeating or undereating. Instead, consume just enough nutrients in the diet to power the activities of life. Overconsumption and underconsumption inhibits the ability to have a fully functional life. Eating the right amount of the right things gives you plenty of energy to live a relaxed and happy life.

Yogi Bhajan recommended eating until the stomach is three-quarters full (half-full of food, one-quarter full of liquid) and one-quarter empty (KRI, 2011). Avoid being so crammed full of food that there is no space. Without the space it takes a huge amount of additional *praana*, or energy, to digest food.

In modern society, stuffed with large portions of tempting but unsatisfying carbohydrates, it is easy to disconnect from what it feels like to be full. We must re-train the digestive tract and the brain to interpret the signals of fullness, and develop the body's fullness radar.

One of the best practices to start retraining the fullness radar is to eat slowly. Digestion happens during the parasympathetic or relaxed state of the nervous system. Stress simply does not allow for optimal digestion. The digestive process will continue to happen on a survival level, but it won't deliver the most nutrition, energy, or *praana* out of the food if you eat quickly.

When we eat slowly and consciously, it gives the brain time to process incoming information. There are two different ways that the brain understands fullness. One is a chemical signal that enough nutrients have been consumed, and the other is a volume signal that indicates a large enough volume of food has been eaten. It takes a little while for the brain to register these types of fullness. The desire to stop eating begins only when the brain registers *both*

> *"Don't underfeed your body, but please don't overfeed.*
> *What is the proof that you are underfeeding your body or overfeeding? If you cannot sleep you are underfeeding your body and if you cannot get up you are overfeeding."*
>
> © The Teachings of Yogi Bhajan, May 27, 1974

Digest This! Men and Women Digest Differently

Because of the additional space taken up by the uterus and the complex cycle of female hormones, men and women experience noteworthy differences in their digestive systems. A woman's stomach and colon take more time to empty and thus women have more risk of constipation (a longer than twenty-four hour transit time) and stomach upset. However, women have a lower incidence of heartburn because the seal at the bottom of the esophagus is stronger in women and they secrete less stomach acid than men. (Legato, Singh, 2015).

signals. If food is coming in too quickly the brain cannot register fullness until it's too late. If the food that comes in is low quality or processed, the brain does not get the chemical signal that enough nutrients are present. This is why it is so easy to overeat junk food. Eating high-quality food and eating it more slowly are the primary ways to re-train the brain and body to understand fullness (Furman, 2003).

Nirmal's Food Experiments

I think of my diet as an experiment. I have tried the green diet suggested in the Kundalini Yoga teachings, and I know how I feel when I do that (crabby at first, then bright and clear). I have tried eating wheat and being off of wheat. I had terrible seasonal allergies until I cut wheat out of my diet; now they're gone. I used to eat meat, but I don't anymore because it just stopped feeling good in my body.

All in all, my diet is an experiment for my body. I want to choose food that makes me feel alive, healthy, and clear, but I have to try different options and really pay attention to how I feel in order to figure out what foods will get me there. Easier said than done, as the adage goes; but I remember when I first noticed that going wheat free made my allergies disappear. Still, I had to prove it to myself. Every six months or so I would convince myself that I could eat that sandwich or pizza or cereal, and the next day I would pay the price with runny nose, itchy eyes, and sneezing fits!

Intestinal Flora There are a huge variety of bacteria and enzymes in the digestive tract. These elements play an important role in helping to digest food. It is important to have a high count of healthy flora in the gut in order to have the most effective digestion process.

Medication—especially antibiotics—and poor diets can lead to a very low flora count. This creates a ripple effect of problems. If flora count is low, even after switching to a super healthy diet, the mechanisms to break down and absorb all the good nutrients are not present or have been damaged. This is why people take probiotics—to restore a healthy flora balance in the gut.

It's a Brave New... *er*, Bacteria

Recent studies on mice have revealed that the bacteria in the gut can influence feelings of anxiety and/or courage. When intestinal bacteria from the guts of anxious mice were transferred into the guts of fearless mice, those mice then became anxious. This worked just as well in reverse; when the gut bacteria for brave mice were transferred into their anxious counterparts, those mice became visibly less anxious and more fearless (Stein, 2013).

Acid Alkaline Balance Scientists use pH to measure acidity and alkalinity in the body. A very slight alkaline pH (7.4) is considered ideal for the human body (pure water has a neutral pH of 7). The lungs and kidneys work together to maintain pH homeostasis. Processed food and animal proteins create additional acidity, which forces the body to work harder to maintain the appropriate internal environment.

Everything that happens in our bodies is based on complex chemical reactions. In any chemical reaction if the substances are not at the appropriate pH it requires more energy to make the reaction happen, if it can happen at all. When we eat slightly more acidic food than desirable, our bodies must work a little bit harder on each reaction to get the desired results. If we support our body in keeping neutral pH everything happens with more ease.

We create more acidity when we eat a diet high in processed foods and animal products. These foods tend to make the body acidic because of the long digestion process and the amount of acid it takes to get broken down.

Effects of a neutral or base pH:
- *Clearer skin*
- *More energy*
- *Less gas*

The Navel Chakra

The Navel Chakra is the source of fuel, heat, transformation, and willpower. Steady, healthy digestion sets the stage for physical strength, mental acuity, clear focus, and powerful creation in this life. It includes the Navel Point which is just behind and four finger widths below the actual belly button. The umbilicus is the original source point for energy, *praana,* and nutrition. The Navel Chakra however is a broader energetic zone that is our nourishment center.

The Navel Chakra encompasses the intestines, abdominal organs, abdominal muscles, and lower back muscles, and it extends from the solar plexus to below the belly button. When this energy center is balanced and strong we experience a zest for life and an ability to get stuff done. There is a sense of accomplishment, confidence, effectiveness, and sustained energy. When the Navel Chakra is weak or imbalanced, there is a lack of energy to complete projects and a tendency to become harsh or brash.

The Chinese Medicine Perspective

Much like the Western perspective, the digestive system from the Chinese medicine perspective is considered the very core of life; it is how *all* aspects of life, not just food, are processed. If digestion is troubled, there will be gas and bloating on a physical level, and emotionally there is a sense of fatigue, stress and overwhelm.

Our thoughts and feelings are actually a part of the digestive process. In other words, how we *feel* and how we *metabolize* are interconnected. This intricate interrelationship varies widely across individuals. Even though anatomically each person has the same basic physical process of digestion, each person also has a vastly different energetic makeup. The capacity to process emotions and food is affected by karma, genetics, relationships, and lifestyle.

Because every constitution is unique, every diet will be unique to the individual. The right diet for one person could be completely different from the right diet for another. Each person has different digestive strengths and weaknesses.

Overeating and the Aura

Almost everyone has had an experience where they eat comfort food in order to feel better after a bad day. We feel uncomfortable, but also small. This small feeling comes from the impact of the emotions on the Seventh Light Body, called the Aura, which consists of energy permeating and surrounding the Physical Body. The Aura's energy is intricately connected to emotions and is impacted by the subtle exchanges of energy that happen while petting a beloved dog, walking down a busy city sidewalk, basking in sunlight, sharing a laugh with a friend, grieving the loss of a beloved pet and yes, emotional overeating. In fact just about any experience that affects your emotions or brings you around energies considered separate from your own, which means just about every human experience, affects the Aura!

> IF YOUR DIGESTION IS JUST RIGHT, YOU WILL FEEL SHARP, PERCEPTIVE, AND ON TOP OF YOUR GAME.

When the Aura is strong and large, there is a feeling of safety, strength, and power. A strong Aura is less affected by weaker or negative energies around it. The Aura may shrink when we have a challenging talk with a boss or a fight with a friend. These challenging interactions pop the energy bubble of the Aura, in turn leading to the small or desperate feelings. It's important to find ways to regularly nourish yourself so that your Aura can be strong. Self-care, time in nature, meditation, and plenty of good rest is essential. Not only will you feel light and uplifted when your Aura is strong, but those around you will also feel an uplifting effect.

When your Aura is weak, it may be tempting to reach for calories and stimulants like coffee or soda to give you a temporary boost in energy. These kinds of energy sources lead to a false sense of expansion, and do not contain the vital *praana* your Aura truly needs in order to expand and feel strong. The pain of a weakened Aura is only masked by these empty energy sources that fill you up in the moment but let you down in the long run. The body has to work overtime to process the calories and toxins present in many of these sources of false vitality, which diverts energy that could otherwise be used to strengthen the Aura and restore the body. A cycle of depletion can launch, which leads to consuming more empty calories to experience a temporary buzz of energy, and a pattern of overeating may develop. Masking your true energetic needs with addictive low-energy foods leads to a silent disconnect. Instead of trying to beat your low-energy feelings with questionable foods or other substances, consider using yoga, meditation, and mindfulness to connect to your true energetic needs and help strengthen your Aura.

A Strong Aura Leads to Healthier Food Choices

When depression, overwhelm, sadness or food cravings kick in, try some quick Aura fixers instead of junk food. These simple activities can increase feelings of safety and connection which will allow you to be with your experience rather than run away from it.

Here are some examples of quick Aura fixers: cold shower, Ego Eradicator, Breath of Fire, Jumping Jacks.

TIPS AND TECHNIQUES FOR A STRONG DIGESTIVE SYSTEM

Aasanas and Exercises

Elbow Stimulating Postures stimulate the meridian of the *Large Intestine*.
Examples: Arms out to the sides flapping, bringing the backs of the hands to touch behind the head
Powerful Leg Postures stretch and stimulate digestive meridians in the legs.
Examples: Frog, Rock Pose, Crow Squats
Abdominal Pressure Postures supports peristalsis.
Examples: Plow, Sufi Grind, Tuck Pose, torso twists of all kinds
Vigorous Movements help to quicken transit time.
Examples: Sufi Grind, Sat Kriya, dancing

Left Nostril Praanayam

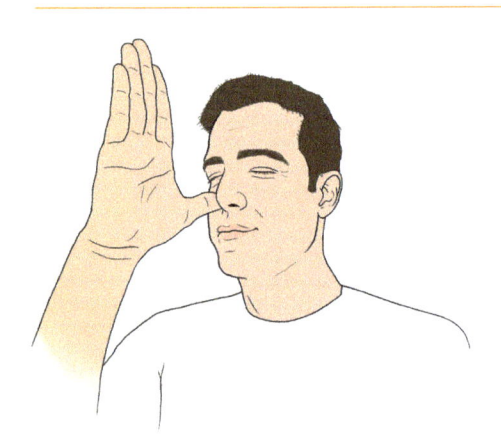

Left nostril breathing activates the ida nerve ending in the left nostril, which relates to calmness and relaxation. Left nostril breathing is associated with the moon energy, which has subtle qualities of being changeable, feminine, yin, giving, and cool. Breathing through the left nostril for even five minutes can calm the mind, support healthy digestion, and lower blood pressure.

Sit in Easy Pose. Close off the right nostril with the right thumb, and stretch the other fingers straight up like antennas. The left hand rests on the left knee in Gyan Mudra. With eyes closed focus your eyes at the Third Eye point. Begin to breathe long and deep through the left nostril. Continue for 3–11 minutes.

Transformational Energy Points

Stomach 36: Walk Three Miles

One of the most energizing points, it helps the body convert food into energy, thus giving you strength and stamina and earning its name "walk three miles (5 kilometers)".

Location: On the outer lower leg. When kneeling on the heels in Rock Pose, this is the point that takes the most pressure along the leg.

Effects: Balance the earth element, profound support to digestive functions.

Yoga for this Point: Rock Pose

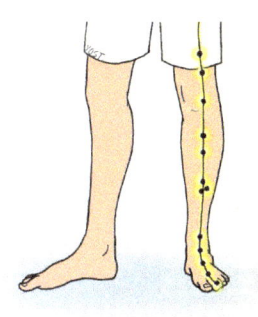

Plants, Herbs, and Food

Vegetarian Diet The yogic diet is a whole food, mostly plant-based diet. Eating less processed food and proteins from animal sources reduces the inflammation and cholesterol levels in your blood and helps to create greater vitality in the body. Besides the positive effects on your personal health and vitality, a vegetarian diet also helps the planet. Researchers at the University of Chicago found that a vegetarian diet has a greater impact on reducing greenhouse gas emissions than driving a hybrid car. Their findings were based on the amount of methane gas emissions produced by animals raised for their meat and the pollution produced by the transportation and cooling of meat products (Eshel et al. 2006). Of course, while reducing polluting gasses is one factor, buying pesticide-free produce and sustainably-produced products will further increase the planet-friendly factor of your vegetarian diet.

The largest portion of food in the diet should come from vegetables. Vegetables have very little fat, tons of fiber, and millions of nutraceuticals and antioxidants to give *praana* and life force to your body.

> AFTER A MEAL, GIVE YOUR DIGESTION A YOGIC BOOST BY SITTING IN ROCK POSE AND PRACTICING LEFT-NOSTRIL BREATHING.

Knowing more about how your body works on both the physical and subtle levels will naturally guide you to make better food choices.

Eat Fruit Sugar comes in many forms. Processed sugar can sneak into your diet all too easily if you don't know how to watch out for it; these hidden sugars often become a source of craving and addiction. If your consumption of processed sugar has become a problem point in your diet, tame your sweet tooth by filling up on fruits. Yogi Bhajan once taught a Kundalini Yoga kriya that included an exercise of eating fruit. He ordered hundreds of dollars of fresh fruit (plums, peaches, nectarines, melons, and more) and instructed students to "OD on fruit!" (Bhajan, 1994c). There were several other kriyas he taught where he recommended less extreme fruit consumption, like having a piece of fruit at the end of the kriya.

Fruit is the original fast food; it can be taken anywhere, stores easily and often comes in its own compostable wrapper. Fill your cupboards, fridge and freezer with good quality fruits and learn to prepare them in healthy ways. Eating an apple outright may seem boring or unappetizing to you at first, so play with recipes that prepare apples in healthy interesting ways that will peak your palate and your curiosity (like the one on page 196). Focus on adding fruit to your diet daily and see if you can satisfy your sweet tooth in a way that heals your body instead of sabotages it.

Tips to Reconnect with the Sensation of Fullness

- Drink a glass of water about 30 minutes before you eat a meal
- Sit down to eat at a real place setting: porcelain plate and flatware
- Put your fork or spoon down between each bite and chew thoroughly
- Turn off the TV and focus on your meal
- When you're halfway through the portion you've served, take a three-minute break and check in with how your stomach feels:
    - Ask yourself, *Am I still hungry?*
    - If you want to continue eating, is it because you are hungry or is it for another reason?

Choose Higher Quality Food The simplicity of a yogic diet supports a relaxed experience at mealtimes. The simpler the food, the less energy the body has to expend to process it, which lowers the chances of an irritated or inflamed digestive system. The gut is strengthened by the simplicity of the yogic diet. With easier to digest foods coming in, your gut is able to make better choices about what to absorb and what to pass through the digestive tract. In this way, the gut is a reflection of the broader choices you make in relationship to food.

Our modern culture gives us the luxury of many food choices. You can be vegan, carnivore, lacto-vegetarian, ovo-lacto vegetarian, or whatever floats your food boat. You have the blessing of lots of information, research and your own experience, and then deciding freely what food paradigm to accept for yourself. We no longer have the survival challenges of 150 years ago—long cold winters, no food storage, and eating meat as a necessity rather than a choice. Take advantage of this luxury and find the diet that supports your most vital life.

Fasting Fasting can be done in many ways and for various reasons (better health, spiritual development, medically mandated fasting prior to procedures, etc.). As mentioned earlier in the digestive system chapter, Yogi Bhajan's teachings recommend that you give your digestive system one day each week to rest (KRI, 1983). A weekly fast can take lots of forms from nothing but water and tea to consuming only green vegetables for an entire day once per week. A weekly fast is not recommended for pregnant or menstruating women, and any dietary change should always be checked with your doctor to ensure it does not interfere negatively with a condition or medical issue you may be facing. Otherwise, consider an occasional day of rest for your digestive system and see how you feel after trying it for a few weeks. If it is working well, you should notice an increase in your energy and a lessening of any general digestive troubles such as gas, bloating, and constipation.

Balanced Food Rules Try to be balanced about food rules. Find a diet that works for you and realize that it may be different from what works for others. Also remember the social and cultural implications of what we eat. You don't have to be so rigid that you can't eat in community and enjoy a meal with others. Remember that pleasure and happiness are important to healthy digestion.

Making Dietary Changes The secret to helping resolve destructive food habits is to focus on adding healthier foods to your diet rather than taking away unhealthy foods. The body is made up of food that was eaten in the past. If you make an abrupt change in diet that involves cutting out certain foods, your body can interpret that, on a subtle level, as a rejection of who you are. If you've lived on French fries, soda, and hot dogs your whole life and abruptly stop eating them, it can feel as though you are losing yourself. This feeling of deprivation, familiar to anyone who has gone on an intense diet, is fueled by a sense of separation from the very stuff that you are made of.

Focus on adding healthier foods to the diet and finding ways to improve the quality of the food you eat. Instead of cutting out dessert, try switching to baked apples. This mindset aligns with the expanded consciousness of a yoga and meditation practice. The goal is not to berate yourself into eating better. The goal is to expand your strength and sensitivity and invite higher quality food in.

It is common to slip off the healthy diet wagon and revert to old eating habits. It takes time to create a change in the body and for the body to not only accept, but even begin to crave, new healthy foods. One great way to stimulate digestion and stay on track with healthier food is through herbal teas. If you find yourself slipping off the healthy food wagon and veering toward processed foods, grab a hot herbal tea on your way down to cushion the fall. The hot water is beneficial for sluggish digestion, and the plant medicine in the tea keeps your body oriented toward real food. Ginger tea is the most obvious, inexpensive, and tasty tea that supports digestion and nerves.

Japa's French Fry Affair

When I first got onto a yogic path in life, I loved fast food. French fries were my passion. They helped me feel grounded and alive (or at least that's how I, somewhat yogically, justified my French fry fondness). But, honestly, I was also emotionally attached because of my family's fast-food outings growing up. There was an element of nostalgia for me as I indulged my French fry romance. When I met Yogi Bhajan, he immediately gave me what I considered at the time a very strange recipe containing root vegetables. I noticed that when I ate it, I no longer craved French fries. You can find this very same recipe for Beets and Potatoes on page 196 of this chapter. It is a salty and grounding meal that builds the blood, and helped me successfully transition off of fast food.

Probiotics are the friendly bacteria living in the gut that help to break down food. They are found naturally in sauerkraut, yogurt, and kefir. The sour quality of these foods is known for reducing heat or inflammation. Probiotics can also be taken in capsule form.

Healthy Fats Processed and shelf-stable oils that are clear are stripped of all their nutrients. They do not benefit the body. It is possible that their lack of nutrients actually *strips* the body of valuable minerals as they pass through. Your body is better able to absorb and process fats from whole foods like avocados, nuts, or unrefined oils that are not shelf stable and need to be refrigerated. When purchasing oil, hold the clear glass bottle up to the light and turn it upside down: Are particles floating through the oil? There are visible particles only in unrefined oils. These particles are minerals that are needed to keep your body strong (Pitchford, 1990).

Healing Properties of Kitcheree This rice and bean soup is easily digested, tonifies the blood and *Qi* energy, harmonizes the digestion, and is cooling and nourishing. It is said to strengthen the blood and increase energy, so it is often eaten to help speed up recovery from cold or flu. The cooling, moistening and strengthening properties help to reduce inflammation.

Peppermint A simple way to help digestion is to have a cup of peppermint tea after dinner. This soothes and supports the digestion and allows for better sleep. Overeating or poor digestion can often affect sleep. The body cannot rest well if it is busy digesting (Khalsa, K. P. S., n.d. 2008).

RECIPES FOR THE DIGESTIVE SYSTEM

APPLES

Apples are a great antidote to constipation among other digestion complaints and are generally cleansing. Baked apples support all the doshas, but because of their astringent quality, Vata should be careful not to overindulge.

BAKED APPLES

This is a very light and nourishing dessert or breakfast. As an added bonus, it can also help to relieve constipation and strengthen the blood.

- ✓ 4 to 5 apples, cored and chopped
- ✓ 3 tablespoons (15 ml) butter or ghee
- ✓ 1 teaspoon (5 ml) cinnamon
- ✓ A pinch of lemon peel
- ✓ 1 pinch of salt
- ✓ A splash of vanilla

Cut apples and place in a shallow baking dish.

Cut up the butter and mix in with the apples, sprinkle remaining ingredients on top, and cover with foil, bake for 30 minutes at 325 degrees.

Serve warm with ice cream or cold for breakfast with yogurt.

(Bhajan, 2011).

YOGI BHAJAN'S BEETS AND POTATOES

Balances *Vata* and increases *Kapha*.

This recipe is recommended for recovering junk food addicts or new vegetarians.

- ✓ 6 potatoes
- ✓ 2 beets
- ✓ 1–2 tablespoons (15-30 ml) peanut oil
- ✓ 1 tablespoon (15 ml) turmeric
- ✓ 1 cup water (240 ml)
- ✓ 1 teaspoon (5 ml) black salt

Clean beets and potatoes and then steam them for 45 minutes to one hour until both are soft. Once cooled, slip off the skins on the beets but leave potato skins on. Cut the beets and potatoes into bite sized pieces. Put 1–2 tablespoons (15-30 ml) of peanut oil into a frying pan and heat. Add turmeric and sauté for one minute.

Add the beets and potatoes to the pan and stir. Add 1/4–1/2 cup of water (60-120 ml) and mash the potatoes a little bit, letting the color of the beets mix together. Add 1/8–1/4 tsp (1-2 ml) of black salt* to the entire mixture and stir together.

Serve on toasted pita bread with feta or goat cheese.

*Black salt is a very sulfurous smelling salt that Yogi Bhajan specifically recommended for various health applications. A simple search of "Black Salt", or "Sulfur Salt" as he sometimes called it, in the online database of his teachings, The Yogi Bhajan Library of Teachings™ *(www.libraryofteachings.org)* will turn up many examples.

KITCHEREE (MUNG BEANS AND RICE)

Good for all doshas (Pitchford, 1990). Experiment with spices to balance your body type. To cool *Pitta*, add cumin, coriander, or fennel. To support *Kapha*, add onions, garlic, ginger and/or chili. To soothe *Vata*, add cardamom, fennel, black mustard seeds and lots of ghee (Morningstar, 1995).

Mung beans and rice is a famous dish in Kundalini Yoga culture. It is known for being easily digestible, a good source of protein, and generally nourishing and healing. Rice is the most common grain, although millet, quinoa, or other grains can also be used. The traditional recipe for kitcheree includes lots of spices and veggies (you can find recipes in lots of Kundalini Yoga books). But even an extremely simple version is a profoundly nourishing and Qi-building food.

Try this incredible and simple crockpot treat; prep time is only 5 minutes!

Soak the mung beans overnight and rinse your grain well. Put the rice and beans in a crockpot and cover with water. Cook on low 6–8 hours. Make sure there is enough water to keep the beans and rice covered; it's better to use a little too much water than too little. When you come home in the evening just add ghee, Bragg's liquid aminos, salt and pepper to taste. It is so easy and so satisfying!

Add a spicy masala for more flavor and heat (see the Nervous System chapter, page 129).

Yogi Eating Tips Recap

- ✓ Participate in community meals.
- ✓ Only eat until you are three-quarters full (half food, quarter liquid).
- ✓ Eat only what can be eliminated in 18–24 hours.
- ✓ Eat a whole foods, plant-based diet.
- ✓ Drink plenty of water.
- ✓ Use your teeth (and saliva) to help your digestive system out; chew food thoroughly!

"And whatever little portion you have put in your mouth like a kiss get it in and then chew it. Chew it totally, freely, openly..."

© The Teachings of Yogi Bhajan, August 13, 1992

Balance the Navel Chakra

The Navel Chakra is out of balance when we are too harsh with words, aggressive, brash, completely passive, depressed, uninterested, or uninspired. It is indicated by digestive problems or abdominal pain.

To Balance the Navel Chakra
- Wear yellow
- Wear or meditate with a tiger's eye stone
- Practice Stretch Pose
- Practice Breath of Fire (see page 102 for instructions)
- Eat a whole foods diet and cook and serve food to others
- Roll the closed eyes up as if looking out through the Third Eye point.
- Tap or massage the abdomen

Affirmations for the Navel Chakra

I am steady in my sense of self, personal power, and leadership. My soul is aligned with my willpower and higher calling in life. I enjoy the give and take of life and the flow of being with others.

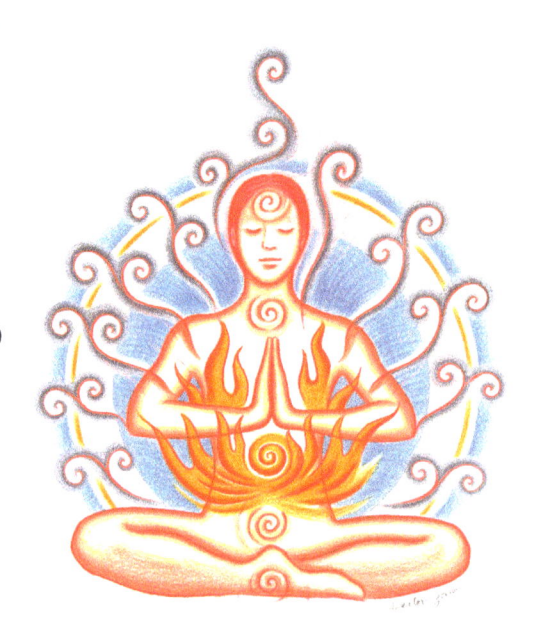

Balance the Aura

If you keep ending up in compromising situations, not meeting the right people, or feeling clumsy, your aura may be out of balance.

To Balance the Aura
- Wear white
- Wear or meditate with any kind of quartz stone
- Practice arm swings
- Dance
- Practice Celestial Communication, a form of moving meditation in Kundalini Yoga as taught by Yogi Bhajan®

Affirmations for the Aura

I am safe in the serenity of my electromagnetic field. I am protected and guided. I am in exactly the right place at exactly the right time.

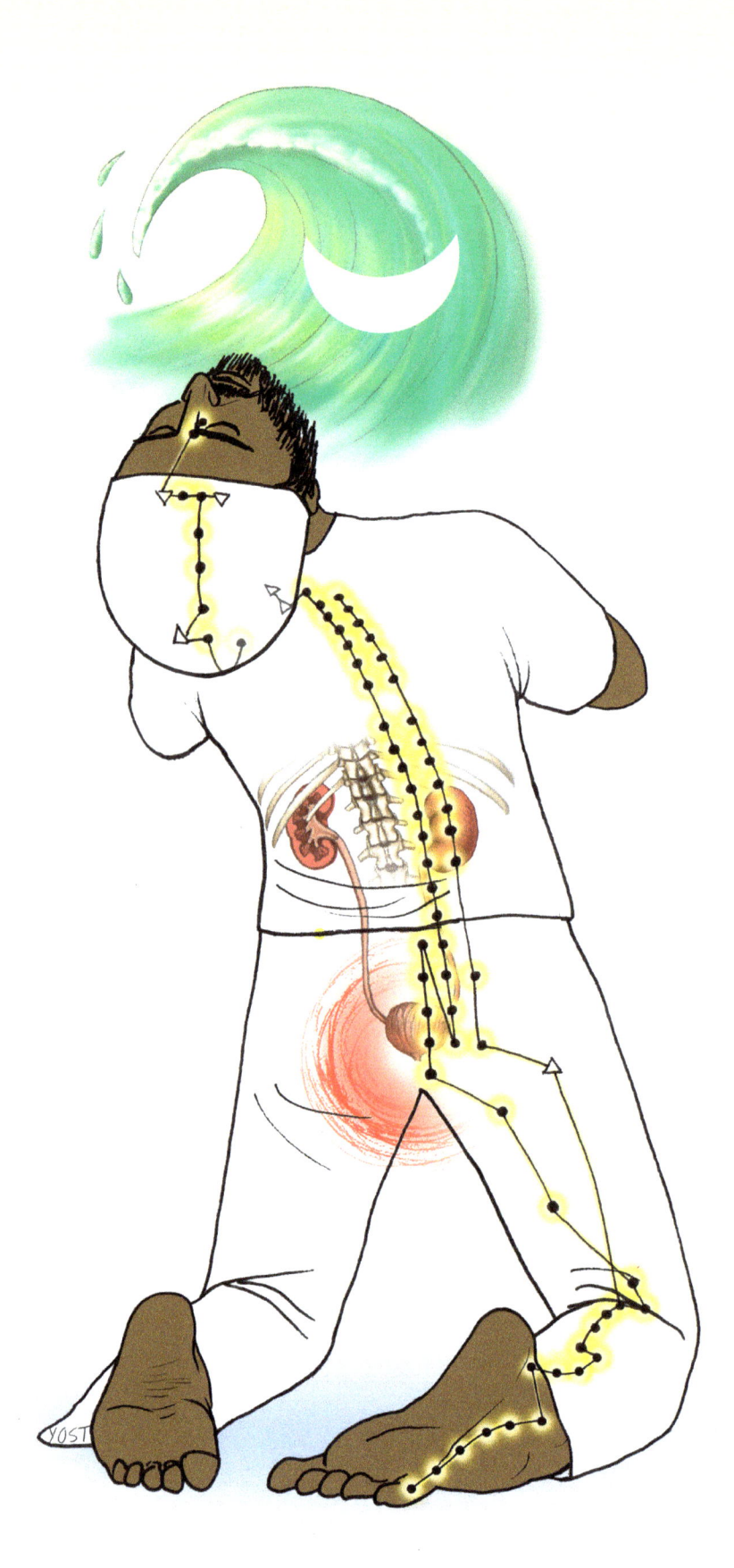

10.0 Camel Pose

Camel Pose offers a wonderful stretch and release for the entire front side of the body. The urinary system houses our capacity for fearlessness.

Notice the subtle anatomy structures: the Root Chakra represented by the red swirl around the bladder, the water tattva shown above as a crashing wave and the longest meridian the *Urinary Bladder*; sweeping over the entire backside of the body.

Notice the physical anatomy structures: The kidneys partially protected under the bottom of the ribcage, ureters and bladder move and filter water through the body.

The Urinary System

The experience of fear and fearlessness is built on the foundation of the urinary system. The kidneys and adrenal glands operate as functional units that send courage into the body via the hormones during moments of stress or pressure. They also create a safe, steady space for recuperation and purification. In times of relaxation, the kidneys contribute to the overall health or strength of the skeletal system and filter the blood. A disciplined lifestyle that supports the health of the kidneys can, over time, contribute to a person's overall feelings of security, bravery, and courage.

Happiness is tied to the ability to courageously move beyond fears. We do that by building a supportive network of friendships and community ties. Working in an ongoing way to build trust with others helps to support and grow the kidney function.

The urinary system is one of the primary waste-removal systems in the body along with the lungs, skin, and lower digestive organs. It is responsible for monitoring and balancing the water in the body and maintaining chemical balance in the blood.

"It isn't the life that matters; it's the courage that you bring to it."

© The Teachings of Yogi Bhajan, May 29, 1993

Strong Relationships
↓
Healthy Kidney
↓
Fearlessness

PHYSICAL ANATOMY PERSPECTIVE

Components of the Urinary System

- Kidneys
- Bladder
- Urethra
- Pelvic Floor

Benefits of a Strong Urinary System
Efficiently removing waste products from the body frees up energy to focus on other things and helps a person feel clear, focused, and fresh.

Primary Purpose
The primary purposes of the urinary system are to help regulate the water and chemical balance of the body and to excrete waste.

The Functions of Water in the Body

A discussion of the urinary system would not be complete without first understanding the general importance of water. Water is everywhere, and it's not just there looking pretty—it puts in a hard day's work supporting all forms of life on earth. About three-quarters of the Earth's surface is covered with water, and the human body is about 60–70 percent water. Water is nourishing for all of the cells and tissues of the human body, and it is necessary for most chemical reactions—trillions each second!—that occur there. Even if water is not a direct reagent, it is the medium in which many of these reactions take place.

How the Body Maintains Water Balance

Water is not only a critical element for most reactions in the body; it is also used for maintaining blood pressure, lubrication, and the exchange of energy within cells. The body fluids must be continually replenished with water from food and drinks. After eating and drinking, water flows through the digestive system to the large intestines, where it is absorbed and transferred to the rest of the body to do its many jobs. Eventually it passes through the kidney and a small portion is excreted as urine. Urine is mostly water but also contains salts that the body no longer needs and a waste product called urea that gives urine its potent smell.

- *Blood is 92% water*
- *The brain and muscles are 75% water*
- *Bones are about 22% water*

Kidneys

The kidneys are bean-shaped organs about the size of a fist; they are located deep in the body, behind the diaphragm—one on each side of the spine—in front of the thick muscles of the back, around the level of the elbows. The eleventh and twelfth ribs protect the top half of each kidney. Each kidney has an adrenal gland resting on top of it.

THE KIDNEYS PROCESS ABOUT 33 GALLONS OF FLUID PER DAY! 99 PERCENT OF THIS FLUID IS SENT INTO THE BLOOD, AND ONLY A SMALL PERCENTAGE IS EXCRETED AS URINE.

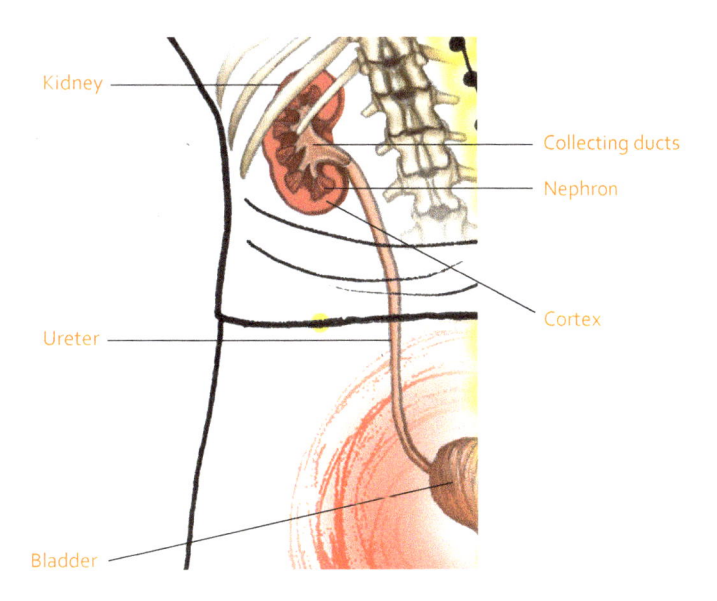

The blood passes through the kidneys as a normal part of its pathway around the body. Inside are tiny filters, called nephrons. The nephrons sort through the blood contents and decide which salts and how much water to return to the bloodstream and what should be removed from the body.

The kidneys continuously filter the blood. With each beat of the heart, about 25 percent of cardiac output travels to the kidneys for cleaning. This process regulates blood pressure and the acid/alkaline balance of the body by controlling levels of water, salt, and electrolytes in the blood. The kidneys contribute to the ongoing support of healthy bones by managing phosphorus and calcium levels in the blood.

Variations from One Body to Another

The position and shape of the bladder is slightly different in men and women. Women share space in the pelvic cavity with the uterus, thus the space for the bladder is smaller and more anterior. Even within the body the location and size of the kidneys is not symmetrical. The left kidney is usually slightly bigger and higher than the right because of the large space inside the abdominal cavity occupied by the liver on the right side of the body.

Bladder

> IN YOGIC TEACHINGS WE ARE ENCOURAGED TO URINATE BEFORE THE BLADDER HAS STRETCHED TO CAPACITY.

The bladder sits on the pelvic floor above a net of ligaments and muscles attached to the pelvic bones. Once passed through the kidneys the products and excess water move through the ureter and into the bladder. The bladder can hold the fluid until there is about 1–2 cups (240-480 ml), then it passes down the urethra and out of the body as urine.

Subtle Ramifications of 'Holding It'

"Because any time you hold the urine in, the bladder meridian totally upsets your system. Do you know that? And you know what a bladder meridian is? It hits the pituitary and it ruins your thinking. For you, it is a joke. For your system, it's a disaster. So try to understand that life is a gift. And every breath you cannot buy. So any moment you live, you breathe, it should be healthy, happy, holy. Everybody has nine holes. If you control what comes in and what goes out, it is holy. There is nothing special about it." (Bhajan, 1993)

The Urinary System

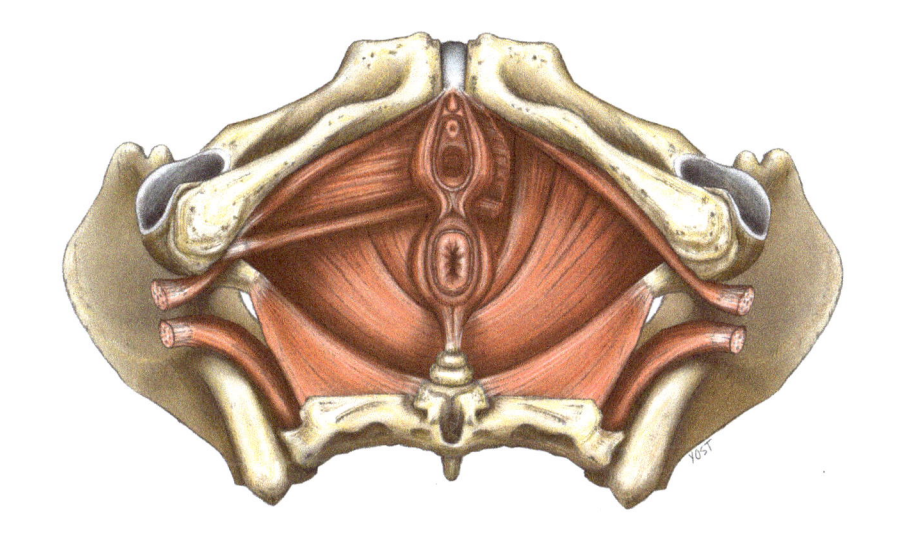

10.2 Pelvic Floor Muscles

Muscles of the pelvic floor engaged in Root Lock.

Pelvic Floor

The bladder sits directly on the pelvic floor muscles. These muscles must be toned and active to support the urinary system properly. The pelvic floor consists of several muscles that run between the sit bones and the pubic bone. When the floor is strong it aids in proper alignment of the pelvis and low back and supports the uterus, prostate, ovaries, and urinary bladder. The pelvic floor can be strengthened naturally by everyday activities: walking long distances, squatting while eating, or preparing food. In today's culture, with more time spent sitting in chairs, it is necessary to actively strengthen the pelvic floor. When the pelvic floor is strong there is less risk for conditions like a prolapsed bladder.

"We have to have a system that we can change our energy, we have x amount of energy for the day and we have to distribute it equally. And we should have the strength when things are rough we can push, when things aren't we can relax. It should be in our own strength. Start living healthy, happy, and holy. You have the right to control what goes in you or comes out of you. And with your head, this conscious eye, Third Eye, you must control yourself."

© The Teachings of Yogi Bhajan, December 3, 1989

Exploring Physical and Subtle Human Anatomy

Relationship to Other Systems

Kidneys and the Adrenal Glands The kidneys and adrenal glands are often talked about in the same breath because of their physical proximity. The health of one of these systems profoundly impacts the other. Any yoga pose or lifestyle practice that massages or stimulates the kidneys will do the same for the adrenals. The adrenal glands are a huge part of the survival response in life or death situations, which is another reason why the emotion of fear is linked to the kidneys (see page 159 for more information on the adrenals).

Urinary System and Reproductive System The urinary and reproductive systems are closely linked by physical proximity and subtle anatomy. Sometimes they are known as one system; the genito-urinary system. Male anatomy shares the same physical structure for ejaculation and urination. Women have separate physical pathways for sexual function and urination. In terms of subtle anatomy, the challenging aspects of the Root Chakra and Negative Mind merge into a single shadowed aspect of these combined systems: insecurity and self-doubt. The yogi achieves victory over this shadow by relating consciously to what comes into and out of the body.

The Urinary System

SUBTLE ANATOMY PERSPECTIVE

Water *Tattva*: Energetic and Symbolic Properties of Water

Just as a discussion of the physical anatomy of the urinary system would not be complete without first understanding the role of water in the human body, a discussion of the subtle anatomy of the urinary system would not be complete without understanding the water *tattva*'s connection to the flow of life on earth. Water is incredibly adaptable, changing shape to fit whatever container it is in, changing form depending on the environment. But water is also incredibly strong, the current of water flowing through a river can, over time, melt away even rigid rock formations. When there is enough water in the body you have the capacity for flexibility, fluidity. You connect with the impermanence of life; everything continually changes and flows. When we are properly hydrated, we can experience that flow and begin to open up to the process; we begin to trust and surrender to that flow.

Challenges to the Urinary System

Staying hydrated is one of the nicest things you can do for your urinary system and your body in general. Consuming enough water is critical to survival. Blood chemistry can quickly get out of balance when dehydration sets in. It can create a backlog of hormones that lead to feelings of overwhelm and disconnect. The nervous system is dependent on a constant supply of fresh lubricating fluid to keep it safe and nourished. Do not wait until thirst sets in before drinking water, because by then dehydration has already begun.

Contemplative practices often result in an expanded awareness of the sensations, needs, and experiences of the Physical Body, including developing sensitivity to the role water plays beyond basic survival. Eight glasses a day may be enough for survival, but more water may be needed to create this fluid sense of consciousness. Drinking water is critical to keeping an elevated state of mind. Too many toxins in the bloodstream can lead to depression, overwhelm and extra stress. If water is seen as a connection to subtlety and the subtle self, then drinking lots of water is a way of sustaining that connection and flow between the Light Bodies and the Physical Body.

> HAVE YOU EVER NOTICED THE SNAPPINESS AND SHORTNESS THAT CAN SET IN WITH DEHYDRATION? WHEN THE WATER TATTVA IS DEPLETED THERE IS NO COOLING SYSTEM FOR THE BODY, HEATING UP EMOTIONS AND RESULTING IN OUTBURSTS. STAYING WELL-HYDRATED SUPPORTS EMOTIONAL STABILITY.

The Dehydration-Anxiety Connection

Every year around summer solstice there is a large gathering of yogis in the mountains above Española, New Mexico. It is in the high desert, about 6,000 feet (1,800 meters) above sea level and very dry, hot, and windy. Often people will forget to drink enough water, especially if they are new, and then they will suddenly burst into tears or lash out at the people around them. They cannot process these extra high levels of anxiety due to their lack of hydration and overwhelm. Better hydration allows for the ability to flow with the challenges of life and maintain grace even in uncomfortable situations.

> *"Give me the tranquility to live in peace against all even and odds. Bless me; bless me to be bountiful, beautiful, and blissful. May the peace prevail; may the prosperity prevail; may the power of the consciousness lead the way to reality for all of us. May we live in love, win, and be victorious for our own consciousness and self-love. God bless us; we bless our consciousness and our own self in peace. Sat Nam."*
>
> © The Teachings of Yogi Bhajan, May 21, 1992

The Pelvic Floor and Subtle Energy Flow

We already learned how key the muscles of the pelvic floor are from a physical perspective (see page 205); from a subtle perspective, a strong pelvic floor supports the movement of energy in the body. In yoga, the capacity to circulate the energy in the body is key to obtaining the desired results from your practice. Our primary energy, the kundalini energy, naturally rests behind the Navel Point in the bowl of the pelvis and relies on good pelvic alignment and musculature for its balance and positive flow. When the spine is aligned, there is a clear pathway for this energy to move from the Navel Point, down to the first two chakras and then up to the crown of the head. If the pelvis is either tipped forward or back it is like a kink in a hose, making it more difficult for the energy to move and flow.

The Urinary System and the Negative and Positive Mind

The Negative Mind is also known as the protective mind; it is discriminating, works to keep us safe and is able to see the downside of any situation. When the Negative Mind is over-developed, fear and aversion to risk rule. When balanced, the Negative Mind protects us from danger without limiting opportunities of healthy risk (Khalsa, 2010).

The Positive Mind is also called the projective mind; it is fearless; it sees the bright side of any situation and generates unlimited possibilities. When overdeveloped the Positive Mind can create a pattern of over promising and under-delivering; disappointment sets in when reality doesn't match the dreams and ideals of the positive projection. When balanced, the Positive Mind is calm, contained, and inspires expansion and boldness. It allows for the impossible to become possible (Khalsa, 2010).

The kidneys and adrenals are closely linked with the functioning of the Negative and Positive Minds because of their role in secreting stress hormones. When they are functioning optimally the kidney/adrenal unit responds to dangerous situations quickly by creating a burst of strength and action in the body. During times of rest, a healthy kidney/adrenal unit gently filters blood and contributes to the stability of the body. The goal is not to get rid of the Negative Mind, but to know when to let it protect us from real dangers in life, just like the goal is not to rid the world of all toxins, but instead to use the kidneys to filter them out.

The Root Chakra

The primary energy of the Root Chakra is about grounding, our connection to the earth, and our sensation of security. The First Chakra is the energy center located at the very bottom of the spine, including the tailbone, legs, and parts of the pelvic bones. The physical location of this chakra also correlates with the urinary system, the bladder, the colon, and rectum. These are the structures in our body that eliminate unneeded elements. The dense network of pelvic floor muscles creates stability and strength and supports these organs.

When the Root Chakra is weak, fears become paralyzing. The state of chronic fear starts a downward cycle: grasping at the strings of life to create the illusion of control, stubbornness, insecurity, and a hesitancy to take chances. Activating the sense of security and contentment from within heals the Root Chakra. The *maya* of the material world can be intoxicating and addictive; there is always a desire for more, even though there is no amount that will fulfill and satisfy. Letting go of seeking fulfillment in the outside world is crucial to Root Chakra balance. When the Root Chakra is balanced, you experience feelings of being grounded and secure. This security allows you to open up to new things in life, and it becomes easier to let go of objects, experiences, and thoughts. A balanced Root Chakra permits change to be less stressful and painful.

> *"Leap and the net will appear."*
> —Gaelyn Foley, author

Chinese Medicine and the Kidneys

> **Women's Health Tip**
>
> *Take 1–2 tablespoons (30 ml) of sesame, flax, or evening primrose oil daily to help the body maintain fluidity and support an easier menopause.*

In Chinese medicine the *Kidneys* and the adrenal glands are seen as one functional unit. They are considered to be the root of life, energy, and longevity in the body. The entire yin and yang balance of the body is controlled by the *Kidneys*.

The yin and yang symbol represents the opposing energies in the world. It acknowledges that each type of energy tends to carry a little bit of the opposite polarity within itself. The body's constant process of inhaling and exhaling, storing and flushing, building and throwing out, living and dying, can be seen in the visual picture of the yin and yang symbol. The pairs of opposites that are at play in our bodies are in constant magnetic motion.

The *Urinary Bladder* meridian is paired with the *Kidney* meridian and together they represent the water element. *The Urinary Bladder* meridian, easily the longest in the body, runs from the eyes, over the top of the head, down the entire back of the body to the little toe. The Kidney meridian runs up the inside of the leg and inches its way up along the connection of

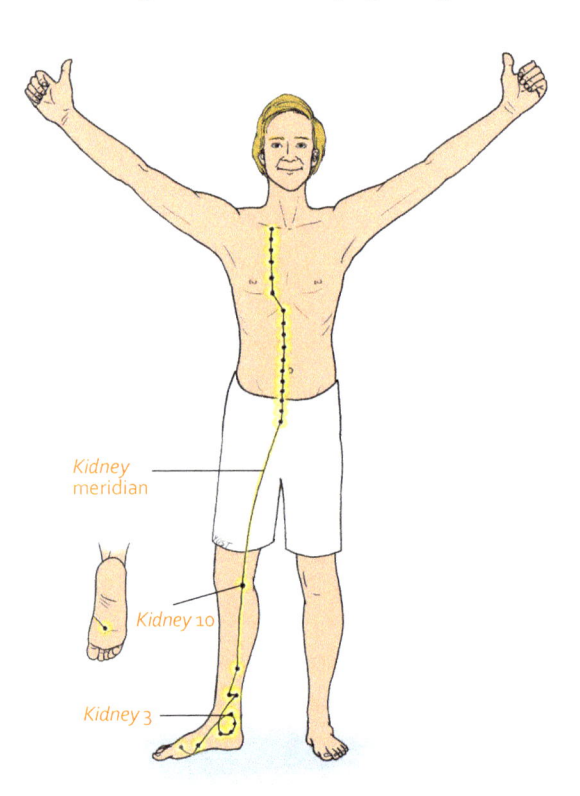

10.3 The *Kidney* Meridian

The Kidney meridian runs up the inside of the leg and inches its way up along the connection of the ribs to the breastbone.

Kidney meridian

Kidney 10

Kidney 3

The Urinary System

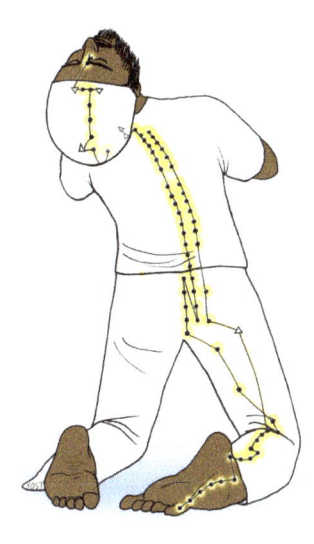

10.4 Urinary Bladder Meridian

the ribs to the collarbone. They intersperse through the entire body and impact the function of all the internal organs. In the same way that the earth is covered by a vast network of water and is greatly affected by the movement and tides, the Urinary Bladder and Kidney meridians exert a huge influence on the overall state of the body. Any postures that extend the spine influence the flow of the water element through these paired, meridian structures. Their physically intertwined impact on the torso and the rib cage is profound and influences the Heart Chakra as well as our feelings of expansion and connection to the soul.

Right and Left *Kidney* Functions

The accumulated life force energy from our ancestors comes to rest in the *Kidneys*, specifically the left *Kidney*. The left *Kidney's* yin is responsible for all of the liquid substances in the body. It is responsible for the nourishing secretions in the body such as mucus, sweat, urine, sexual fluids, and saliva. The left *Kidney* is sometimes thought of as a type of trust fund. This is our deep reserve of energy, stretching back through generations. To maintain healthy function it is ideal to avoid dipping into the energy of the left *Kidney*.

Instead, on a day-to-day basis it is preferable to use the energy from the right, yang *Kidney*, which acts like a checking account. The right *Kidney* is responsible for all metabolic activity in the body and is energetically located below the Navel Point, where it smolders and moves energy in the body. The yang *Kidney* helps the bladder to move and discharge urine, helps in the creation of digestive fire and manages the intake of breath into the *Lungs*. The right *Kidney* is nourished by the daily effort of healthy living.

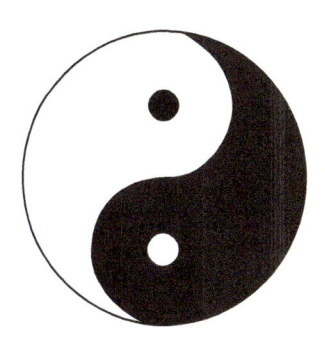

10.5 Yin and Yang

Balanced energy is foundational to many perspectives and goes by different names:

Physical —> Homeostasis
Yogic —> Praana and Apaana
Chinese —> Yin and Yang

Exploring Physical and Subtle Human Anatomy

TIPS AND TECHNIQUES FOR A STRONG URINARY SYSTEM

The urinary system plays a major role in overall health and vibrancy. It makes vital connections between water, sunlight, and the body; and is essential to good blood chemistry in the body. Also, the far-reaching influence of the *Urinary Bladder* and *Kidney* meridians (profoundly affect various other systems, including glands like the all-important pituitary gland) make a healthy urinary system of even greater importance.

At a subtle energy level, the urinary system is supported by a personal practice that involves meditations and exercises especially designed to release fear and stress, and find deep, internal silence. From a dietary standpoint, taking care of organs like the kidneys becomes very important to supporting urinary health.

Aasanas and Exercises

Extensions in the lower back compress the kidneys and adrenals
Examples: Camel Pose, Cat-Cow
Massaging the abdomen stimulates energy of *Urinary Bladder* and First Chakra
Examples: Rocking Bow Pose
Pelvic Floor exercises help the pelvic floor muscles to release tension held in the pelvis.
Example: Butterfly Stretch Pose, Body Drops

Root Lock (*Moolbandh*)

Root Lock (*Moolbandh*) is a basic, yet crucial, skill to learn and apply in the practice of yoga. Yogi Bhajan described Root Lock as pulling up on the rectum, sex organs and navel. It is ideal to have a light Root Lock engaged almost all of the time. With skill and conscious effort we can learn when and how intense of a Root Lock to engage throughout our practice of yoga, meditation, and even in our daily life. The purpose of the locks is to create stability and relaxation, not tension. When you engage the anal sphincter and the muscles of the sex organs, you create a sense of lifting your pelvic floor. By lifting the pelvic floor you stabilize the pelvis. The *transverse abdominis*, the deepest layer of the abdominal muscles, also engages when applying Root Lock, creating a protective relationship to the lower back.

Transformational Energy Points

Conception Vessel 1: Meeting Place of *Yin*

Location: In the perineum

Effects: One of the most restorative points in the body. Balances the mind and redirects energy toward personal growth and development, soothes sexual anxiety.

Yoga for this Point: Mahaa Mudra

Fun Facts: Due to its private location it is rarely accessed in acupuncture treatments, which makes it a rare meditative gem when we sit on the heel at the perineum.

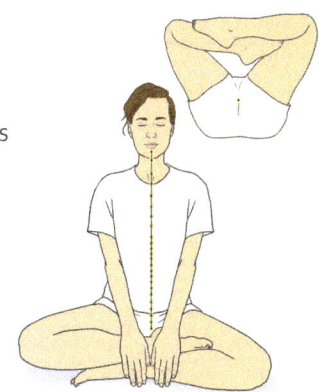

To refine Root Lock, practice engaging the deep core muscles, the *transverse abdominis*, and the pelvic floor, *without* also engaging the gluteus (buttocks) or the external abdominal muscles. It can be hard to isolate these deeper muscles because they are not seen or felt externally.

Upon closer inspection of Root Lock, we find three distinct aspects at play:

- **Rectum or Anal Sphincter:** It is ideal to squeeze the rectum without engaging the entire gluteal group of muscles; it can take some training to unlearn previous habits. The focus is on having a sense of lifting up on the sphincter itself. When engaging Root Lock, there should not be much visible external movement in the buttocks.
- **Sex Organs:** For women this is the same as engaging the Kegel muscles. Draw the muscles of the vagina in and up. Overall this creates a sense of tone and lift to the pelvic floor. Visualize the triangle of the pelvic floor and imagine pulling the center of that triangle up toward

The intent of Root Lock is to activate and bring awareness into the deepest parts of your physical and subtle self.

Effects of Root Lock (*Moolbandh*)

- Energetically seals the effects of an exercise
- Balances the energy of the three lower chakras
- Protects and supports the pelvis and lower back
- Strengthens the internal core muscles
- Stirs and awakens the kundalini

10.6 Incorrect and Correct Alignment
Posture affects the flow of energy through the body. Like putting a kink in a garden hose, energy flow is inhibited when our postural alignment is off (left) and it is supported when we are well-aligned (right).

"*Center of understanding, in our body, nervously is controlled by the navel point. So your eyes, ears, and tongue, throat, is controlled by navel point, whatever you hear, whatever you see, and whatever you say, is controlled by this navel point.*"

© Teachings of Yogi Bhajan, February 5, 1991

STAYING HYDRATED IS THE MOST IMPORTANT THING TO DO TO KEEP THE KIDNEYS HEALTHY. DRINK ENOUGH WATER TO MAKE YOUR URINE A LIGHT YELLOW COLOR.

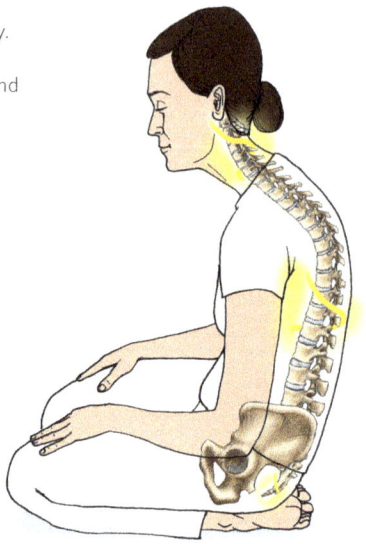

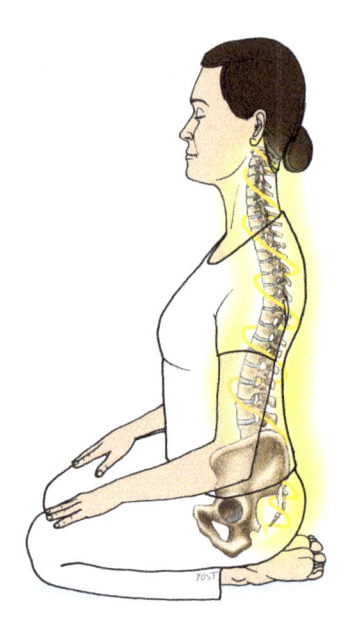

the belly button. Men are often told to pull up on the sex organs. They are also engaging the muscles of the pelvic floor, which feels like an activation just behind and above the scrotum.

- **Navel Point:** Root Lock is about engaging the deepest muscles in the body. There is not a gross external movement when the Navel Point is engaged. The deepest layer of abdominal muscle, the *transverse abdominis*, is engaged during Root Lock, which creates a girdle-like feeling. The outer layers of the abdominal muscles, *rectus abdominis* or the *obliques*, are *not* actively engaged, but they follow along with the movement of the transverse abdominis.

Plants, Herbs, and Food

Electrolytes are the minerals sodium, potassium, magnesium, and calcium. Because of the kidneys responsibility for maintaining the electrolyte balance of the blood, they interact with the mineral stores of the skeletal network and have a vast impact on the bones. These minerals come from the foods and fluids we eat and are essential for the stable functioning of our cells and organs. Foods like root vegetables, beans, and sea vegetables are rich in minerals and help the body to collect the appropriate amounts to circulate in the blood and store in the bones.

The Urinary System

Food-Based Remedies

Yogi Bhajan recommended several food-based remedies to help the urinary system. The following information hails from *Foods for Health and Healing* (KRI 1983).

- **For urinary problems** a fast of beet greens is sometimes effective. Also helpful in urinary disorders are coconut and melons.
- **To cleanse the urinary tract** drink a mixture of 2 parts spinach juice and 1 part carrot juice. Drink a minimum of 1 quart per day.
- **To increase urination** try grapefruit juice. It is a natural diuretic. Pineapple juice also stimulates urination because of its high chlorine content.
- **To cleanse the kidneys** drink 1 cup of milk (240 ml) twice a day with 4 cups (960 ml) of water and some honey. The best time to cleanse the kidneys is during the full moon.
- **To stimulate the kidneys** in order to eliminate wastes, the following foods are effective: pineapple, watercress, coconut, rice, and curry on rice. A 28-day diet of Mung Beans and Rice is also beneficial to the kidneys (see our Mung Beans and Rice recipe on page 197).

Yogi Bhajan often recommended "P fruits" for urinary system health, such as pears, plums, peaches, papaya, persimmons.

Gokshura Tea

Good for Something Goatheads

Ask anyone who's spent some time in the Southwest United States if they think there is any good use for goatheads and the answer will surely come back as a resounding "No!" A common weed with thorny fruits, goatheads are the bane of anyone careless enough to step on one. But beyond this apparent negative quality, goatheads are actually a powerful Ayurvedic remedy known as *gokshura*. They are used traditionally to encourage fertility and prevent and soothe bladder or kidney infections. Postpartum use is said to support recovery from childbirth.

Generally tridoshic (balances all doshas); Bring 1 tablespoon (15 ml) gokushura (goatheads) to a boil in 2 cups of water (480 ml), then simmer uncovered for 30 to 45 minutes. Drink this tea daily. For a tastier treat and to support prostate health, simmer the tea with goat milk, then blend in some sesame seeds and raw honey to taste (Morningstar,1995).

Exploring Physical and Subtle Human Anatomy

Yogic Lifestyle

Sunlight Everyone knows the incredible feeling of relaxation that comes from spending a day at the beach. Being in the sunlight allows the skin to produce vitamin D. The vitamin D that is created in the skin absorbs into the body and floods the vitamin-D receptors in the kidneys. This allows them to regulate levels of calcium, which in turn creates a feeling of calm, balances the blood, maintains healthy bones, and build immunity.

The kidneys are the organs most impacted by time in the sun. The yogic lifestyle advises a healthy relationship with the sun. One way to cultivate that relationship is to let the hair dry naturally in the sun. This practice can awaken the pituitary. Yogi Bhajan also advised spending summer solstice every year in the bright, turquoise sky of New Mexico. He established a Kundalini Yoga event around the solstice for this purpose. Many of those in attendance followed (and continue to follow) his recommendation to wear white clothing. Spending a week in white clothing when the sun is at the most direct angle allows energy to penetrate and build the meridians and acupuncture points of the body.

We recommend techniques for balancing the Root Chakra as a general tonic for urinary system health. These can be found in *Balance the Root Chakra* box at the end of Chapter 3, page 59.

Mantra

Chattra Chakkra Vartee
Chattra Chakkra Bhugatay
Suyambhav Subhang Sarab Daa Sarab Jugatay
Dukaalang Pranaasee Dayaalang Saroopay
Sadaa Ang Sangay Abhangang Bibhutay

You pervade all the four directions, the Enjoyer in all the four directions. You are self-illumined, united with all and beautiful. Destroyer of the torments of birth and death, you are forever merciful. You are the everlasting giver of indestructible power.

This is a mantra used to remove fear, anxiety and phobias and creates victory in every situation.

11.0 Mahaa Mudra

As the life nerve is stretched in Mahaa Mudra, there is expansion in our longevity and creativity through the elongation of the sciatic nerve and the gallbladder meridian. The reproductive system reminds us of the flexibility needed to be patient and creative with our gender polarity.

Notice the subtle anatomy structures: The swirl of the sacral Chakra that holds sexuality and creativity and the Arclines that allow our intuition to shine.

Notice the physical anatomy structures: The ovaries, uterus and testes are compressed in this posture, allowing for cleansing and rejuvenation.

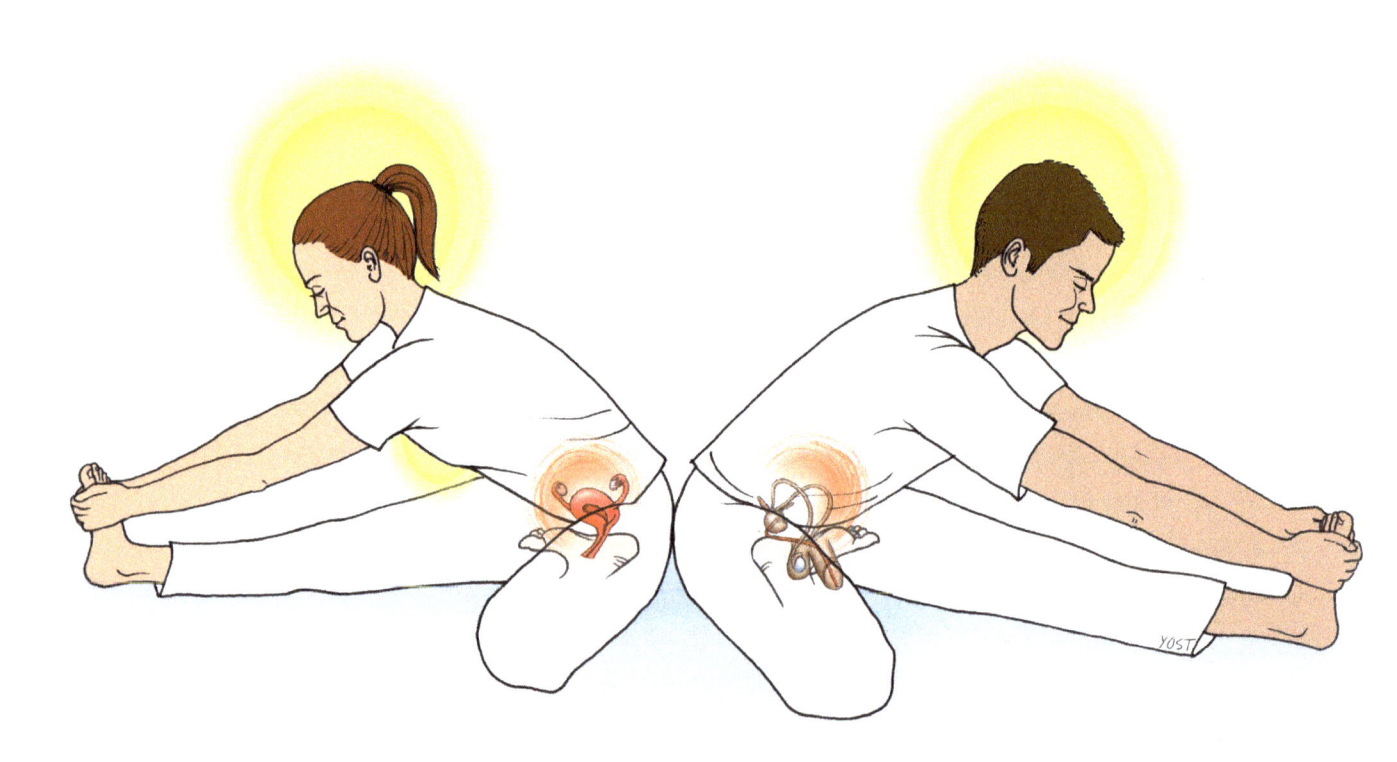

The Reproductive System

As human beings we yearn to leave a legacy and expand beyond time and space. This desire is a central motivating force behind an optimally functioning reproductive system. The complex relationships between sex organs, energy centers, and hormones mimic the cycles of creation. Producing children is only one way the consciousness of reproduction manifests itself. Every creative or expansive act in life, whether it is starting a foundation, inventing something new, crafting a beautiful piece of art, or having a child is born out of the foundation of the physical and subtle aspects of the reproductive system.

> *"We are born of a woman, that is the mother. We are grown by a woman, that is the mother and that's the Shakti, it's a point of relevance how you treat yourself sensually, sexually. There is nothing in sex and there is nothing without sex.... We have to learn today that sexuality...it's a matter of pituitary, it's the sixth Chakra, Agia Chakra, it's a whole balance of life.... In between, there lies a real sensitivity of creativity and pituitary commands the second Chakra, the sensuality, the sexuality, the humanity....It's a honorable subject, it's a graceful subject, it's a subject of reality, conception, aggravation and reality of going through vitality confrontation and raising the issue. Actually, all what you have is sex."*
>
> © The Teachings of Yogi Bhajan, May 28, 1993

PHYSICAL ANATOMY PERSPECTIVE

Components of the Reproductive System

Female
- Ovaries
- Fallopian Tubes
- Uterus
- Vagina
- Labia
- Clitoris
- Breasts

Male
- Testes
- Penis
- Prostate

Benefits of a Strong Reproductive System
The reproductive system encompasses much more than the ability to produce babies. The yogic understanding of gender and sexuality originates in the divine masculine and the divine feminine; a polarity that exists regardless of gender, sexual expression, or sexual orientation. Each individual has both masculine and feminine energies. Staying open to the expansiveness of this polarity allows for a richer experience of life.

Primary Purpose
The primary purpose of the reproductive system is to produce the next generation of humans. It builds sexual energy, which fosters an exciting, healthy, and active sex life. Finally, the reproductive system houses the energy of creativity and longevity in all its forms.

The Female Reproductive System

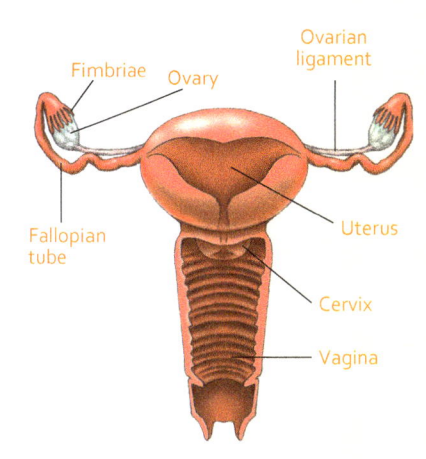

The female reproductive organs are located within the protective basin of the pelvis. From behind, they are fully shielded by the sacral bone and in front, by the rim of the pelvis. The body is elegantly designed to ensure the continuation of the species by protecting this crucial system. The position of the reproductive organs also parallels a more inward, in-depth, and complex interplay of hormones and possibilities in the female system.

Ovaries are paired reproductive organs that produce both hormones and eggs. Like the testicles, they are both an endocrine gland (producing hormones) and a gonad (producing eggs). At birth, each ovary contains 1 to 2 million immature eggs or follicles. These oocytes, or eggs, slowly degrade throughout a woman's lifeti me. During adolescence the ovaries begin the process of maturing an oocyte for possible fertilization. Every month, a hormonal cascade results in the ripening of multiple eggs and culminates in the release of one egg that moves into the fallopian tubes.

Fallopian Tubes Once the egg has matured and left the ovary it slowly moves down the fallopian tubes into the uterus. There are tiny hair-like projections, called cilia, which line the walls of the fallopian tubes and help to sweep the egg forward. If an egg is fertilized by a sperm it usually happens in the fallopian tubes.

The Uterus or womb, is a major reproductive organ in women; it is responsive to hormones and is where the fertilized egg (now called a blastocyst) implants and where a viable fetus will develop and grow throughout a pregnancy. Each month the uterus responds to hormones and builds up an endometrial lining in anticipation of pregnancy. This lining is shed every month if pregnancy does not occur. At the bottom of the uterus is the cervix which opens into the vagina.

The Vagina acts as the birth canal and the passage that menstrual flow takes as it leaves the body. During birth a woman's uterus contracts and the vagina expands significantly to allow the passage of a baby into the outside world.

11.1 Female Reproductive Organs
The female reproductive organs are located within the protective basin of the pelvis.

"Anything creative in you, which comes through thought, body, mental action, is called sex. And in sex, all senses must move."

© The Teachings of Yogi Bhajan, November 12, 1993

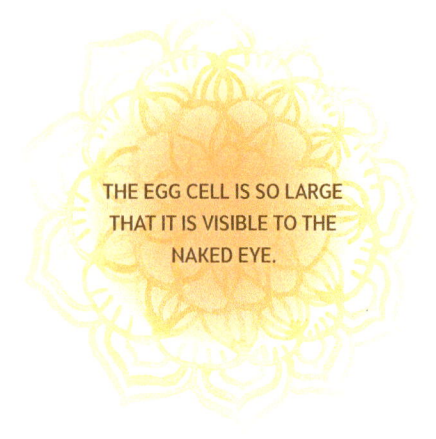

THE EGG CELL IS SO LARGE THAT IT IS VISIBLE TO THE NAKED EYE.

The vagina is also involved in sexual intercourse and plays a significant role in pleasure in human sexuality. It responds to sexual arousal by secreting fluid, which aids in sexual intercourse.

Labia The labia are the external lips of the vagina and act as a protective barrier to the ecosystem that is the female reproductive system. They are one of the erogenous zones of a woman and cover the clitoris, the primary source of sexual pleasure for a female.

Breasts While both males and females have breast tissue, their enhanced development during puberty in girls constitutes them as a secondary sex characteristic. Breasts are responsible for lactation and milk production after pregnancy. They can also be an erogenous zone in women and play a role in sexual pleasure and arousal.

Menstrual Cycle Every month a woman's body creates the possibility for a new human being to form within her. Throughout the month the uterus creates a thick nest of nourishment for the egg. If the egg is not fertilized, the lining sheds during the monthly menstrual cycle. The menstrual cycle is a natural cleansing process.

It is normal for the period to be slightly different every month as an organic reflection of the woman's changing state of being. The cycle is orchestrated by constant, delicate fluctuations of the two main hormones—progesterone and estrogen—throughout the month.

The Power of Pregnancy A woman can conceive children from the onset of puberty until menopause, typically in the early fifties. At birth each ovary contains approximately one million egg cells. In fact, the ovaries contain more eggs than will be used during the menstrual years; by the time menstruation begins the number of eggs has already decreased to approximately 400,000. The quality of the egg cells also decreases over the years with increased likelihood of nonviable cells (Resolve, 2014).

Human reproduction is a complex and sensitive process. Inside the uterus the microscopic sperm finds its way to the tiny egg and implants itself to form the zygote. In the yogic teachings, the sperm circles the egg eight times before penetrating. In some ways this mirrors the dance of Shiva/Shakti or the

The menstrual cycle is often referred to by Yogi Bhajan as the moon cycle, because the phases often correspond to phases of the moon.

male/female dynamic; the zig zag of the sperm can be felt in the way that a man communicates, and the circular qualities of a woman are represented by the stillness of the round egg that waits for the transformation of conception.

The cells begin to divide and the embryo sends out a hormonal message to the mother's body to stop the uterine walls from shedding. This message is the embryo's statement of survival that begins the symbiotic relationship to grow for nine months in the womb.

During pregnancy, a woman has the capacity to connect with the being in her uterus and to help it transform and release karmas before it is even born. The frequency and projection of the woman's mind and spiritual practice can help to build *sattvic* (saintly) energy for the fetus. This energy will help that soul to live to its highest destiny after birth (Khalsa, 2007).

In the yogic tradition the embryo is a part of the woman's body until four months have passed. On the 120th day, the soul then enters the fetus, and the destiny begins for that soul's journey in the physical body. A woman is advised to take time to pray, meditate, and prepare herself for the soul's entry before the 120th day. Her frequency attracts a soul with high caliber; and her conscious process of bringing the heavens into earthly form is a sacred act. The elevation and expansion of the human race comes through the prayer of the mother (Khalsa, 2007).

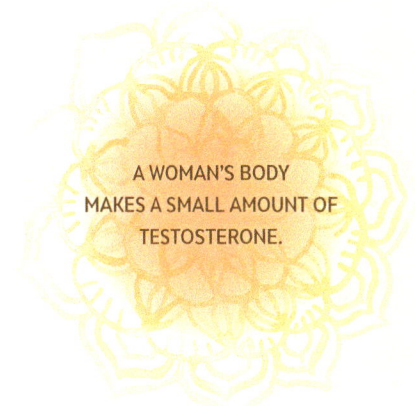

> A WOMAN'S BODY MAKES A SMALL AMOUNT OF TESTOSTERONE.

Generations within Generations

When a female is born, she already has all of the eggs she will ever have already stored in her ovaries. If a woman is pregnant with a female baby, then, she has within her half of the genetic material for her potential future grandchildren. In the yogic tradition it is believed that the effects of our meditations and healing efforts can affect seven generations into the future. When a woman prays and projects positivity during her pregnancy, she is installing that blessing not only in the offspring currently in her womb, but in the next generation as well.

The fact that a sperm can find such a tiny egg in the comparatively vast space of the uterus is a bit like the chance of a meteor finding its way through the cosmos, surviving passage through the atmosphere, and actually landing on the Earth's surface, thus becoming a meteorite.

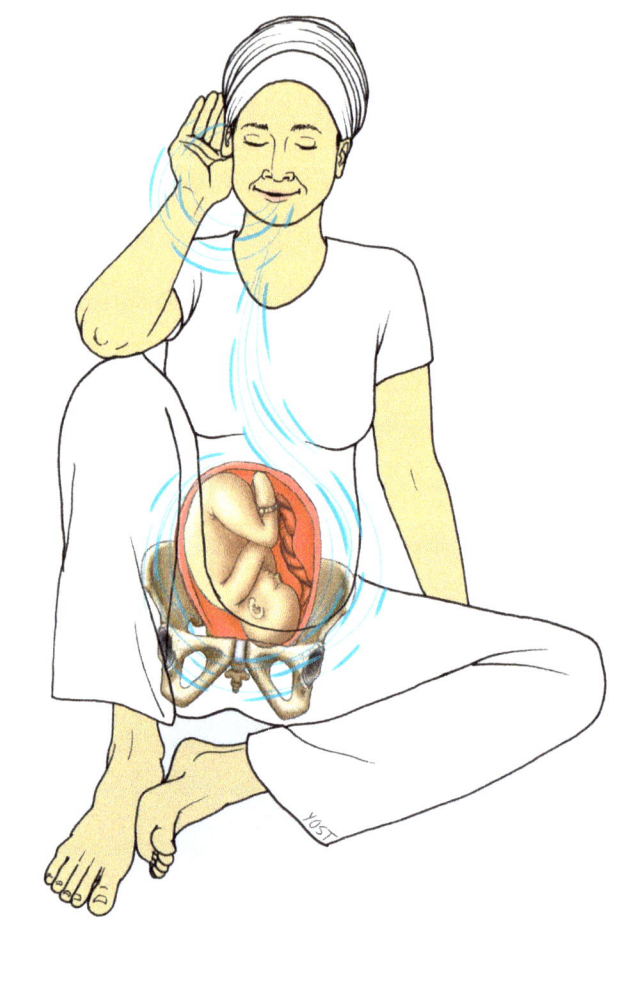

11.2 Pregnancy

During pregnancy, a woman has the capacity to connect with the being in her uterus and to help it transform and release karmas before it is even born.

The Original Scar

In Ayurveda it is believed that at the moment of conception, your parents' genetic constitutions met and created a specific and unique new identity and constitution that is you (Lad, 2009). The egg and sperm merged, and your destiny, body type, and genes rolled into the blueprint for your Physical Body. This blueprint is stored at your Navel Point—four finger widths below the belly button—and is a connection to your source energy. The belly button is the original scar on your body showing your separation from ether and your incarnation into a physical being.

Challenges to the Female Reproductive System

Menstrual Irregularities
There are a variety of ways the menstrual cycle can be challenging including:
- Cycle too long
- Cycle too short
- Excessive bleeding
- Too little bleeding
- Cramps
- Emotional PMS (Premenstrual Syndrome) symptoms

Premenstrual Syndrome (PMS) PMS is difficult for many women to manage because the complexity of the hormonal cycle is usually added to the stress of career and family life. The yogic lifestyle simplifies food choices and creates a regular exercise routine that helps calm the menstrual cycle.

Fertility Issues
What happens when nothing is happening? This can be an especially challenging issue for couples who want to conceive but are unable to for some reason. Yogi Bhajan suggested women struggling with fertility swim every day, relax as much as possible, and drink a special tea of equal portions chamomile, comfrey, and peppermint. But infertility can be incredibly complex. Factors such as a woman's age, past infections or hormonal imbalances can dramatically affect the potential for conception. The health of a man's sperm is also affected by genetic and lifestyle factors.

Pregnancy and All Systems
In pregnancy the womb contains all systems of the developing fetus. Understanding the progression of the fetus gives insight into the subtle relationships between various structures in the body. In weeks 3–8 of pregnancy, three layers of cells form. These three layers of tissue will eventually give rise to all of the structures in the human body.
- **Endoderm:** Internal organs, such as the digestive tract and respiratory pathways
- **Mesoderm:** Connective and structural tissues, such as muscle and bone
- **Ectoderm:** Nervous system and skin

> THE 120TH DAY OF PREGNANCY IS WHEN THE YOGIS SAY THE SOUL ENTERS THE FETUS. THIS ALSO HAPPENS TO BE AROUND THE FIRST TIME A WOMAN TYPICALLY FEELS THE BABY'S FIRST MOVEMENTS WITHIN HER.

> *"Pregnancy is a gift, it's not a guarantee."*
> © The Teachings of Yogi Bhajan, December 4, 1989

Seeing the shared ancestry helps to illuminate the relationships in the fully formed human body. Both the nervous system and the skin, for example, arise from the ectoderm, highlighting the close relationship between physical touch and mental states. It also shows the commonality that makes both the digestive organs and the lungs equal parts of the immune system.

A conscious pregnancy creates a nurturing, safe, and healthy environment for all these systems to develop. This blessing radiates out to future generations.

Japa's Fertility Story

For seven years my husband and I tried to have children. As a woman, it was very painful to me that I could not get pregnant. I felt labeled by my diagnosis of unexplained infertility. It was frustrating to me that everyone kept telling me to relax. I desperately wanted a child and was trying everything I could to facilitate that process. Really, I tried everything!

Finally I realized that this was a process of completely letting go and trusting God. I knew it was my destiny to have a child, either through my body or someone else's. After seven years, my husband and I decided to pursue adoption. We made the commitment, told all of our friends, and started praying. Miraculously, within two weeks, we got a phone call about a baby boy. Within six weeks we held our ten-month-old baby in our arms. It was a startlingly fast adoption process, and I believe it was through the accumulated prayers of our community and our surrender that he came to us so quickly.

The Male Reproductive System

Testes are the male reproductive gland; they parallel the ovaries in the female system and are also paired. Beginning in puberty and for the rest of a man's life, the testicles make sperm and testosterone on a daily basis. Similar to the female system, the testicles rely on a complex interplay of hormones to produce sperm. Sperm is the only human cell with flagella (a tail) which is what propels the sperm forward to meet the egg. The head of the sperm contains enzymes to help penetrate the egg and it contains 23 chromosomes (½ of the DNA code). Sperm is produced and stored in the testicles. Their position, outside of the body, is more vulnerable but it allows the sperm to remain cool, which is important for its viability.

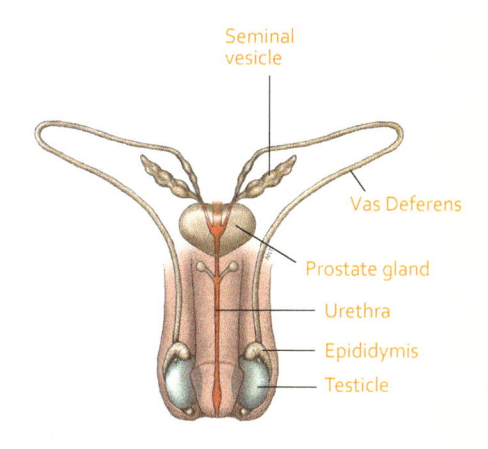

The Penis is the male's primary sexual organ and also contains the end of the urethra. It is used during sexual reproduction as a passage way for sperm. Urine is also released through the urethra.

Prostate Gland An important reproductive structure inside the male body is the prostate gland. This gland is responsible for vital enzymes and fluids that help the sperm survive in the acidic environment of the vagina and enter the uterus.

Challenges to the Male Reproductive System

Males' difficulty with sperm health can negatively influence conception. Diet, lifestyle factors and prior drug use can create sperm with less motility and function. In sexuality, men can have difficulty maintaining an erection for many reasons. The ability to get and maintain an erection is both voluntary and involuntary, and is heavily influenced by the health of the nervous system and other factors. Prostate health is another concern for men, especially as they age. When the prostate becomes enlarged it can interfere with normal urination.

11.3 Male Reproductive System
The male reproductive organs are more exterior than their female counterparts.

IF THE OVARIES AND UTERUS DROPPED OUT OF THE BODY THEY WOULD RESEMBLE THE TESTICLES AND PENIS. IN FACT, IN UTERO THE MALE AND FEMALE GENITALIA START AS THE SAME STRUCTURES.

SUBTLE ANATOMY PERSPECTIVE

Humanology

When teaching about Humanology—the lifestyle components of Kundalini Yoga—Yogi Bhajan would refer to men and women as being different species. He would talk about the innate differences in function, capacity, and roles for men and women. These teachings fit in with new findings about the brain, roles of hormones, and other physiological differences between the sexes. It's not as simple as one sex being better than the other. It's just that women and men *are* quite different. Humanology teachings do not create rigid roles or force limitations on either gender, instead they create a basis for understanding gender differences.

Further, everyone has both masculine and feminine energy within them. Someone who is genetically and anatomically identified as a woman may express 30 percent female energy or 90 percent female energy; it varies according to each individual. Understanding the Humanology teachings as a way to identify and work with the energies within us makes it a broad and applicable philosophy regardless of anatomical sex or gender identity.

Kundalini Yoga's Humanology Teachings in a Nutshell

Yogi Bhajan used the term 'Humanology' to encompass his teachings on lifestyles and lifecycles, relationships, communication, prosperity and success. In short, Humanology is the study of being human. Kundalini Yoga, sometimes referred to as the Yoga of Awareness, can be used as a tool for discovering what it means to be human because it brings you into a deep state of self-awareness (Bhajan, 2010).

These polarities exist within everyone but will be expressed in different ways in different people. They may play out within the structure of a heterosexual, traditional gender-roles marriage, or they may be expressed in the internal relationship of the divine masculine or feminine within, or the natural polarity that exists in any couple, regardless of sex or gender.

The Reproductive System

Subtle Qualities of the Masculine and Feminine Polarities

Masculine
- Direct
- Authoritative
- Fire
- Power
- Building
- Sun Energy
- Explosive
- Penetrating
- Zig zag

Feminine
- Indirect
- Cooperative
- Water
- Restoring
- Nurturing
- Moon Energy
- Sustainable
- Introspective
- Circular or Oval

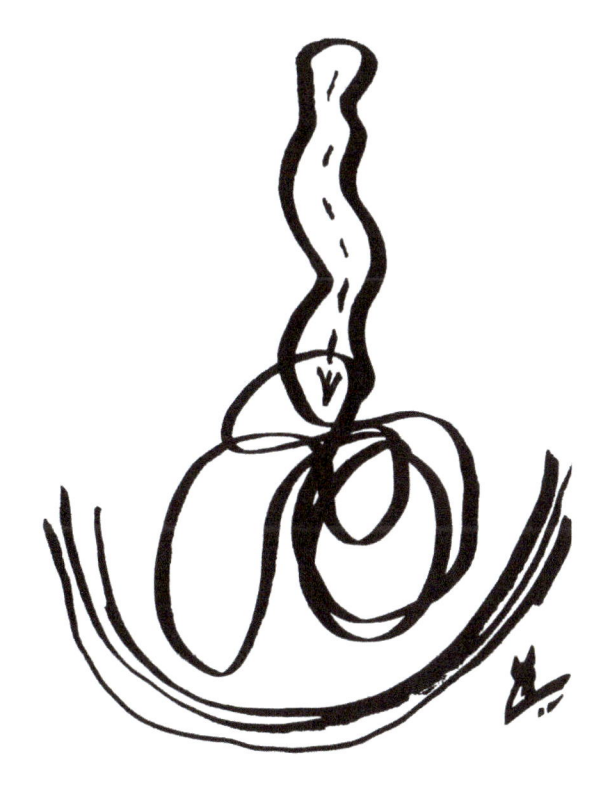

"A male spermatozoa is zig zag and the egg is oval. So geometrically there are two figures, which join together, the zig zag speeding head arrow is spermatozoa and the oval egg which moves. It's not round. So those two figures in faculty creates the human life and you work it out. Look at your life, either your life is zig zag or it is oval."

© The Teachings of Yogi Bhajan, December 20, 1994

11.4 Yogi Bhajan's Illustration
A representation of the male and female energies

Exploring Physical and Subtle Human Anatomy

The Sacral Chakra

The Second Chakra is the energy center associated with the organs of reproduction. It is located about the level of the sacrum. The Sacral Chakra has the powerful capacity to influence the exchange of energy with others. This energy can be directed toward sexual pursuits, spiritual awakening, or creating a life of substance. Kundalini Yoga postures and exercises target the Second Chakra in a unique way. The repetitive and sometimes quick nature of the exercises stimulates the Second Chakra by tapping into a movement pattern similar to that of sexual intercourse. This differs from other styles of yoga because instead of long, slow, or fluid movements, Kundalini Yoga repeats short, quick movements for extended periods of time. The repetitive motion is like the invigorating nature of a percussive massage compared to the soothing nature of long, slow massage strokes.

Japa's Spinal Flex Story

The first time I went to a Kundalini Yoga class, there was a female teacher demonstrating Spinal Flex. It was so clearly sexual in nature that my puritanical side was shocked. A part of me felt like she shouldn't be doing this in public. Over time I've come to appreciate how the sexual appearance of spinal flex is about tapping into the creative potential of the Sacral Chakra.

The Sacral Chakra is often neglected unless it is for personal hygiene or sexual stimulation. In our culture there is very little relationship with the genitals outside of sexuality. Practicing a yoga exercise that brings focus to the reproductive organs creates a new relationship with the Second Chakra and its energies. The Second Chakra is naturally about connection and expansion; awakening the Second Chakra allows for the opportunity to connect with the divine. This creates a doorway for the rest of the body to experience expanded consciousness and have a relationship with the divine energy.

There is a polarity in some cultures around sexuality. It can range from a complete shutdown and shaming around sexual expression to a complete focus on sexuality that reaches the point of obsession. The Second Chakra can hold cellular memories that revolve around deep issues of shame, fear of

The Ethics of Touch

Trauma and confusion around touch and sexuality is one reason Kundalini Yoga teachers refrain from touching or adjusting students during classes. The student must be allowed to have their own space to heal and transform. Yoga teachers may not know the emotional history of the students in their classes, and it is important to create a safe and comfortable space for the students to go through their process. A student can have a powerful experience without the risk of being triggered by touch, sexuality, or intimacy.

---

abandonment, or confusion around sex and sexuality. The practice of yoga and meditation creates a safe and neutral way to access and begin to heal these shadows without putting ourselves or other people at risk.

Activation of the Second Chakra through yoga postures encourages a healthy connection with both divine and sexual energy. Creating meaningful, passionate and authentic sexual and personal relationships starts with a healthy Second Chakra. It is a continuous practice to put that connection with divine energy first. In order to have a healthy relationship with the self, first cultivate a healthy relationship with the divine.

Celibacy and the Spiritual Path

Some spiritual traditions advocate complete celibacy. While this can certainly be a legitimate practice, it is not the suggested lifestyle in Kundalini Yoga as taught by Yogi Bhajan®; instead we practice a "householder" lifestyle, which means having meaningful work in the world and a family life at home. Partnership is encouraged so that trust and consciousness can be developed in a mutual experience of ecstasy. When approached with intention and clarity, sex can be both awakening and just plain fun.

Although at times, abstaining from sex can be used to support health in the reproductive system. Some dietary remedies for male potency, for instance, may ask the man to refrain from sex before and after the diet or cleanse. Allowing the reproductive system time to rest and repair, especially when it is facing some kind of imbalance or crisis, may call for occasional abstinence.

> *"Any such sex act, which is creatively controlled by your own psychological rhythm, will give you more energy, more expansion."*
>
> © The Teachings of Yogi Bhajan, November 12, 1993

> SACRED SEX DOES NOT MEAN BORING VANILLA; IT MEANS AN EXPERIENCE OF EXPANSION THAT CONNECTS YOU WITH YOUR DIVINE TRUTH AND INNERMOST NATURE.

Ojas

Ojas is the primal fluid of life. It slows the aging process, lubricates the spine, prevents the graying of hair, and loss of teeth. Plentiful *ojas* helps to maintain the health of the reproductive organs and glands and is essential for one's quality of life and longevity.

For men *ojas* is exemplified in the sperm. Men lose *ojas* during sex, which means a loss of *praana* and life force through the seminal fluid. In a committed relationship, the woman's strong Arcline and Aura help buffer a man from the impact of his lost *ojas*. If they are conceiving a child, then he is giving his *ojas* to her to build a life together.

The capacities to create a child and produce milk are products of a woman's *ojas*. These creative processes require a lot of energy. For women, the relationship with *ojas* is the inverse of a man's. Her *ojas* is increased during sexual intercourse. Healthy sexuality moves her energy and opens her connection to the divine. Women, of course, do have the possibility of becoming pregnant with sexual intercourse. And women assume an enormous outpouring of *ojas*, energy, life force, and physical risk when they carry a pregnancy to term. For women, practicing sexual restraint was originally about decreasing the opportunities for pregnancy and allowing for conscious and purposeful conception.

Sex is considered beneficial for both men and women because of its relaxing qualities. In the yogic tradition, it is considered to be beneficial to be discriminating in your choice of sexual partners. Within a committed relationship all sexual acts that both parties enjoy and agree to are encouraged (Khalsa, 1998).

The Reproductive System and the Arclines

Sexual union is the closest experience we humans have to connecting with the divine. When approached with sacredness the merging of masculine and feminine energies during sex can be a moment of release, awe and transformation. This merging happens regardless of the sex or gender of the participants. The world of sexuality and play is vast and creative, and when each partner is treated with reverence and respect, it allows for the subtle anatomy of the body to be supported and nurtured.

"Sex is given to you for longevity. If sex does not produce longevity, it will produce destruction, it will produce disease."

© The Teachings of Yogi Bhajan, September 20, 1989

The Reproductive System

Because of the secretions of the pineal and pituitary glands that occur during lovemaking, a person can appear to glow after sex. This glow is the unseen subtle anatomy of the Arcline or halo that exists over and around the head from ear to ear. It is enhanced through meditation, service, pure, devotional love and sex. Every sexual encounter leaves an imprint on a woman's Arcline. Besides the physical fact that women have breasts, they also have a subtle anatomy feature at the heart center—the Arcline from nipple to nipple (Bhajan, 2010). A woman is equipped with this extra Arcline to allow her to hold the space for creating and nurturing the next generation. The protection of the second Arcline allows her to access deep wells of compassion, love, and service. This Arcline also holds the memory of past loves and sexual relationships (Khalsa, 2007).

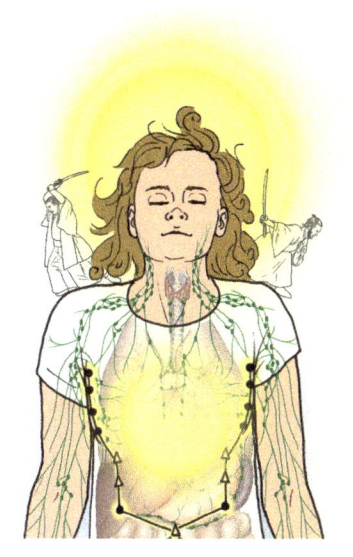

11.5 The Arclines

Breast Health and the Arcline

Breasts are an important secondary sex characteristic for women and are mirrored by the subtle anatomy of the Arcline. Breasts have a role in feeding children, if the woman chooses to have any, and the Arcline represents the vast potential of a woman to create healing, compassionate communities and families.

The lifestyle of Kundalini Yoga helps to clear the baggage of previous sexual encounters. Practices like cold showers, drinking the detoxifying spices in Yogi Tea, and vigorous yoga kriyas all help to clear the breasts, lymphatic fluid, and Arcline and contribute to a woman's health.

The Reproductive System and the Subtle Body

The Subtle Body is the Light Body connected to the reproductive system because of its capacity to exist beyond space and time, and to leave a legacy. The Subtle Body carries the soul to the heavens at the time of death. While alive, it allows for the experience of mastery and calmness when nurtured with a steady spiritual discipline. The Subtle Body shows its power in silence and the ability to communicate without speaking. When a married couple have been together for many years, sometimes just a look or a nod can be all the communication that's needed to tell the other person what is happening.

> WHEN THE SUBTLE BODY IS STRONG, YOU DON'T HAVE TO SAY A LOT BECAUSE YOUR PRESENCE CONVEYS ALL.

TIPS AND TECHNIQUES FOR A STRONG REPRODUCTIVE SYSTEM

The amount of creative change that the reproductive system is capable of requires extra nurturing and care to stay healthy. When your reproductive system is strong and supported you feel expansive, creative, and potent. We are able to create meaningful relationships and feel like we are living for a purpose. It is perhaps not an understatement to say that a strong reproductive system, as the foundation of your creative potential, allows you to leave a lasting impact on the world.

Aasanas and Exercises

Exercises that exert pressure on the sexual organs bring blood flow and energy, and are cleansing and rejuvenating for the Second Chakra
Examples: Spinal Flex, Locust Pose, Sat Kriya
Pelvic floor exercises build strength in the muscles that support reproductive organs.
Examples: Crow Squats, Butterfly Pose, Root Lock

Transformational Energy Points

Conception Vessel 4: Life Gate

Location: Three finger widths below the belly button

Effects: Source of profound transformation. Uncovers deep inner strength and peace. Balances masculine and feminine energy.

Yoga for this Point: Bow Pose, Locust, Camel, Sat Kriya, Stretch Pose

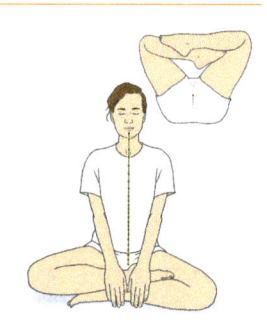

Yoga Restrictions during Pregnancy

During pregnancy, do not put additional stress or excessive heat into the belly. Because of pregnancy hormones the ligaments around the low back and pelvis are especially susceptible to overstretching or injury. Once stretched these ligaments do not generally return to their proper length. This can lead to low back problems after the pregnancy. Inverted or upside-down postures should also be avoided to keep energy centered in the uterus.

Postures and Exercises to Avoid During Pregnancy
- Breath of Fire
- Root Lock
- Anything pumping the navel
- Anything lying flat on the belly
- Anything with a hyper-extended (sway) back
- Twists focusing on the lower back
- Inversions (Shoulder Stand and Plow Pose)
- Anything that gets heart rate above 130 bpm
- Avoid lying flat on the back; especially after the first trimester, when the weight of the pregnant uterus slows the return of blood to the heart and reduces blood flow to the fetus.

RECIPES TO SUPPORT THE REPRODUCTIVE SYSTEM

DATE AND SESAME MILK

Increases Kapha, reduces Vata (heavy, sweet), reduces Pitta (sweet).

- ✓ 1 ⅔ (420 ml) cup of milk (cow, almond, or your preference)
- ✓ 2–3 tablespoons (30-45 ml) of sesame seeds
- ✓ A thumb (2 cm) of ginger

Sweetener: maple syrup, honey or a few dates, pits removed

Blend all of these ingredients and heat the drink if preferred warm.

(Khalsa, Y. 2008)

OTHER HEALING FOODS AND HERBS FOR THE REPRODUCTIVE SYSTEM

For Men

- **Food:** figs, saffron, pistachios, dates
- **Herbs:** ginseng

For Women

- **Food:** all fruit, mango pickle, eggplant, raspberry
- **Herbs:** nettle, dang gui, rehmannia

Plants, Herbs, and Food

Sesame Seeds and Sesame Oil Sex creates movement, flow and expansion in the psyche and body, just like a vigorous workout session or yoga series. Plants that create energy for the physical body to produce the sex hormones and circulate them properly are good quality fats like coconut oil, sesame oil, ghee or fresh nuts and seeds. Because of their nourishing and rejuvenating properties, they are linked to reproductive health and quality of life.

The sesame seed has long been touted as an elixir of life. These tiny gems are full of nutrients like copper, magnesium, calcium, and healthy fats. The tiny sesame seed, rich in fatty acids, also supports the cardiovascular system, boosts immunity, reduces inflammation, balances hormones, and nourishes eyes, skin, and hair. A wonderful energy drink can be made with sesame seeds to restore sexual vitality at any time but especially after sex.

Mantra

Ong Namo Guru Dev Namo

Meaning: I call on the subtle divine wisdom, the divine teacher within.

This mantra connects one with the spiritual family of Kundalini Yogis around the world and with the Golden Chain of teachers that have shared this knowledge. It heals the longing to belong.

The Reproductive System

*Ardas Bhaee Amar Das Guru Amar Das Guru Ardas Bhaee.
Ram Das Guru Ram Das Guru Ram Das Guru Sachee Sahee*

Meaning: All prayers and miracles will be heard and answered.
This is a special mantra that allows for healings, blessings, and completion.

Balance the Sacral Chakra

When the Sacral Chakra is out of balance you may experience addictions (to sex, drugs, alcohol, shopping, etc.). You may also feel depressed, frustrated creatively, stuck in life, and judgmental of others. Some people with Sacral Chakra imbalance suffer chronic yeast infections.

To Balance the Sacral Chakra
- Wear Orange
- Wear or meditate with a Carnelian stone
- Do Frog Squats
- Dance
- Enjoy a healthy sex life!

Affirmations for the Sacral Eye
I bask in the pleasures of life. I glow with the ecstasy of my beautiful body and the integrity of my soul. I create beauty, meaning, and joy.

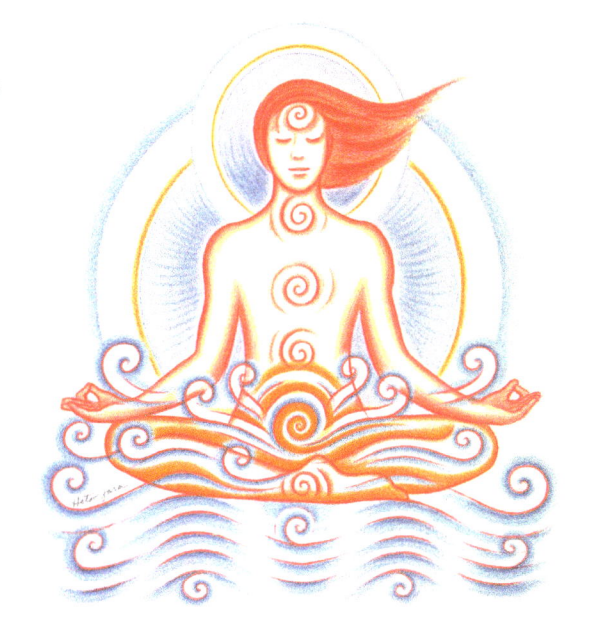

Exploring Physical and Subtle Human Anatomy

APPENDICES

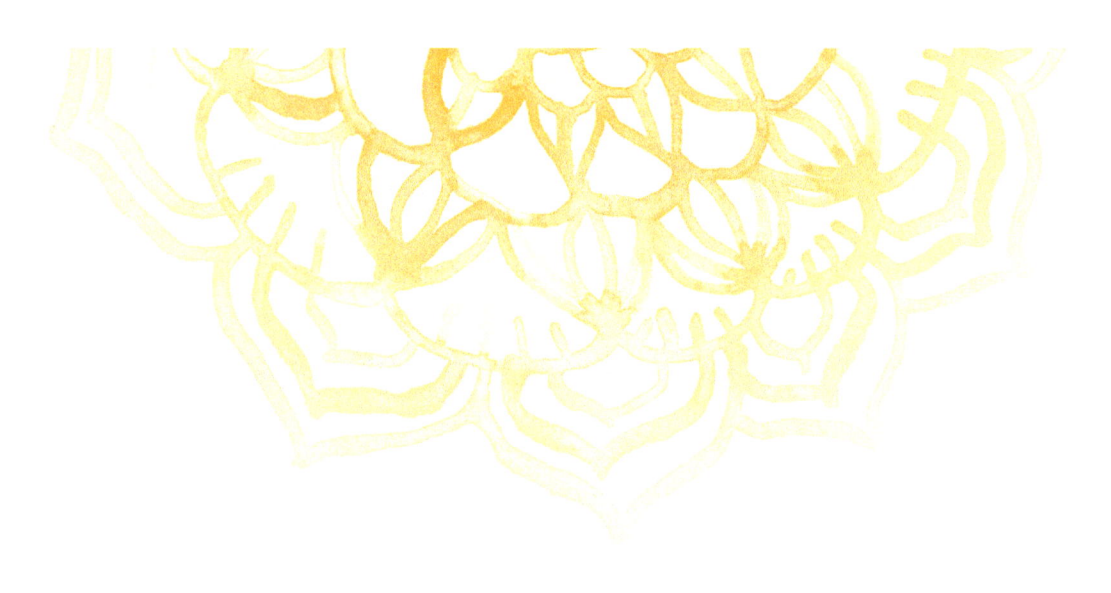

Before You Begin

Beginning Your Practice–Tuning-In

The practice of Kundalini Yoga as taught by Yogi Bhajan® always begins by tuning-in. This simple practice of chanting the Adi Mantra 3-5 times aligns your mind, your spirit and your body to become alert and assert your will so that your practice will fulfill its intention. It's a simple bowing to your Higher Self and an alignment with the teacher within. The mantra may be simple but it links you to a Golden Chain of teachers, an entire body of consciousness that guides and protects your practice: ***Ong Namo Guroo Dayv Namo,*** which means, ***I bow to the Infinite, I bow to the Teacher within***.

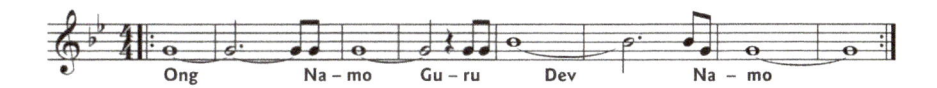

[Musical notation: Ong Na-mo Gu-ru Dev Na-mo]

How to End

Another tradition within Kundalini Yoga as taught by Yogi Bhajan® is a simple blessing known as *The Long Time Sun Shine* song. Sung or simply recited at the end of your practice, it allows you to dedicate your practice to all those who've preserved and delivered these teachings so that you might have the experience of your Self. It is a simple prayer to bless yourself and others. It completes the practice and allows your entire discipline to become a prayer, in service to the good of all.

> *May the long time sun shine upon you*
> *All love surround you*
> *And the pure light within you*
> *Guide your way on.*
> *Sat Nam.*

Other Tips for a Successful Experience

Prepare for your practice by lining up all the elements that will elevate your experience: natural fiber clothing and head covering (cotton or linen), preferably white to increase your auric body; natural fiber mat, either cotton or wool; traditionally a sheep skin or other animal skin is used. If you have to use a rubber or petroleum-based mat, cover the surface with a cotton or wool blanket to protect and support your electromagnetic field. Clean air and fresh water also helps support your practice.

Practice in Community

Studying the science of Kundalini Yoga with a KRI certified teacher will enhance your experience and deepen your understanding of kriya, mantra, breath and posture. Find a teacher in your area at http://www.3HO.org/ikyta/. If there isn't a teacher in your area, consider becoming a teacher yourself. There are Aquarian Teacher Trainings all over the world. Go to www.kundaliniresearchinstitute.org for more information.

Breath & Bandhas

Kundalini Yoga incorporates profound praanayams throughout its practice. Understanding and mastering the breath is an important part of successfully practicing any Kundalini Yoga kriya. We have provided the descriptions of three of the most basic praanayams in the practice of Kundalini Yoga but as you work through the meditations and kriyas in the 21 Stages of Meditation, please read the instructions for the breath carefully.

Long Deep Breath

To take a full yogic breath, inhale by first relaxing the abdomen and allow it to expand. Next expand the chest and finally the collarbones. As you exhale, let the collar bones and chest relax first, then pull the abdomen in completely.

The diaphragm drops down to expand the lungs on the inhale and contracts up to expel the air on the exhale.

As you inhale feel the back area of the lower ribs relax and expand. On the exhale be sure to keep the spine erect and steady.

Breath of Fire

This breath is used consistently throughout Kundalini Yoga kriyas. It is very important that Breath of Fire be practiced and mastered. In Breath of Fire, the focus of the energy is at the solar plexus and navel point. The breath is fairly rapid (approximately 2 breaths per second), continuous and powerful with no pause between the inhale and exhale. This is a very balanced breath with no emphasis on either the exhale or the inhale, but rather equal power given to both.

Breath of Fire is a cleansing breath, renewing the blood and releasing old toxins from the lungs, mucous lining, blood vessels, and cells. It is a powerful way to adjust your autonomic nervous system and get rid of stress. Regular practice expands the lungs quickly. See the Appendix for more complete directions on this powerful praanayam.

Cannon Breath

Cannon Breath is a powerful continuous and equal inhalation and exhalation through the mouth, similar to Breath of Fire, but through rounded lips instead of through the nose. Very cleansing, this breath is invigorating, energizing and rejuvenating.

To consolidate the energy at the end of a kriya, many will call for a Cannon Fire exhale, which means we suspend the breath on the inhale and then use a single strong exhale through the mouth like a Cannon.

Bandhas

Bandhas or locks are used frequently in Kundalini Yoga. Combinations of muscle contractions, each lock has the function of changing blood circulation, nerve pressure, and the flow of cerebral spinal fluid. They also direct the flow of psychic energy, *praana*, into the main energy channels that relate to raising the Kundalini energy. They concentrate the body's energy for use in consciousness and self-healing. There are three important locks: *jalandhar bandh, uddiyana bandh,* and *mulbandh*. When all three locks are applied simultaneously, it is called maahaabandh, the Great Lock.

Jalandhar Bandh or Neck Lock

The most basic lock used in Kundalini Yoga is *jalandhar bandh,* the neck lock. This lock is practiced by gently stretching the back of the neck straight and pulling the chin toward the back of the neck. Lift the chest and sternum and keep the muscles of the neck and throat and face relaxed.

Uddiyana Bandh or Diaphragm Lock

Applied by lifting the diaphragm up high into the thorax and pulling the upper abdominal muscles back toward the spine, *uddiyana bandh* gently massages the intestines and the heart muscle. The spine should be straight and it is most often applied on the exhale.

Applied forcefully on the inhale, it can create pressure in the eyes and the heart.

Mulbandh or Root Lock

The Root Lock is the most commonly applied lock but also the most complex. It coordinates and combines the energy of the rectum, sex organs, and navel point.

Mul is the root, base, or source. The first part of the *mulbandh* is to contract the anal sphincter and draw it in and up. Then draw up the sex organ so the urethral tract is contracted. Finally, pull in the navel point by drawing back the lower abdomen towards the spine so the rectum and sex organs are drawn up toward the navel point.

Pronunciation Guide

This simple guide to the vowel sounds in transliteration is for your convenience. Gurbani is a very sophisticated sound system, and there are many other guidelines regarding consonant sounds and other rules of the language that are best conveyed through a direct student-teacher relationship. Further guidelines regarding pronunciation are available at www.kundaliniresearchinstitute.org.

a	hut
aa	mom
u	put, soot
oo	pool
i	fin
ee	feet
ai	let
ay	hay, rain
r	flick tongue on upper palate

Kriya Analysis

One benefit of studying anatomy from both the physical and subtle perspectives is that it brings a depth of understanding to your practice or teaching of Kundalini Yoga kriyas and meditations. Yogi Bhajan was sometimes very explicit about exactly how kriyas would affect the body. In other instances, there is very little information about what is happening behind the scenes. These are the times that you can use your intuition and your practical knowledge to figure out for yourself how or why a particular aasana is affecting the body.

> "We have seventy-two thousand nerve endings, which are controlled by the secretion of the pituitary. The impulsation is directed by the pineal, it is nurtured by the gland system called thyroid, it is strengthened by the two big boxes in the chest called lungs. Its impulse energy is controlled by the kidneys, its back and forth measurement is controlled by the adrenals, and its perpetual strength is controlled by the sexual glands; this is the relationship in this order."
> ©The Teachings of Yogi Bhajan, April 9, 1991

This quote reveals the way that kriyas affect different physical aspects of the human body. Moving through a series of postures or exercises in a specific order creates specific effects on the body and builds a frequency of change in the subtle anatomy.

Just like the human being is magically more than the sum of her parts, a kriya in the Kundalini Yoga tradition, especially when practiced in a group, has a magical depth beyond any list of effects. Remember to view kriyas as a whole and to take into account your own personal experience of the *whole* rather than getting lost in the details of each posture. Practicing kriyas moves us through an intricate pressurization of different muscle groups that connect with the internal organs and help to eliminate inflammation, bring stimulation, or balance the frequency of the interior of the body.

Below are a few examples applying anatomical thinking to kriyas in order to extrapolate additional benefits.

Kriya for Balancing the Chakras and Corresponding Organs

© The Teachings of Yogi Bhajan, July 17, 1984

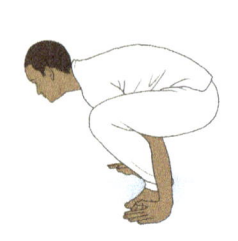

1) Chair Pose with Breath of Fire: Begin in a standing position. Place your feet shoulder-width apart. Squat down so the thighs are parallel to the ground. Reach toward the toes, placing the palms on top of the feet by bringing the hands through the inside of the legs, around to the outside. Be sure to keep the back straight and only lift the head and look forward. Five minutes.

Musculoskeletal: Squatting postures build the muscles of the thighs and Navel Point. This posture also engages Root Lock to protect the low back

Respiratory/Pranic Body: The slight compression of the lung space, plus the Breath of Fire creates an intense pressure which quickly distributes *praana* through the body

Chinese Medicine: Eyes open releases the *Liver* meridian

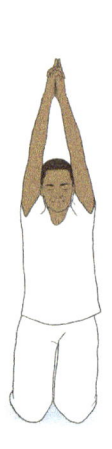

2) Sat Kriya: Sit on the heels and stretch the arms straight over the head so that the elbows hug the ears. Interlock the fingers except the index fingers, which point straight up. Begin to chant Sat Naam emphatically in a constant rhythm about eight times per ten seconds. Chant the sound *Sat* from the Navel Point and solar plexus and pull the navel all the way in and up, toward the spine. On *Naam* relax the belly. Continue very powerfully. To end, inhale and squeeze the muscles tightly from the buttocks all the way up the back, past the shoulders. Five minutes.

Digestive: Navel pull supports peristalsis and moving food through the digestive tract

Lymphatic/Immune: Arms overhead supports lymphatic drainage from the arms.

Drishti: Eye focus stimulates upper glands to secrete

Kriya Analysis

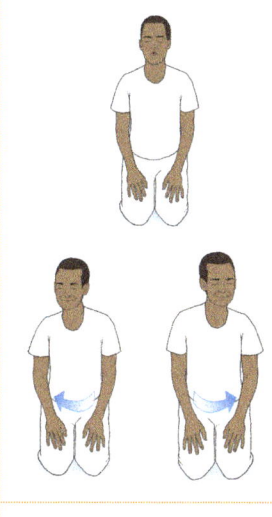

3) Sitting in Rock Pose on your heels, rest the hands on the thighs.
a) Begin Sitali Pranayam, inhaling in short sips through a curled tongue until the lungs are full of air.
b) Rotate the hips around in a circle. Hold the breath and rotate to the left for 1/2 the duration of the held breath. Then hold and rotate to the right for 1/2 the duration of the held breath.
3 times.

Digestive: Rock pose compresses acupuncture points in the legs which support digestion.

Respiratory: Holding the breath in or out can help to build and expanded lung capacity

All Systems: This is an easy posture that disperses the energy and allows for integration of the effects of first two postures

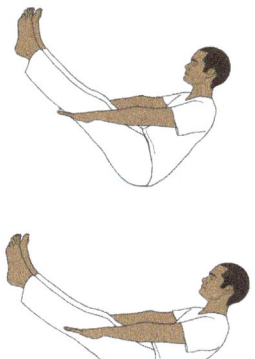

4) In Victory Pose with your feet off the ground at a 60° angle and your torso raised off the ground at a 60° angle
(a), inhale. In a motion like a sit-up, drop the torso and legs down to 45° (b), exhale, and then back up to 60°. 5 minutes. If done properly, this is the equivalent of 8 hours of exercise.

Musculoskeletal: This posture is an intense abdominal strength builder when done correctly.

Lymphatic: The movement at the hip joint massages the lymph nodes in the groin.

Radiant Body: The Radiant Body gets polished by successfully moving through challenging poses.

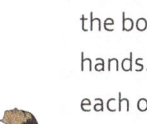

5) Lie on the back and bring the hands to the Navel Point. The left hand is closest to the body and the right hand is over the left. There is about 2 inches between the body and also between the hands. Rotate the hands around each other in a clockwise direction, maintaining the 2-inch separation between the hands, and keeping the hands over the Navel Point. Long deep breathing. 3 minutes.

Aura: By moving the hands in the space around the body you can clear blocks or congested energy areas

Chinese Medicine: Energy flow is faster around the hands and feet and influences change in the interior of the body through meridian entry/end points located on the fingertips.

Exploring Physical and Subtle Human Anatomy

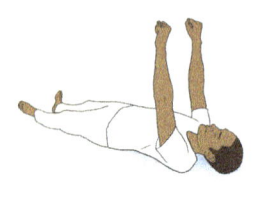

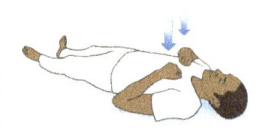

	6) Remain on your back and extend your arms up to 90°, straight above you. Make fists of your hands and with great tension, pull your fists into your chest. Release and repewat 2 more times.	**Circulatory:** Moving the arms with great tension puts a bit of healthy stress on the chest and heart **Lymphatic:** Squeezes lymph fluid from muscle tension, cleansing **Heart Chakra:** This movement can help to activate and clear out stagnate energy
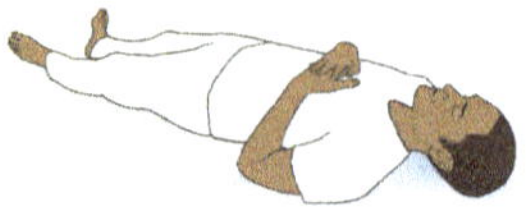	**7) Rest on the back** with the left hand on the heart and the right hand over the left. Long deep breathing—whispering Ham Dam Hari Har. Hari Har Ham Dam. This is the meditation of the celestial angels. God is my breath, breath is my God. 5 minutes.	**Endocrine:** Chanting balances the glands in the brain via the vibrations of the skull **Ether Tattva:** whispering balances this *tattva* **Subtle Body:** all meditation supports the Subtle Body
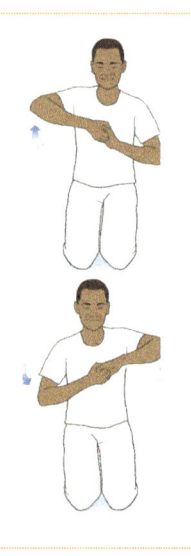	**8) Sitting in Rock Pose**, place hands in Bear Grip. Left palm faces out from the chest with the thumb down. Place the palm of the right hand facing the chest. Bring the fingers together. Curl the fingers of both hands so the hands form a fist, where the fingers of one hand are hooked around the fingers of the other hand. The arms keep a steady pull at the heart. Move your elbows up and down, quickly. 11 minutes.	**Heart Chakra:** The steady pull of the hands creates a healing tension at the heart **Lymphatic:** The rapid movement of the arms supports lymph fluid moving through the nodes in the armpits **Chinese Medicine:** entry point for *Heart* meridian is in the center of armpit
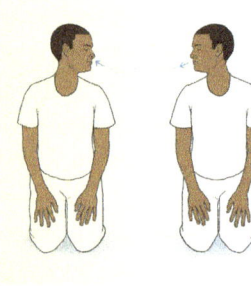	**9) Remain sitting on your heels,** place your palms on your thighs and begin inhaling turning your head to the left, and exhaling turning your head to the right. 3 minutes.	**Lymphatic:** Moving the neck pushes lymph through the nodes **Throat Chakra:** By activating the muscles of the neck you can strengthen the throat chakra **Vagus Nerve:** activates and soothes the vagus nerve

Kriya Analysis

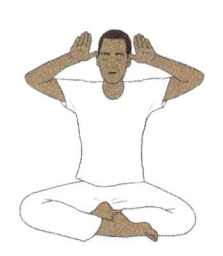

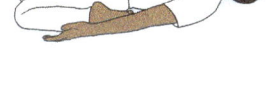

	10) Come sitting in Easy Pose and bring the hands up to the face with the thumbs pressing on the temples. The fingers will be about 2 inches from the face. Roll the eyes up to the Third Eye Point, creating a pressure. Now chant, Har Wahe Guru, Har Sat Nam. This mantra allows you to feel no pain at the time of death. 5 minutes.	**Mind:** There are acupuncture points at the temples that help to soothe the mind, relieve headaches and can help to combat addiction **Drishti:** Eye focus stimulates the Crown Chakra and upper glands
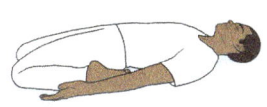	**11) Prepare to sit on your heels** but let your hips rest between your heels, touching the ground. Relax back down on your back with your hands by your sides. Do this as long as possible. Do not do so long that any part of your body falls asleep.	**Musculoskeletal:** This intense posture stretches the psoas muscle, one that is chronically tight on most people. **Urinary System:** tweaks the *Urinary Bladder* Meridian, the longest in the body
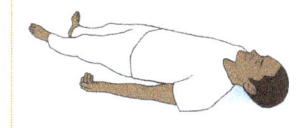	**12) Then relax on the back.** 11-62 minutes.	**Heart Chakra:** Deep relaxation creates a gentle resting time for the heart center. **All Systems:** restores all systems, allows for integration of all subtle and physical changes initiated by Kriya

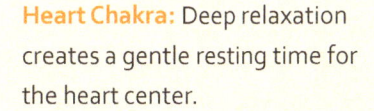

Comments on this kriya: You must stimulate your Navel Point once a day. If you do Breath of Fire, it will cleanse your lungs, make them strong, you will have deep breathing all day, you will have good oxygen in your bloodstream, and you will be young and healthy for a long time. If you do it 5-15 minutes every day, it is the best way to keep the blood purified. It's a direct blood purification system.

Exploring Physical and Subtle Human Anatomy

Body Adjustment to Elevate the Spirit

© The Teachings of Yogi Bhajan, July 2, 1984

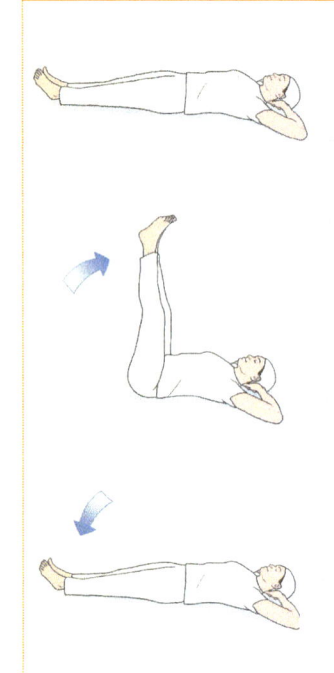

1. Lie down flat on the back with the hands clasped under the neck. Keeping the heels together, raise both legs to 90 degrees as you inhale. Be sure to press your lower back into the floor before and during the lift and lift from the navel. Lower the legs as you exhale. Do not bend the knees. But if you don't have the abdominal strength to keep the legs straight, use your hands to provide leverage for your back by placing them on the floor under your buttocks. You can start with 54 repetitions and, with practice, build up to 108 repetitions.

Musculoskeletal: strengthens the abdominal muscles

Digestive: pressure into the abdomen supports the digestive process.

Immune: Lymph system is flushed in the groin and legs

Chinese Medicine: Important meridian points on legs and feet are cleared through this movement.

Circulatory: Supports venous return to the heart

Kriya Analysis

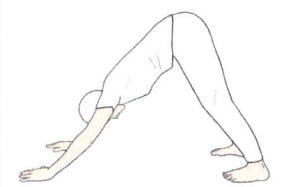

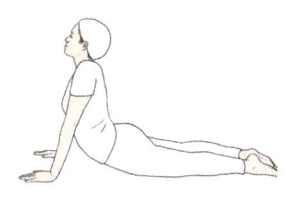

2. Come into Triangle Pose. The palms of the hands and the soles of the feet are on the ground, with the feet about hip-width apart. Create a straight line between your wrists and your hips, and from your hips to your heels. Pull the chin in and elongate the back of the neck. Roll the armpits toward each other. Smoothly begin to move the body into Cobra Pose. In Cobra Pose your palms are flat on the ground and your body is arched up through the upper back. The feet are together. The shoulders are pressed down and the neck is long. Move smoothly from Triangle to Cobra to Triangle, etc. Do not bend the knees. Keep the arms straight if you have sufficient strength and flexibility, otherwise you may keep the arms bent with the elbows in toward the sides of the body. You can start with 21 repetitions and build up to 52 repetitions with practice.

Nervous: These postures create a safe stretch for all of the tissues around the nerves in the body, helping the nerves to fire more efficiently. Also the shifting of the torso from upside down to right side up helps to flush the cerebrospinal fluid around the brain and spinal cord.

Chinese Medicine: Stretches all meridians on arms, legs, and back

Musculoskeletal: Builds significant arm strength

Earth *Tattva*: Challenging physical posture is grounding and strengthens this *tattva*

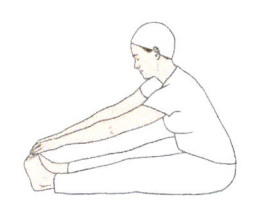

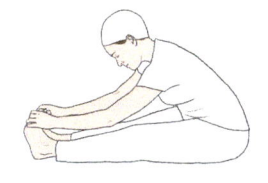

3. Sit with your legs straight out in front of you. Flex the feet and engage the leg muscles as you reach forward from the navel and grab on to your toes (or as far down your legs as you can reach). Inhale in this position, and exhale as you lengthen the spine and bend farther forward. The head stays in line with the spine. Try to get the belly to the thighs rather than the head to the knees. Move up and down, inhaling up, exhaling down. Repeat 108 times.

Musculoskeletal: Stretches the hamstrings, a chronically tight area for many people.

Life Nerve: Stretches the sciatic nerve and urinary *Bladder* meridian

Exploring Physical and Subtle Human Anatomy

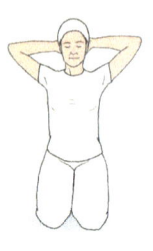

4. Sit in Rock Pose* and interlace the fingers behind the neck. Twist the torso and head to the left and right. Repeat 108 times to each side.

Lymphatic/Immune: Twisting postures help to move the lymph fluid through the lymph vessels and nodes.

Aura: This vigorous movement creates a flushing action for the aura, moving out old stagnant energy

Chinese Medicine: activates and flushes the *Spleen* through a meridian point beneath the armpit

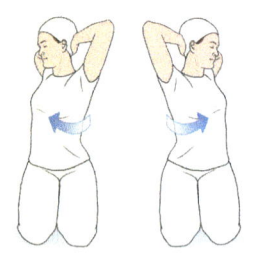

5. Come onto your hands and knees. Relax the spine down and raise the head up on the inhalation (Cow Pose). Open the heart and raise the chin up without scrunching the back of the neck. On the exhalation, arch the spine up and lower the head (Cat Pose). Move steadily and smoothly between the two positions; follow the breath. Repeat 108 times.

Musculoskeletal: This is a complete movement for the spine; it helps keep all segments relaxed and mobile

Chinese Medicine: tweaks all the organs through the Shu points, located above the paraspinal muscles

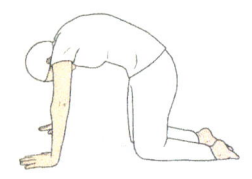

6. Come into Rock Pose and roll the head around on the neck rapidly in one direction 52 times, and then in the opposite direction 52 times.

Lymphatic/Immune: Moving the head pressurizes the lymph nodes in the neck

Digestive: Compresses *Stomach* meridian in leg

Throat Chakra: promotes energy flow

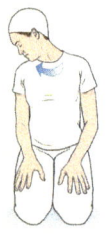

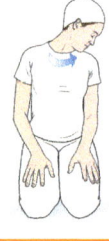

Kriya Analysis

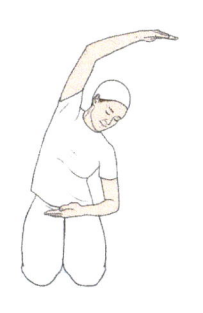

7. Still in Rock Pose, bend at the waist from side to side. As you bend to the left, your right arm will arch over your head, stretching in the direction of the bend. Then stretch to the right with your left arm reaching over your head. Repeat 52 times to each side.

Yogi Bhajan's Notes: This exercise is for the liver, spleen, and colon and to eliminate gas

Liver: Side bends pressurize the liver, helping move blood through the organ and support its role of detoxifying, clearing hormones, and balancing the blood.

Fire *Tattva*: Still in Rock Pose, this posture balances digestive fire by compressing and slowing blood flow in legs, pressing on digestive meridians and allows for blood to pool in torso

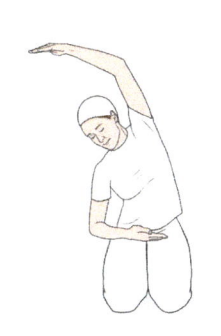

8. Remain in Rock Pose and reach one arm forward as if reaching out and grabbing energy. Then pull it back in, while reaching forward with the other arm. The movement is rapid and fluid. The shoulders and trunk move slightly in a churning motion. Chant *Sa* as one arm reaches forward, *Ta* as you pull that arm back and the other arm reaches forward, *Na* as the first arm reaches forward again, and *Ma* as the second arm reaches forward again. Continue for 5 minutes.

Lymphatic System: Pushes lymph fluid and cleanses chest area

All *Tattvas*: Physical movement coordinated with breath and *Bij* mantra balances all *tattvas*

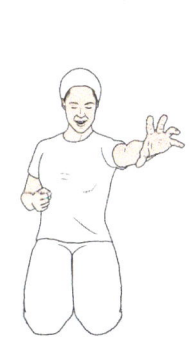

Exploring Physical and Subtle Human Anatomy

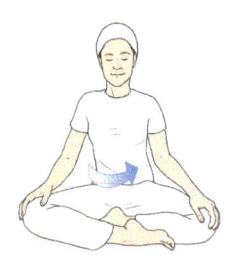

	9. Sit in Easy Pose with your hands on your knees. Begin grinding your trunk in a circular motion, in a counter-clockwise direction. Continue for 3 minutes.	**Digestive:** Churning motion of the torso supports moving food through digestive tract **Spine:** Gentle motion of the spine helps to release blocks or muscle tightness **All systems:** gentle posture allows for integration of changes from previous postures
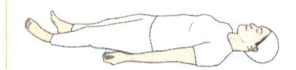	**10. Lie down flat on your back.** Close your eyes and relax to the sound of the gong. Continue for 10 minutes. Get ready for a journey into your inner self and float in space. You will gain a tremendous amount of energy.	**Endocrine:** Deep relaxation as a counterpoint to vigorous exercise allows the glands to feel refreshed **Lymphatic/Immune:** Full body rest give the immune cells an opportunity to coordinate and creates the most efficient immune response

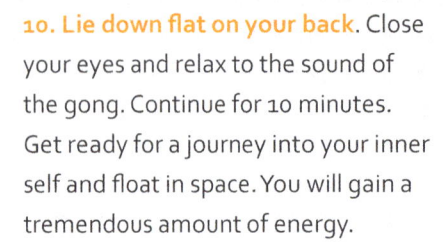

Comments from Yogi Bhajan on this kriya: This set will keep you out of trouble. This is how you can elevate your spirit by adjusting your body. This kriya has been published in the KRI manual ***Fountain of Youth.***

Meditations for the Nervous System

Meditation for Release of Cold Depression
As taught by Yogi Bhajan, December 17, 2000

Interlace your fingers so that the fingertips press into the cavities between fingers on the back of each hand. The index fingers are straight up, pressed together along their length. Thumbs cross each other comfortably. Hands are held at chest level. Eyes are open and focused at the tip of the nose.

Play the CD, *Wahe Guru, Wahe Jio*, by Sangeet Kaur. (This is the same version on the *Raag Sadhana* CD). Chant the mantra from your Navel Point, creating a mental focus in this way:

At the sound of *WHAA*, focus at the Navel Point
HAY, focus at the chest
GUROO, focus at the lips
Continue for 3–31 minutes.

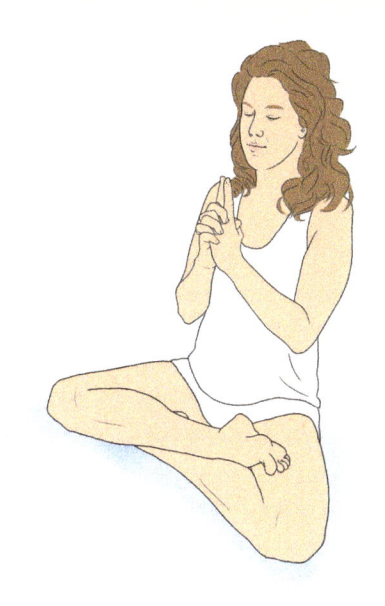

To end, inhale and hold. Listen to the sound of the mantra. Exhale. Then inhale again, hold, and give all the cold depression to God. Exhale. One last time, inhale, hold, and feel the preciousness of life. Let it go through your exhalation, so that at the end of life, you may give it with ease. Relax.

Fountain of Youth and in Aquarian Times, July 2006.

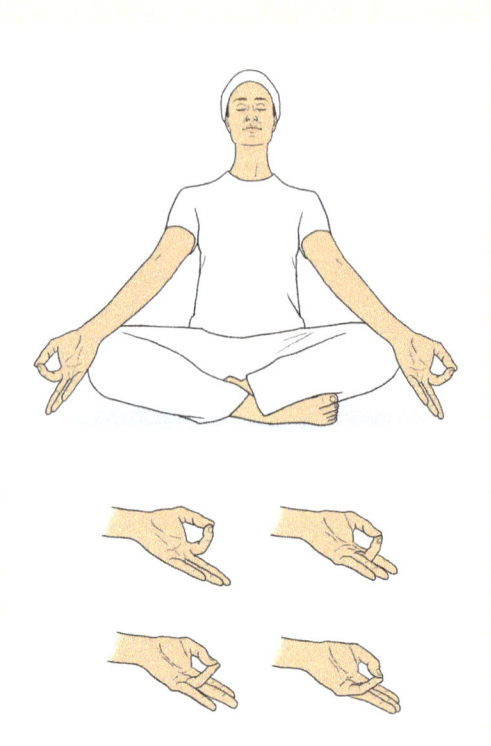

Kirtan Kriya

Sit straight in Easy Pose.

Eyes: Meditate at the Brow Point.

Mantra: Produce the five primal sounds (panj shabd):
S, T, N, M, A, in the original word form:
SAA: Infinity, cosmos, beginning
TAA: Life, existence
NAA: Death, change, transformation
MAA: Rebirth

Each repetition of the entire mantra takes 3 to 4 seconds. This is the cycle of Creation. From the Infinite comes life and individual existence. From life comes death or change. From death comes the rebirth of consciousnes to the joy of the Infinite through which compassion leads back to life.

Mudra: This mantra can be done in many different mudras. Most common is to begin in Gyan Mudra. The elbows are straight while chanting, and the mudra changes as each fingertip touches in turn the tip of the thumb with firm pressure.

On SAA, touch the first (Jupiter) finger On TAA, touch the second (Saturn) finger On NAA, touch the third (Sun) finger On MAA, touch the fourth (Mercury) finger.

Voice: Chant in three languages of consicousness: Human: normal or loud voice (the world) Lovers: strong whisper (longing to belong) Divine: mentally; silent (Infinity)

Time: Begin the kriya in a normal voice for 5 minutes; then whisper for 5 minutes; then go deep into the sound, vibrating silently for 10 minutes. Then come back to a whisper for 5 minutes, then aloud for 5 minutes. The duration of the meditation may vary, as long as the proportion of loud, whisper, silent, whisper, loud is maintained.

Meditations for the Nervous System

To End: This sequence will take 30 minutes. Follow with one 1 minute of silence. Then stretch the arms over your head and spreading the fingers wide, shaking them out, circulating the energy, inhaling and exhaling 3 times. Relax.

Comments: Each time the mudra is closed by joining the thumb with a finger, the ego "seals" the effect of that mudra in the consciousness. The effects are as follows: 1st finger: Gyan Mudra Knowledge; 2nd finger: Shuni Mudra Wisdom, intelligence, patience; 3rd finger: Surya Mudra Vitality, energy of life; 4th finger: Buddhi Mudra Ability to communicate. This meditation brings a total mental balance to the individual psyche. Vibrating on each fingertip alternates the electrical polarities. The index and ring fingers are electrically negative, relative to the other fingers. This causes a balance in the electromagnetic projection of the aura.

Practicing this meditation is both a science and an art. It is an art in the way it molds consciousness and in the refinement of sensation and insight it produces. It is a science in the tested certainty of the results each technique produces. Meditations have coded actions to their reactions in the psyche. But because Kirtan Kriya is effective and exact, it can also lead to problems if not done properly. Yogi Bhajan said at Winter Solstice 1972 that a person who wears pure white and meditates on this sound current for 2-1/2 hours a day for one year, will know the unknowable, and see the unseeable. Through this constant practice, the mind awakens to the infinite capacity of the soul for sacrifice, service, and creation.

Checkpoints For Kirtan Kriya: If during the silent part of the meditation, the mind wanders uncontrollably, go back to a whisper, to a loud voice, to a whisper, and back into silence. Do this as often as you need to.

Some people may experience headaches from practicing Kirtan Kriya. The most common reason for this is improper circulation of prana in the solar centers. To avoid or correct this problem, meditate on the primal sounds in the "L" form. This means feel there is a constant inflow of cosmic energy into the solar center, or Tenth Gate. Imagine the energy of each sound moving through the Crown Chakra, and out through the Third Eye Point as it is projected to Infinity. This energy flow follows the energy pathway called the Golden Cord—the connection between the pineal and pituitary glands. You may also want to try covering the head with a natural fiber cloth.

More Helpful Healing Information

Chakras

Name	Location in Physical Body	Positive Energetic/ Emotion	Shadow Emotion/ Imbalanced state	Healing Yoga/ Lifestyle practices
Root (1st)	Tailbone, legs, feet Organs of elimination Digestive System, Urinary System	Security, self-confidence	Scarcity mentality, constipated (in life or actual digestion)	Crow Pose Stand outside barefoot Eat high-fiber diet
Sacral (2nd)	Sacrum, reproductive organs, hips/pelvis Endocrine System	Creativity	Frigid or hyper-sexual, shame	Frogs Dance Enjoy a healthy sex life
Navel (3rd)	Digestive system, abdominal muscles, midback	Power/energy, commitment, ability to follow through	Depression, anger	Stretch Pose Breath of Fire Eat a whole-foods based diet
Heart (4th)	Heart, lungs, ribs, shoulders, arms, thymus gland Circulatory and respiratory systems	Love, compassion, service, forgiveness	Neediness, self-doubt, attachment	Ego Eradicator Serving/volunteering Balanced in both giving and receiving
Throat (5th)	Trachea, esophagus, thyroid, cervical vertebrae, thymus gland Respiratory system	Speaking your truth, Being authentic	Speaking too harshly or afraid to speak up.	Head Rolls Chant Honor your word
Third Eye (6th)	Pituitary gland, brain, forehead, eyes, ears, eyebrows, upper palate, sinuses. Endocrine system	Intuition, insight	Indecisiveness, lack of understanding	Meditate Chant Focus eyes at Third Eye
Crown (7th)	Pineal gland, top of the head, skull, endocrine system	Seat of the soul	Grief, disconnection from God/ community	Focus eyes at crown Chant Listen deeply
Aura (8th)	Surrounding the body, the electromagnetic field Endocrine system	Radiance, protection, act as a magnet to attract souls purpose	Dingy, let in experiences that don't serve your purpose on this planet	Arm swings & pumps Celestial Communication

The Ten Bodies

	Body Name	Main Attribute	Balanced	Weak / Over Strong
1st Body	Soul	The essence of "you," the initiating self	Connected to purpose and destiny, wisdom, leadership	Lost, over-analyze everything, stuck
2nd Body	Negative Mind	Gives discernment and protection	Warns of potential danger, real and imagined	Creates fear, can only see the down side: Debbie Downer
3rd Body	Positive Mind	Opens you to the possibility in every moment	The cheerleader within; rose-colored glasses; encourages healthy risk-taking; supportive	Gullible, head in the sand
4th Body	Neutral Mind	Finds the win-win situation	The meditative mind; exists beyond the polarity of "good" and "bad"; alignment with destiny	Trapped in duality or paralyzed
5th Body	Physical Body	The container for all other light bodies	Embodies strength and courage; teacher aspect	Narcissism and overly concerned with perfection of physical body
6th Body	Arcline	A line of energy that extends over the head from ear to ear; a halo. Women have a second arcline that extends in front of the body from nipple to nipple.	Power of prayer; link arclines to uplift others	Vulnerable, open to other people's misery or sadness. Overwhelmed
7th Body	Aura	Electromagnetic field, divine shield; around the physical body up to nine	If your presence doesn't work, nothing will.	Concerned with controlling or manipulating others, depressed, addicted
8th Body	Pranic	Charging up the energy of the body with the breath	Flexible, able to shift gears between action and relaxation	Shortness of breath, panic that there won't be enough, greediness
9th Body	Subtle	Noticing everything in stillness, creating through the power of subtlety	Mastery through discipline and subtlety; connecting beyond time and space; the power to heal over distance	Overly particular, difficult, finicky, high-maintenance
10th Body	Radiant	What you project out into the world	Clear projection, authentic interactions with the people around you, balanced life, leadership	Black-and-white thinking; my way or the highway, fanatical

Chinese Medicine Concepts

Chinese Medicine Organ Clock

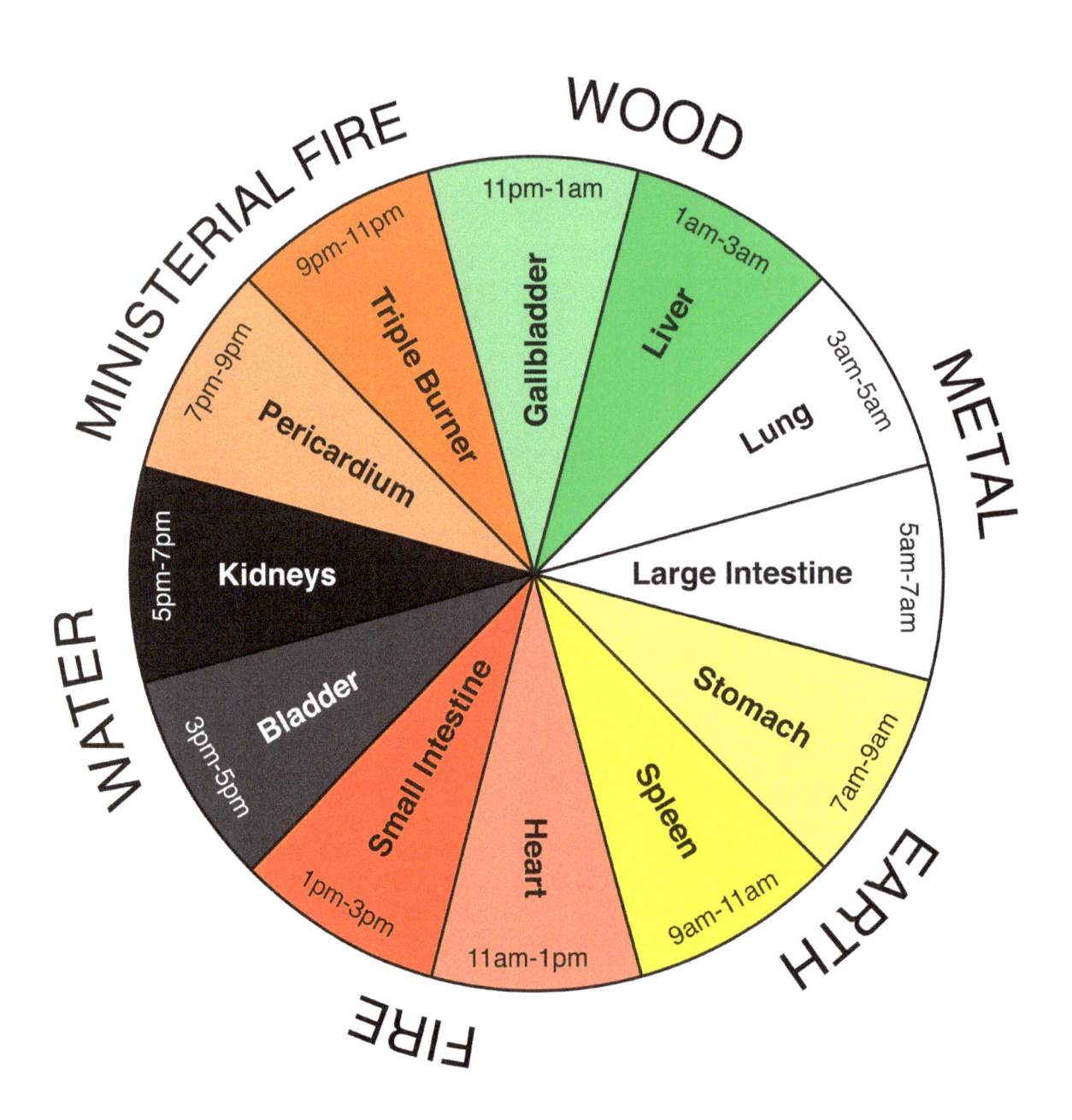

Chinese Medicine Concepts

The Five Elements or Phases in Chinese Medicine

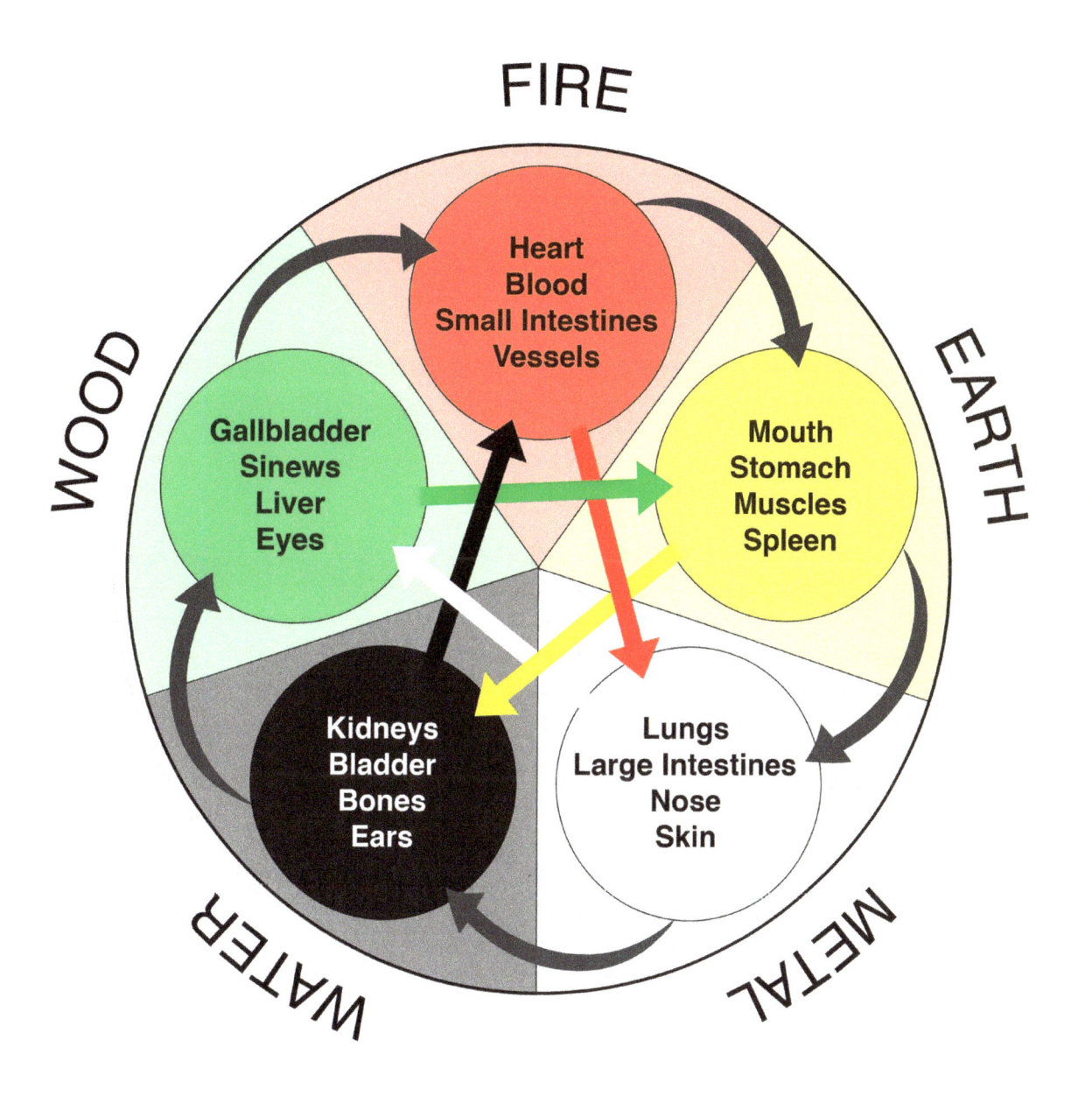

FIRE
- Heart
- Blood
- Small Intestines
- Vessels

EARTH
- Mouth
- Stomach
- Muscles
- Spleen

METAL
- Lungs
- Large Intestines
- Nose
- Skin

WATER
- Kidneys
- Bladder
- Bones
- Ears

WOOD
- Gallbladder
- Sinews
- Liver
- Eyes

Exploring Physical and Subtle Human Anatomy

Supporting Health through the Seasons

Note: Adapted from Kaur, Sat Dharam, Danylak-Arhanic, M., & Dean. (2005). The *Complete Natural Medicine Guide* to Women's Health, pages 258-259.

There are so many systems and ways to support your body that sometimes it can feel overwhelming. One approach to make sure you are taking care of all of the body systems is to align your health focus with the seasons so that you can organically support each system in an integrated way through the year. Below are some ways to divide up the systems and self-care that is coordinated with the Five Elements.

Winter Period
December 20–March 20

Systems/Organs to Support
- Kidneys
- Bladder
- Adrenals
- Bones
- Urinary System
- Reproductive System

Element/Concepts to Work With
The water element represents the emotional self. This is a time of going inward to set your foundation for the year. This is also a time to work with eliminating fear.

Habits to Adapt
- Cut back on or eliminate caffeine (switch to Yogi Tea)
- Avoid sugar
- Drink lots of water: two and a half liters of fresh water daily
- Eat beans, minerals, root vegetables, and seaweed
- Go to bed early in the winter—before ten o'clock to replenish kidney *Qi*
- Practice Root Lock
- Take Vitamin D
- Incorporate weight bearing exercise, slow deep stretches, and longer meditations

Supporting Health through the Seasons

Spring Period
March 21–June 20

Systems/Organs to Support
- Liver
- Gallbladder
- Joints and Tendons
- Nervous System
- Musculoskeletal System

Element/Concepts to Work With
The wood element represents our ability to grow and strengthen. This is a time to clear stagnation and anger from the physical and energetic bodies and build the courage to move forward. Liver detoxification helps encourage relaxation and feelings of courage.

Habits to Adapt
- Try a liver flush for a few weeks. Some people find this flush beneficial for helping to boost immunity.
- For joint health: add turmeric to your diet.
- Include meditations, kriyas, or journaling practices to release anger.
- Incorporate vigorous physical workouts.

Summer Period
June 20–July 21

Systems/Organs to Support
- Heart
- Small Intestine
- Circulatory system
- Endocrine System

LIVER FLUSH RECIPE

- ✓ Half grapefruit
- ✓ 2 oranges
- ✓ Half lemon
- ✓ 4 sprigs of parsley
- ✓ 1 clove of garlic
- ✓ 1 to 2-inch (3-4 cm) piece of ginger
- ✓ A pinch of cayenne
- ✓ 1 to 2 cups (240 ml to 480 ml) water or apple juice
- ✓ 2 tablespoons (30 ml) olive oil or flax seed oil
- ✓ 1 teaspoon (5 ml) turmeric (optional)

Blend all ingredients, adding the 2 tablespoons (30 ml) olive oil or flax seed oil last; add water or apple juice to thin if needed.

Exploring Physical and Subtle Human Anatomy

Element/Concepts to Work With

The fire element is all about transformation and creativity. Now is the time to bring in new creative adventure and reshape what is not working.

Habits to Adapt

- Stay cool, calm, and joyful.
- Continue the vigorous workout you adopted in the spring, 30–40 minutes cardio per day.
- Eat herbs and plants that build the blood: Green food, nettles and fresh seasonal vegetables.
- Take good care of your teeth because of the connection to cardiovascular health.
- Meditate to calm the mind and keep the creativity elevated.
- Remember to give to yourself as part of your overall practice of being a giving person.
- Develop the Crown Chakra and Third Eye for insight.

Late Summer Period
August 21–Sept 20

Systems/Organs to Support

- Stomach
- Spleen
- Pancreas
- Muscle
- Digestive System

Element/Concepts to Work With

The earth element is about nurturing yourself; focus on your feelings of self-worth, self-care, and self-nurturing. Let the critical parts of yourself be healed.

Habits to Adapt

- Increase anti-inflammatory diet: vegetables, fruit, and whole grains.
- Consider adding in digestive enzymes and probiotics.
- Eat lots of kitcheree; perfect your own recipe for it.
- Avoid processed foods with trans fats and polyunsaturated fats
- Allow for healthy fat intake to soothe intestinal lining: ghee, coconut oil, hemp oil, sesame oil, 3-6-9 omega oil blends.

Fall Period

September 21–December 20

Systems/Organs to Support
- Lungs
- Large Intestines
- Skin
- Respiratory and Immune System

Element/Concepts to Work With

The metal element, through the lungs and large intestine, is about letting go of grief and taking in purifying energy through air and good quality food. It can also mean letting go of attachments to material possessions, decluttering a physical space as well as the mind through meditation. It is an element of structure and boundaries, so keep developing disciplines to support your development.

Habits to Adapt
- Fall is another perfect time to increase cardio or vigorous workouts.
- Continue to balance the body' pH with alkaline fresh foods.
- Hydrotherapy. Add in cold showers, saunas/steam rooms and a daily, oil massage to cleanse the lymph (Kaur et al, 2005).

Body Systems Guided Visualization

You may want to record yourself reading this guided visualization or ask a trusted friend to read it aloud to you. Or listen to the recording on our website *enlightenedbodies.com*

Come into a meditative posture. Prepare for a guided visualization of your body systems. Let go of grasping for understanding and allow the subconscious mind to absorb the information. Breathe deeply and feel every breath settling you more and more into your own body.

Notice the beat of your heart. Tune into the subtle rhythm in the chest. Imagine you are riding on a drop of blood inside your heart. Feel yourself being propelled and pushed out into the arteries. As you leave the heart and begin to travel through the body, you deliver nutrients and oxygen to the tissues of the body. The body cells receive your nutrition and respond by giving you toxins and carbon dioxide. You slide back into the veins, travel back to the heart and then to the lungs where you drop off the toxins. Release those things which your body is no longer using.

Stay in the lungs for a few moments. Feel the gentle rhythm of the inhalations and exhalations. Feel the alternate power of expansion and contraction. Allow yourself to absorb and be full of oxygen. Then, continue to travel on the blood stream, passing back to the heart and out again to the body tissues.

This time you separate from the blood and stay behind in the spaces between the cells. You rest in the spaces, as clear, lymphatic fluid. Feel how the gentle rhythm of the breath and subtle movements of the body massage the tissues around you. This gentle movement presses you into a lymphatic vessel and eventually a lymph node. Here, you rebuild your supply of white blood cells and allow old cells to be broken down. You return to the bloodstream clear, refreshed, and protected.

Feel the perfect balance of heart, lungs, lymph, blood, and breath.

Body Systems Guided Visualization

Now draw yourself into the center of your brain. Feel the pulsing of the nervous system that begins here. Tap into the electric current of a single nerve pathway. You stretch from the brain, down the spinal cord and exit out between the vertebrae of the spine. Feel the electricity, which travels down your length, and out to the body. Feel the gentle, soothing rhythm of the nervous system pulsing. Feel the dynamic loop of information from the brain out to the body and from the body back to the brain. Feel yourself forming a perfect circuit.

Travel deep into the center of the brain. Here you find spaces filled with fluid, and you find the glands of the brain. Become the pituitary gland. Feel yourself creating a little drop of hormonal bliss. Imagine you are dropping this bliss into the blood stream where it will travel though the body and spread into all tissues of the body. Feel how this drop of bliss affects every part and action of the whole body.

Finally, bring yourself into the digestive tract. Feel that you are the tube that spans from the mouth, to the stomach, to the intestines, and finally to the anus. Feel the sensitivity of your walls and the delicate balance of chemicals within. Observe your perfect intelligence in absorbing nutrients and your discerning selection of which elements won't serve you, allowing those things to move through. Feel how you are affected and stimulated by the rhythm, relaxation, and movement of all the other systems. Feel how you simultaneously serve and support those same systems.

Feel all of your body systems working together, protecting you, balancing you, and supporting each other and the body as a whole. Take a moment and feel the beautiful and complex simplicity of this perfect body.

Kriyas for Each Body System

Kundalini Yoga Kriyas for the Musculoskeletal System

Kriya for Elevation	*Aquarian Teacher Yoga Manual*
Surya Namaskar (Sun Salutations)	*Aquarian Teacher Yoga Manual*
Physical Body Kriya for Self-Healing	*Waves of Healing*
Heal Your Back Kriya	*Heal Your Back*
Basic Spinal Energy Series	*Kundalini Yoga Sadhana Guidelines, 2nd Edition*
Flexibility and the Spine	*Kundalini Yoga Sadhana Guidelines, 2nd Edition*

Kundalini Yoga Kriyas for the Circulatory System

Har Aerobic Kriya	*I Am A Woman*
Movement Relaxation Series	*I Am A Woman*
Kriya for the Lungs and Bloodstream	*Kundalini Yoga for Youth and Joy*
Love is Love Meditation	*Transformation, Vol. 2*
New Lungs and Circulation	*Aquarian Teacher Yoga Manual*

Kundalini Yoga Kriyas for the Respiratory System

New Lungs and Circulation-	*The Aquarian Teacher Yoga Manual*
Kriya for Lungs, Magnetic Field and Deep Meditation	*Kundalini Yoga Sadhana Guidelines, 2nd Edition*
For Health and Openness	*KRIYA*
Meditation to Conquer Self-Animosity	*The Aquarian Teacher Yoga Manual*
Breathwalk	*Breathwalk*

Kundalini Yoga Kriyas for the Immune System

Kriya for Disease Resistance	*Aquarian Teacher Yoga Manual*
Wake Up the Body to Handle Stress and Strain*	*Owner's Manual for the Human Body*
Kriya to Relieve Inner Anger	*Owner's Manual for the Human Body*
Self-Renewal	*Physical Wisdom*
Mahan Jaap	*Meditation Manual for Intermediate Students*
Kriya to Build Yourself to Act, Not React	*Transformation, Vol. 1*

*This kriya may sometimes be referred to as the "Fish Fry Kriya" because of exercises that involve lying on the belly and jumping like a fish.

Kundalini Yoga Kriyas for the Nervous System

The Brain Doctor	*Transformation*, Vol. 1
Withstanding the Pressures of the Time	*I am a Woman Yoga Manual*
Seven Wave Sat Nam Meditation	*Aquarian Teacher Yoga Manual*
Sodarshan Chakra Kriya	*Aquarian Teacher Yoga Manual*
Meditation for Cold Depression	See appendix, page 249 for instructions
Smiling Buddha Kriya	*KRIYA*

Kundalini Yoga Kriyas for the Endocrine System

Kriya for the Glands	*KRIYA*
Wahe Guru Kriya	*Aquarian Teacher Yoga Manual*
Glandular System Tune Up	*Owner's Manual for the Human Body*
Pituitary Gland Series	*Aquarian Teacher Yoga Manual*
Two Meditations for Opening the Higher Centers	*KRIYA*

Kundalini Yoga Kriyas for the Digestive System

Healthy Bowel System	*Aquarian Teacher Yoga Manual*
Nabhi Kriya	*Aquarian Teacher Yoga Manual*
Apana Kriya	*Kundalini Yoga Sadhana Guidelines, 2nd Edition*
Metabolic Change	*Kundalini Yoga for Youth and Joy*
Left Nostril Breathing	See instructions on page 190

Kundalini Yoga Kriyas for the Urinary System

Stress Set for the Adrenals and Kidneys	*Aquarian Teacher Yoga Manual*
The Kidneys	*Kundalini Yoga for Youth and Joy*
For Endless Courage and Endurance against the Entire Universe	*Kundalini Yoga Sadhana Guidelines, 1st Edition*

Kundalini Yoga Kriyas for the Reproductive System

Sat Kriya Workout	*Aquarian Teacher Yoga Manual*
Kriya for the Instinctual Self	*I Am A Woman Yoga Manual*
Releasing Premenstrual Tension and Balancing Sexual Energy	*Aquarian Teacher Yoga Manual*
Transforming the Lower Triangle to the Higher Triangle	*Aquarian Teacher Yoga Manual*
Grace of God Meditation	*I Am A Woman*

Glossary

3HO: The Healthy, Happy, Holy Organization (3HO) is an international community of people from all walks of life, all religions, all economic backgrounds, and all countries, who practice Kundalini Yoga, meditation, and the yogic teachings of Yogi Bhajan in order to manifest Health, Happiness, and Holiness (wholeness) in their daily lives and the lives of others.

Aquarian Age: An astrological age that began in 2011; a time period of elevated consciousness

Chakras: Energy centers in the body through which the Kundalini Energy flows and rises. They are four dimensional in nature and connect the Subtle Body with other realms. There are eight chakras in the Kundalini Yoga tradition.

Elevated: Taking the high road; seeing the big picture and acting in a way that reflects connection to higher consciousness or a deed that is good for humanity.

Elements (Tattvas): the substances that create the universe; from the Ayurvedic, yogic, and Oriental Medicine traditions, these substances move in a cyclical fashion. All life is formed from the elements or *tattvas*. Each *tattva* contains certain qualities that shape a person's constitution and how her or his metabolism works. They are slightly different in name in each tradition, but the qualities are very similiar. Ayurvedic/Yogic: Earth, Water, Air, Fire, Ether. Chinese: Earth, Water, Wood, Fire, Metal

Enlightenment: A profound sense of alignment with the higher self and the divine in all things; being connected to happiness, peace, and light; creating within oneself a connection to authenticity and truth; and having the capacity to be the lighthouse.

God: The **G**enerating, **O**rganizing and **D**estroying or Delivering force that permeates all.

Ida/Pingala: *Ida* and *pingala* are energy pathways that spiral through the right and left sides of the body ending at the nostrils. They represent and tap into different energies within the body. The *ida* connects to the left side of the body, ending at the left nostril; it captures the energy qualities of the moon and the divine feminine. It is calm and restorative. The *pingala* is on the right side and embodies the energies of the sun and the divine masculine; it is direct and active. All of these energy channels are cleared and activated by the practice of Kundalini Yoga.

Karma: The law of cause and effect regarding mental, moral, and physical actions. Ego attaches us to and identifies us with objects, feelings, and thoughts. These attachments create a bias toward certain lines of action. Instead of acting, you begin reacting. Karmas are the conditions required in order to balance or complete these tendencies. Though necessary, karma is not dictatorial or fatalistic. It is the mechanism that allows the finite experience of existence to maintain and stabilize itself. We all have free will and can take actions to redirect the momentum of a karma. We can transform it or neutralize it using meditation, *jappa*, good deeds, or intuition to remove your sense of ego and the identification with that past line of action.

Kriya: A series of yogic postures and exercises placed together to have a specific impact. The Sanskrit root *kri-* indicates action and the addition of *ya* indicates a complete action.

Kundalini Energy: The uncoiling of your essential consciousness, your creative potential, the energy of consciousness, the energy of the soul itself. Literally it means "the curl in the lock of the hair of the beloved."

Maya: The illusion of the reality of sensory experience of one's self and the world around us. Usually thought of as what takes us away from, or blinds us from, perceiving God.

Meditation / Prayer / Contemplative Practices: Practices that traditionally help a person develop the ability to align with inner peace; a way of connecting with a higher power. These practices include yoga, meditation, self-reflection, chanting, therapy, journaling and energy healing among others.

Meridians: In Chinese medicine, every organ has a meridian that extends from the internal organ to the surface of the body. This channel is not necessarily a physical structure but an energetic opening to influence the health of the organ. Points along the meridian can be stimulated to influence the corresponding organ.

Naadis: Channels of flow for the *praana*. There are 72,000 *naadis*, of which 72 are vital. Of those 72, three major *naadis* are important for the understanding of Kundalini Yoga: *ida*, *pingala*, and *sushmuna*.

Ojas: The primal fluid of life in Ayurveda. It slows the aging process, lubricates the spine, and prevents the graying of hair and loss of teeth. Plentiful *ojas* helps to maintain the health of the reproductive organs and glands and is essential for one's quality and longevity of life.

Praana/Apaana: *Praana* and *apaana* are the two primary forces of the body. *Praana* is the life-force energy that governs all restorative and building functions, such as inhaling and absorbing oxygen or eating and absorbing food. *Apaana* is the eliminating or destructive energy that regulates all elimination of waste in the body.

Praanayam: The practice of controlling the breath. Specific praanayam or breathwork techniques include Breath of Fire, One Minute Breath or Long Deep Breathing.

Soul/Higher self: The part of you that is connected to a greater power and is part of everything.

Sushmuna: The *sushmuna* is the central energy channel and runs between these two pathways.

Ten Bodies (also called the 'Ten Light Bodies' in this book): The Ten Bodies are capacities of the human psyche. They are: Soul Body (1st), Negative Mind (2nd), Positive Mind (3rd), Neutral Mind (4th), Physical Body (5th), Arcline (6th), Aura (7th), Pranic Body (8th), Subtle Body (9th), and Radiant Body (10th).

The Universe/Infinite/Divine: The unifying force of existence; it is the spark of consciousness in all beings. The grand plan.

Glossary

Yoga/yogic: Anything having to do with the lifestyle and community and practice of yoga, specifically Kundalini Yoga practices. Generally a vegetarian diet, lifestyle oriented to reducing or eliminating compulsive behaviors and creating a peaceful community that is supportive and oriented toward alignment with a higher purpose and helping to create peace.

White Tantric Yoga: A special full-day meditation course that balances the chakras to cut through blocks in the subconscious mind. Meditations are usually of 31 to 62 minutes long and are done sitting across from a partner and in long rows.

Resources

Ardekani, B. A., Figarsky, K., &Sidtis, J. J. (2012). Sexual dimorphism in the human corpus callosum: An MRI study using the OASIS Brain Database. *Cerebral Cortex. Available at* http://cercor.oxfordjournals.org/content/early/2012/08/09/cercor.bhs253.fulldoi: 10.1093/cercor/bhs253

BBC News (2006, Feb. 1). Sex chemistry "lasts two years." BBC News. Available at http://news.bbc.co.uk/2/hi/4669104.stm.

Bergoth, E., Remes, S., Pekkanen, J., Kuppila, T., Büchele, G., &Keski-Nisula, L. (2012).

Respiratory tract illnesses during the first year of life: Effect of dog and cat contact.Pediatrics. Originally published online July 9, 2012. Available at http://pediatrics.aappublications.org/content/early/2012/07/03/peds.2011-2825.full.pdf

Bhajan, Y. (1982, Feb. 17) Lecture, Boulder, Co.

Bhajan, Y. (1984, May 1.) Lecture. Los Angeles, CA.

Bhajan, Y. (1988, Feb. 14) Gurdwara Talk. Sterling, VA.a

Bhajan, Y. (1988, Oct. 1). Khalsa Chiropractic Lecture. Oxnard, CA.b

Bhajan, Y. (1988, Oct. 11) Lecture. La, CA.c

Bhajan, Y. (1989, July 24) KWTC Lecture. Espanola, NM.a.

Bhajan, Y. (1989, Nov. 17) Lecture. La, CA.b.

Bhajan, Y. (1989, Dec. 2) Meditation Course. Rome, Italy.c

Bhajan, Y. (1990, Nov. 21) Kundalini meditation Stockholm, Sweden.a.

Bhajan, Y. (1990, May 27) Meditation. Vancouver, BC, Canada.b.

Bhajan, Y. (1991, Mar. 5) Lecture. Chakra Series. La, CA.a

Bhajan, Y. (1991, Sept. 7) Gurudwara, Ross Street. Vancouver, BC. Canada.b

Bhajan, Y. (1992, June 17). Lecture conducted in Albuquerque, NM.a

Bhajan, Y. (1992, June 30), KWTC lecture class. Lecture conducted from Española, NM.b

Bhajan, Y. (1992, Dec. 17) Orlando Meditation Course. Orlando, FL.c

Bhajan, Y. (1993, Sept. 16). Lecture class at yoga west in LA, CA.a

Bhajan, Y. (1993, Dec. 21) Lecture class at Winter Solstice, Lake Wales, FL.b

Bhajan, Y. (1993, Dec. 28). Lecture. Fort Lauderdale, FL.c

Bhajan, Y. (1993, June 8) Lecture. Espanola, NM.d

Bhajan, Y. (1993, Sept. 12) Gurdwara Lecture. Espanola, NM.e

Bhajan, Y. (1994, March 16) Lecture. Espanola, NM.a.

Bhajan, Y. (1994, Jul. 4) Lecture. Espanola, NM.c.

Bhajan, Y. (1994, Aug. 27). Workshop. Monterey, CA.b.

Bhajan, Y. (1995, Nov. 18). Lecture. Wellesley, MA.a.

Bhajan, Y. (1995, May 31) Teacher's Meeting. Amsterdam, Netherlands.b.

Bhajan, Y. (1997, Mar. 23) Gurdwara. Millis, MA.

Bhajan, Y. (1998, Aug.12) Lecture class. Espanola, NM.

Bhajan, Y. (2010). *The Aquarian teacher textbook & yoga manual.* Santa Cruz, NM: Kundalini Research Institute.

Bhajan, Y. (2008). *Man to Man: A Journal of Discovery for the Conscious Man.* Santa Cruz, NM: Kundalini Research Institute.

Black Elk, C. (2014) Oral story. Manderson, SD.

Block, K. I., & Mead, M. N. (2003). Immune system effects of Echinacea, ginseng, and astragalus: A review. *Integrative Cancer Therapies,* 2(3), 247–267. Available at http://www.ncbi.nlm.nih.gov/pubmed/15035888

Buettner, D. (2012). The Blue Zones: lessons for living longer from the people who've lived the longest. Washington, D.C.: National Geographic Society.

Breitling, S. M. (2014). Living, loving, trying: A challenge to us all. *Durham Academy Record,* (Winter), 5.

Bruzek, A. (2014) available at: http://www.npr.org/sections/health-shots/2014/09/18/349514734/life-s-unfair-but-chimps-and-humans-know-when-to-even-the-score

British Lung Foundation. (n.d.). *About your lungs.* British Lung Foundation. Available at: http://www.blf.org.uk/Page/About-your-lungs

Channahoff-Khalsa, D. S. (2004). An introduction to Kundalini Yoga meditation techniques that are specific for the treatment of psychiatric disorders. *The Journal of Alternative and Complementary Medicine,* 10(1). Available at http://www.kundalini-yoga-lausanne.com/download/Shannahoff-Khalsa%20Kundalini%20Yoga%20and%20Psychiatric%20Disorders.pdf

Chopra, Deepak. (n.d) Available at: http://www.chopra.com

Clement-Kruzel, S., Hwang, S. A., Kruzel, M. C., Dasgupta, A., & Actor, J. K. (2008). Immune modulation of macrophage pro-inflammatory response by goldenseal and Astragalus extracts. *Journal of Medicinal Food,* 11(3), 493–498. http://www.ncbi.nlm.nih.gov/pubmed/18800897

Cohen, S. (2002). *Happiness and the immune system.* Available online at http://www.positivehealth.com/article/mind-matters/happiness-and-the-immune-system

Comparison of female and male pelves (n.d.). Available at https://www.boundless.com/physiology/the-skeletal-system/the-pelvic-hip-girdle/comparison-of-female-and-male-pelves/

Cook, E., & Dunifon, R. (2012). *Parenting in context: Do family meals really make a difference?* Ithaca, NY: Cornell University, College of Human Ecology, Cornell Cooperative Extension, Bronfenbrenner Center for Translational Research.

Cuda, Gretchen (2010). Available at: http://www.npr.org/2010/12/06/131734718/just-breathe-body-has-a-built-in-stress-reliever

DiSalvo, D. (2009). Forget survival of the fittest: It is kindness that counts. *Scientific American.* Available at http://www.scientificamerican.com/article.cfm?id=forget-survival-of-the-fittest

Duke, J. A. (2007). The garden pharmacy: Turmeric, the queen of COX-2-Inhibitors. *Alternative and Complementary Therapies,* 13(5): 229–234. doi:10.1089/act.2007.13503.

Duncan, M.H. (1994). Hormone replacement therapy. Cardioprotective effect is genuine. *British Medical Journal,* 309(6948), 191–192. Available at http://www.ncbi.nlm.nih.gov/pmc/articles/PMC2540677/

Eshel, G., & Martin, P. A. (2006). Diet, energy, and global warming. *Earth Interactions,* 10(2006), Paper # 9, 1.

Farhi, D. (1996). *The breathing book: Vitality and good health through essential breath work.* New York: Henry Holt and Company, LLC.

Etherington J1, Harris PA, Nandra D, Hart DJ, Wolman RL, Doyle DV, Spector TD.(1996) The effect of weight-bearing exercise on bone mineral density: a study of female ex-elite athletes and the general population. J Bone Miner Res. Sep;11(9):1333-8. Available at http://www.ncbi.nlm.nih.gov/pubmed/8864908

Furman, J. (2003). *Eat to live.* New York: Barnes & Noble.

Gresham, L.S.K. (2015) Oral story. Ram Das Puri, NM.

Goodman, S. (2002, Nov.). Editorial Issue 82. *Positive Health Online.* Available at http://www.positivehealth.com/article/mind-matters/happiness-and-the-immune-system

Hamzelou, J. (2011). Transsexual differences caught on brain scan. *New Scientist.* Available at http://www.newscientist.com/article/dn20032-transsexual-differences-caught-on-brain-scan

Hawking, Stephen (1988, Oct. 17). Der Spiegel

The Healthy Breast Program. Website: http://www.mammalive.net/healthy-breast-program

Hayes, L. (1984, 1987, 2004). *You can heal your life.* New York: Hay House, Inc.

Holbeich, M., Genuneit, J., Weber, J., Braun-Fahrlander, C, Waser, M., & von Mutius, E. (2012). Amish children living in northern Indiana have a very low prevalence of allergic sensitization. *The Journal of Allergy and Clinical Immunology, 129*(6), 1671–1673. Available at http://www.jacionline.org/article/S0091-6749(12)00519-2/fulltext

Holmes, H. (2008). *The well-dressed ape.* New York: Random House.

Huang, Y., Zaas, A. K., Rao, A., Dobigeon, N., Woolf, P. J., et al. (2011) Temporal dynamics of host molecular responses differentiate symptomatic and asymptomatic influenza a infection. *PLoS Genetics, 7*(8): e1002234. doi: 10.1371/journal.pgen.1002234

Irwin, B. C., Scorniaenchi, J., Kerr, N. L., Eisenmann, J. C., &Feltz, D. L. (2012). Aerobic exercise is promoted when individual performance affects the group: A test of the kohler motivation gain effect. *Annals of Behavioral Medicine, 44*(2), 151–159. Available at http://link.springer.com/ article/10.1007%2Fs12160-012-9367-4

Iyengar, B. K. S. (1966). *Light on Yoga: Yoga Dipika.* New York: Schocken Books, Inc.

Journalism of Courage Archive. (2014). *Children growing up with furry pets are healthier: Study.* Mumbai, India: The Indian Express, Ltd. Available at http://www.indianexpress.com/news/children-growing-up-with-furry-pets-are-healthier-study/981368

Juhan, D. (2007). *Job's body: A handbook for bodywork.* New York: Midpoint Trade Books Inc.

Kaur, S. D. (1990). *A call to women: The healthy breast program & workbook: naturopathic prevention of breast cancer.* Dallas, TX: Quarry Press.

Kaur, S., Danylak-Arhanic, M., & Dean. (2005). *The complete natural medicine guide to women's health.* Toronto, Ontario Canada: Robert Rose, Inc.

Khalsa, D. (2011, April 15) Conscious Communication, Level Two lecture.
Clearwater, FL.

Khalsa, D. (2014) http://www.alzheimersprevention.org/downloadables/Yoga_and_Medical_Meditationtm.pdf

Khalsa, G. K., & Michon, C. (2000). *The eight human talents; Restore the balance and serenity within you with Kundalini Yoga.* New York: HarperCollins Publishers and Narayan, LLC.

Khalsa, G. K.(2003). *Bountiful, beautiful, blissful: Experience the natural power of pregnancy and birth* with Kundalini Yoga and meditation. New York: St.Martin's Press.

Khalsa, G. S. (1993). *Tantric numerology.* Mount Vernon: WA: Radiant Light Press.

Khalsa, G. P. S. (2003). *Divine alignment.* Beverly Hills, CA: Cherdi Kala, Inc.

Khalsa, G. P. S. (2010). *The heart rules: Yoga from the heart.* Beverly Hills, CA: Cherdi Kala, Inc.

Khalsa, G. S.,& Yogi Bhajan. (2000). *Breathwalk: Breathing your way to a revitalized body, mind and spirit.* New York: Random House and Santa Cruz, NM: Kundalini Research Institute.

Khalsa, G.T.K. (1998). *The Art of Making Sex Sacred.* Santa Cruz, NM: Yogi Ji Press.

Khalsa, H. K. (2006). *Praana, praanee, praanayam.* Santa Cruz, NM: Kundalini Research Institute.

Khalsa, H. S. S., D. C. (2013). The Hue-man: In form & function. San Lorenzo, California: Golden Dragon Productions.

Khalsa, K. P. S. (n.d.). *Healing wisdom: Strengthen your resolve with healing herbs and foods.* Santa Cruz, NM: 3HO – Healthy, Happy, Holy Organization. Available at http://www.3ho.org/3ho-lifestyle/health-and-healing/herbology

Khalsa, K.P.S. & Tierra, M. (2008). The Way of Ayurvedic Herbs. Twin Lakes, WI: Lotus Press.

Khalsa, M. K. K. (2005). *Bound lotus manual.* (Los Angeles, CA) Publisher.

Khalsa, N. S. (1994). *The ten light bodies of consciousness.* Anchorage, AL. NSK Productions.

Khalsa, S. (2009). *The Vitamin D revolution: How the power of this amazing vitamin can change your life.* New York: Hay House.

Khalsa, S. S. K. *Overcoming cold depression.* Española, NM: Guru Ram Das Center for Medicine and Humanology. Available at http://www.grdcenter.org/articles/cold-depression.php

Khalsa, S.S.K. (2010, August). KRI Immersion Lecture. Espanola, NM.

Khalsa, S.S.K. (2011, January). Oral story. Espanola, NM.

Khalsa, T. T. K. (2007). *Conscious pregnancy: The gift of giving life.* Española, NM: 3HO Women.

Khalsa, Y. (2011) *The Ancient Art of Self Healing, Second Edition.* Available as an eBook at:kundaliniresearchinstitute.directfrompublisher.com

Kröger, H., Kotaniemi, A., Kröger, L., &Alhava, E. (1993). Development of bone mass and bone density of the spine and femoral neck: A prospective study of 65 children and adolescents. *Bone Miner, 23*(3), 171–182.

Lad,V. (2009). Ayurveda: The Science of Self-Healing. Twin Lakes, WI: Lotus Press.

Mayo Clinic Staff. (2014). *Chronic stress puts your health at risk.* Rochester, MN: Mayo Foundation for Medical Education and Research. Available at http://www.mayoclinic.org/healthy-living/stress-management/in-depth/stress/art-20046037

Moore, K., Persaud, T., Torchia, M. (2013) *Before we are born: Essentials of Embryology and Birth Defects, 8th Edition.* Canada: Elsevier Saunders.

Morningstar,A.,Desai,U.(1995) *The Ayurvedic Cookbook.* Twin Lakes, WI: Lotus Press.

Myelodysplastic Syndromes Foundation, Inc. (2012). *What does my bone marrow do?*Yardville, NJ: Author.

Myss, C. (1997). *Anatomy of the spirit: The seven stages of power and healing.* New York: Three Rivers Press.

National Institute of Dental and Craniofacial Research (NIDCR). (2014). *Heart disease and oral health.* Bethesda, MD: National Institutes of Health, National Institute of Dental and Craniofacial Research. Available at http://www.nidcr.

nih.gov/OralHealth/Topics/HeartDisease/

Novotny, S., & Kravitz, L. (2007). The science of breathing. *IDEA Fitness Journal,* 4(2), 36–43. Available at http://www.unm.edu/~lkravitz/Article%20folder/Breathing.html

Pitchford, P. (1990).*Healing with whole foods: Asian traditions and modern nutrition.*Berkeley, CA: North Atlantic Books.

Ratzburg, C. Melatonin: The myths and facts. Available at http://www.vanderbilt.edu/AnS/psychology/health_psychology/melatonin.htm#Melatonin and the Immune System

Resolve: The National Infertility Association. (2014). The effect of egg quality on fertility. Mclean, VA: Ovascience.

Roach, M. (2003). *Stiff: The curious lives of human cadavers.* New York: W. W. Norton & Company, Inc.

Rogers, Fred. (2003). *The world according to Mister Rogers: Important things to remember.* New York: Hyperion.

Editor: Nicholas J. Schork, University of California San Diego and The Scripps Research Institute, United States of America

Received: January 5, 2011; Accepted: June 28, 2011; Published: August 25, 2011

ScienceForums.net. (2010–2013). *Why do some humans have extra ribs?* Online chat available at http://www.scienceforums.net/topic/52559-why-do-some-humans-have-extra-ribs/

Shannahoff-Khalsa, D. (2006). *Kundalini Yoga meditation: Techniques specific for psychiatric disorders, couples therapy, and personal growth.* New York: W.W. Norton & Company, Inc.

Shannahoff-Khalsa, D. (2010). *Kundalini Yoga meditation for complex psychiatric disorders: Techniques specific for treating the psychoses, personality, and pervasive developmental disorders.* New York: W.W. Norton & Company, Inc.

Stein, R. (2013, November 18). Gut bacteria might guide the workings of our minds. [Radio program segment.] National Public Radio.

Sullivan, P. (2011). Artistry in action. *Yoga Journal.* Available online at http://www.yogajournal.com/practice/2768

Taylor, J. B. (2006). *My stroke of insight: A brain scientist's personal journey.* New York: Penguin Group.

Tortora,G.,Derrickson, B.(2006). *Principles of Anatomy and Physiology.* Danvers,MA:John Wiley & Sons.

Wikipedia. (n.d.) Modeh Ani. Retrieved from: https://en.wikipedia.org/wiki/Modeh_Ani

Weaver, D. E. (2014) Oral story. Chicago, IL.

Whedon, J. M. (2009). Cerebrospinal fluid stasis and its clinical significance. *Alternative Therapy Health Medicine,* 15(3), 54–60.

Yogiji, Siri Singh Sahib Bhai Sahib Harbhajan Singh Khalsa. (2006). The science of hydrotherapy. In Yogi Bhajan, *Kundalini Yoga for youth and joy* (pp. 8–9). Santa Cruz, NM: Kundalini Research Institute. Available at http://www.sikhdharma.org/pages/ishnaan-science-hydrotherapy

Index

120th day, 223,
    soul and, 225

abdominal muscles, 14, 41-45, 53, 187, 212-214, 246
    brain and, 41
    diaphragm and, 45
    movement and, 41-43
    navel chakra and, 14, 187, 254
    root lock and, 53, 212-214
    specific muscles and, 43-45
abhyanga (self-massage), 125
absorption, 64, 86, 89, 176-177, 181, 183
    digestion and, 176-177, 181, 183
    glucose and, 162
    oxygen and, 86
    praana, apaana and, 64, 89
abstinence, 231
acceptance, viii, 72, 75-76, 98, 115, 165
    heart center and, 75-76
    grief and, 98
    neutral mind and, 72
    of self, 165
    relationship of teacher to student and, viii
    sickness and, 115
accident, 163
acid alkaline balance, 187
acquired immunity, 113
acupuncture points, xiii, 20, 25, 28, 38, 52, 145, 216, 243, 245
    joints and, 38, 52
    light and, 26, 216
    meridians and, 20, 25-26, 28, 52
    shu points and, 145
    trauma and, 56
    Yogi Bhajan and, xiii, 25
adaptogenic herbs, 171

addiction, 163, 182, 192, 245
    aura and, 19
    endocrine and, 163
    food and, 182
    permanent habits and, 163
    sacral chakra and, 237
adoption, 226
adrenals, 120, 159, 162, 171, 201, 203, 206, 209-210
    aasana, exercise and, 167
    adaptogenic herbs and, 171
    Chinese *Kidneys* and, 210-211
    fear and, 206
    kidneys and, 201, 203, 206
    positive, negative minds and, 209
aerobic, 78, 100, 264
    circulatory system and, 100
    har aerobic kriya, 264
    physical training and, 100
agonist muscle, 42
air *tattva*, 84, 97, 142
    circulatory system and, 84
    nervous system and, 142
    qualities of, 97
allergies, 54, 80, 104, 116, 186
    black pepper and, 104
    dairy and, 54
    immune system and, 116
    nettle leaf and, 80
    seasonal and, 186
amalaki, 79
anger, 14, 73, 98, 143, 160, 179, 181, 254, 259, 265
anxiety, vi, 13, 74, 78, 80, 149, 184, 187, 208, 213, 216
aorta, 45, 64-65, 71
apana, 266
Arcline, 18-19, 108, 117-118, 232-233, 255, 268
arm swings, 77, 122, 147, 199, 254
armpit postures, 147
arteries, 60, 62, 64-67, 71, 78-79, 262
arterioles, 65, 67
articular cartilage, 39
astragalus, 124, 271
asymmetrical body, 90, 179
atria, 67
atrophy, 29
attachment behaviors, 157, 163
Aura, 11-12, 15, 18-19, 145, 165-166, 188-189, 199, 232, 243, 248, 253-255, 268
autonomic nervous system, 49, 95, 138-139
ayurveda, ii-iii, xii, 9, 21-22, 54, 73, 79, 224, 268, 273

b cells, 111-112, 114
baby pose, 103, 147
bacteria, 55, 68, 94, 114-116, 148, 177, 180, 186-187, 195, 274
bear grip, 122, 244
biceps brachii, 42
bile, 178
birth canal, 221
black pepper tea, 105
bladder, 52, 137, 200, 202-205, 209-212, 215, 245, 247, 258
blastocyst, 221
blood, 40, 61-68, 77-80
    bones and, 31
    inflammation and, 46,
    heart and, 71,
    oxygen and, 86, 245,
    praana and, 103
    immune system and, 110-111, 113-114,

endocrine system and, 151-153, 156, 160-162,
urinary system and, 201, 203-204, 209,
chemistry of, 214
vitamin D levels, 216,
diet and, 260
blue pearl, 168
bone density, 30-31, 54-55, 273
bone marrow, 31, 110, 113, 273
bone-building activities, 30
bones, 29-33, 35, 37, 39, 41-42, 45, 51-52, 55-56, 61, 113, 148, 169, 203-205, 209, 214, 216
    clavicle, 30, 33, 69
    femur, 113
    hips 32-33, 39, 153, bo 254
        humerus, 113
    iliac crest, 32
    illiopsoas, 44
    ilium, 32-33
    ischial tuberosities, 32
    ischium, 32-33
    osteoclast, 153
    pubic bone, 32, 42-43, 45-46
    sacrum, 13, 32, 35-36, 46, 230, 254
    scapula, 33
    sit bones, 32, 45, 205
    sternum, 36, 69
    tailbone, 13, 35-36, 209, 254
bow pose, 167, 212, 234
bowing, 76, 147, 167
brain, 123, 130-133 144, 155-157, 164, 203, 247
    brain chemistry, 138
    cave of brahma, 133
    crown (seventh) chakra and, 15
    drishti, 168-169
    frontal lobe, 131, 169
    gray matter, 134
    left brain, 133
    limbic system, 131
    right brain, 128, 133
    third ventricle, 133
    ventricles, 164
    white matter, 134

breasts, 153, 220, 222, 233
    breast health, 233
breath, 4-5, 47, 63-64, 78, 85-86, 90-92, 101-104, 139-140
    Aura and, 189
    Pranic Body and, 19, 99
    ribcage and, 37
    longevity and, 97
    mouth, nose and, 88
Breath of Fire, 55, 78, 84, 93-94, 102-103, 140, 189, 198, 235, 242, 245, 254, 268
bridge pose, 8, 77
bronchi, 86-87, 89
bundle rolls, 147
butterfly stretch, 212

calcium, 31, 52, 54-55, 153, 158, 204, 214, 216, 236
camel pose, 10, 77, 100, 200, 212
capillaries, 62, 65, 80, 100, 110
cardiac muscle, 41, 71
cartilage, 30, 36, 39
cave of brahma, 133
celibacy, 148, 231
central nervous system, 130, 134
cerebrospinal fluid, 133-134, 147, 274
cervical vertebrae, 35-36, 41, 254
    hands on exploration, 35
cervix, 221
Chakras, vii, ix, xiii, 8-13, 15, 20, 50, 88, 93, 99, 136-137, 139, 145, 150, 208, 213, 242, 254, 267, 269
    First (Root) Chakra, 13, 46, 58, 82, 137, 159, 200, 206, 209, 216
    Second (Sacral) Chakra, 13-14, 137, 218, 230-231, 234, 237
    Third (Navel) Chakra, 14, 137, 139, 159, 174, 187-188, 198, 254
    Fourth (Heart) Chakra, 14, 60, 69, 72, 75, 77, 81-82, 98, 137, 158, 211, 244-245
    Fifth (Throat) Chakra, 14-15, 84, 98-99, 107, 137, 244, 248
    Sixth (Third Eye) Chakra, 1 5, 156
    Seventh (Crown) Chakra, 15, 139, 150, 164-165, 168, 173, 245, 253, 260

Eighth (Aura) Chakra, 11-12, 15, 18-19, 145, 165-166, 188-189, 199, 232, 243, 248, 253-255, 268
chant, 81, 104, 107, 109, 156, 169, 172-173, 242, 245, 249, 251-252, 254
Chinese medicine, iii-iv, xiii, 9, 20-22, 25, 74, 79, 97-98, 120, 137, 164, 188, 210, 242-244, 246-248, 256-257, 268
chiropractic care, 56
Christianity, 73
circulatory system, iii, 14, 18, 60-82, 85, 95, 100, 114, 259, 264
clavicle, 30, 33, 69
clitoris, 220, 222
cloves, 124-125, 149
cobra pose, 42, 44, 52, 77, 100, 122, 138, 247
coccyx, 35-36
cold depression, 142-144, 159, 251, 265
cold showers, 80-81, 233, 261
collective wellbeing, 119
commitment, 70, 117, 226, 254
community, 18, 85, 108-109, 115, 117-119, 124-125, 129, 131, 151, 175, 193, 197, 201, 226,
    digestive system and, 175, 193
    community meals and, 124, 197
    immune system and, 108-109, 115, 117-119
    prayers and, 226
    sadhana and, 151
    sangat, xiv, 118-119, 125
    yoga and, 129
Conception vessel, 213, 234
connective tissue, 30, 39-41, 43, 134
consciousness, 3-4, 9, 50, 52, 72, 133, 148, 163, 165, 194, 207-208, 219, 230-231
    cycles of, 31
    chanting and, 169
    constitutional body type (Ayurveda)
    kapha, 22, 24, 105, 125, 196-197, 236
    pitta, 22-23, 79, 105, 125, 197, 236
    vata, 22-23, 125, 196-197, 236
    contemplation, 9, 17, 72, 131
corydalis, 55

Index

cranial nerves, 136-137
Crown (seventh) Chakra, 15, 139, 150, 164-165, 168, 173, 245, 253, 260
cruciferous vegetables, 171
cycle of consciousness, 31
cycle of intellect, 31
anger, 18, 52, 139, 143, 159, 160, 208-210, 255
    adrenals and, 159
    musculoskeletal and, 52
    nervous system and, 139
    pancreas and, 160
    cold depression and, 143
    negative mind and, 18, 208 - 210, 255

dang gui, 79, 236
dashmula, 149
deep relaxation, 101, 113, 122, 170, 245, 250
    immunity and, 122
dehydration, 207-208
delivery, 115
depression, vi, 14, 123, 130, 142-144, 159, 183, 189, 207, 251, 254, 265, 273
destiny, vii, 5, 9, 11, 17-18, 72, 99, 166, 223-224, 226, 255
diaphragm, 45, 54, 67, 84, 86-87, 90, 92-94, 102, 203
    hands on exploration, 93
diaphragm lock, 54, 93
diastolic pressure, 67
digestion iv, 14, 49, 138, 174-181, 183-199, 254, 260, 266
    digestive organs, 14, 108, 174, 184, 201, 226
    digestive tract, 41, 79, 114, 135, 137-138, 176-178, 180, 183, 185-186, 193, 225, 242, 250, 263
    intestinal flora, 181, 183, 186
    large intestine (colon), 176-177
    motility, 227
dignity, 70
discipline, 19, 74, 151, 164, 233, 255
disease, vi, xv, 11, 29, 47, 64, 76, 109-110, 115, 232, 265, 273
divinity, 70, 74, 85, 173
dopamine, 138

drishti, 138, 163, 167-169, 242, 245
dura, 134

ears, 15, 35, 124, 149, 214, 242, 254
earth *tattva*, 21-24, 51, 191, 260, 267
    Chinese Elements and, definition, 260, 267
    doshas and, 22-24
    musculoskeletal system and, 51
    root chakra and, 209
earthly plane, 3
ectoderm, 225-226
eggs, 184, 221-223
ego eradicator, 82, 84, 100, 147, 189, 254
elder, 109
electrical impulses, 134-135
electronics
    cold depression and 142-143
    overexposure and, 143
electrolyte, 214
elimination, 13, 29, 63, 92, 106, 175-177, 183, 254, 268
emotion, 9, 11, 51, 69, 84, 182, 206, 254
emotional healing, 34
emotional scar, 34
endocrine system, iv, 15, 140, 151-173, 254, 259, 265
endoderm, 225
energy center, 3, 98, 187, 209, 230
energy healing, xiii, 56, 268
enlightenment, 1, 27, 155, 267
enteric nervous plexus, 138
erection, 227
erogenous zone, 222
esophagus, 14, 45, 176-177, 185, 254
estrogen, 152-153, 160, 222
ether *tattva*, 21-22, 128, 142, 224, 244, 267
exhalation, 63, 67, 90, 248, 251
external intercostals, 94
eyes 15, 149, 156, 164, 168, 236,
    drishti and, 156, 164, 168
    navel point and, 214
    onions and, 149
    sesame and, 236

fallopian tubes, 220-221
false ribs, 36

fascia, 30, 39-40, 44, 47-48, 56
fear, 3, 70, 74, 76, 93-94, 131, 158, 179, 201, 206, 208-209, 212, 216, 230, 255, 258
fearlessness, 200-201
femur, 113
fertility, 215, 225-226, 274
fetus, 156, 221, 223, 225, 235
filter, 200-201, 204, 209
fire *tattva*, 21-24, 54, 159, 174, 181, 211, 229, 245, 260, 267
    bhandas and, 54
    Chinese *Elements* and, definition, 260, 267
    digestion and, 174, 181, 211
    doshas and, 22-24
    masculine and, 229
fish fry, 147, 265
five *Elements*, see *tattvas*
floating ribs, 37
food
    black pepper tea, 105
    cruciferous vegetables, 171
    fruit, 79, 104, 124, 192, 236, 260
    garlic, 21, 148-149, 197, 259
    ghee, 57, 105, 149, 196-197, 236, 260
    ginger, 21, 105, 148-149, 194, 197, 236, 259
    grapefruit juice, 215
    kitcheree, 195, 197, 260
    masala, 149, 197
    mung beans and rice, 21, 197, 215
    onion, 21, 148-149
    pineapple ginger juice, 105
    pomegranate black pepper tea, 105
forgiveness, 14, 75, 82, 254
frogs, 52, 167, 254
frontal lobe, 131, 169
fruit, 79, 104, 124, 192, 236, 260

gallbladder, 53, 137, 176, 178, 218, 259
garlic, 21, 148-149, 197, 259
gas exchange, 63, 85, 89, 100
gender identity, 144, 228
ghee, 57, 105, 149, 196-197, 236, 260
ginger, 21, 105, 148-149, 194, 197, 236, 259
ginseng, 124, 171, 236, 271

God 6, 26, 53, 64, 73, 75-76, 85, 93, 168, 177, 208, 226, 244, 268
    balance and, 168
    blessed, 6, 75
    breath is, 85, 244
    defined, 64, 267
    hand(s) of, 76, 93
    fertility and, 226
    food and, 177
golden chain, 109,
golgi tendon, 41, 49
governing vessel, 167
grace, xi, 6, 13, 38, 70, 82, 99, 173, 208, 266
grapefruit juice, 215
gray matter, 134
Guru Pranaam, 147

habits, 31, 101, 135, 163, 193-194, 213, 258-261
half wheel, 77
hands 69, 75-76, 115, 124,
    healing, 75-76
happiness, 6, 70, 77, 123, 125, 137, 148, 193, 201, 267, 271-272
head rolls, 107, 122, 254
healing, xiii-xv, 34, 48, 56, 61, 118, 124, 233, 258
    Heart Chakra and, 69, 75-76,
    mantra, 81-82, 123
    food and, 177, 184, 195- 197, 215, 236,
heart, physical, 31, 36-37, 41, 61-62, 65-67, 70-71, 78-79, 81
    ventricles, 67
Heart (fourth) Chakra, 14, 60, 69, 72, 75, 77, 81-82, 98, 137, 158, 211, 244-245
Heart Meridian, 60, 74-75, 77, 244
heart rate, 78, 134, 137, 139, 235
heart valves, 66-67
hemisphere, 133
herbs, ii-iii, vii, xiii, 21, 26, 54-55, 79, 104, 124, 148, 171, 191, 214, 236, 260, 273
    amalaki, 79
    astragalus, 124, 271
    black pepper tea, 105
    cloves, 124-125, 149
    corydalis, 55
    dashmula, 149

Dang Gui, 79, 236
ginseng, 124, 171, 236, 271
milky oat seed, 80
licorice, 171
nettle Leaf, 80
peppermint, 195, 225
turmeric, 55, 57, 149, 180, 196, 259, 271
hips 32-33, 39, 56, 126, 147, 153, 174, 243, 245, 247, 254
hormones, 63, 110, 141, 152-153, 155-164, 167, 171, 179, 185, 201, 207, 209, 219, 221-222, 227-228, 235-236, 249
    hormone pathway, 154
    hormone secretion, 134
    specific hormones and,
        dopamine, 138
        melatonin, 135, 154-155, 170, 274
        oxytocin, 137, 152, 156
        progesterone, 153, 160, 222
        relaxin, 33
        serotonin, 138
        testosterone, 37, 153, 160-161, 223, 227
householder, 129, 148, 231
Humanology, iii, xiv-xv, 9, 24, 122, 228, 273
humerus, 113
hypertrophy, 29
hypothalamus, 133, 141, 156-157, 162-164, 167-169
hypoxemic blood, 64

ida, 20, 87-88, 190, 267-268
iliac crest, 32
ilium, 32-33
illiopsoas, 44
immune system, iv, vi, 19, 49, 75, 94-95, 103, 108-126, 149, 226, 261, 265, 271
    immune cells, 68, 110-112, 116, 250
        macrophage, 271
        memory cells, 112
    interstitial fluid, 68
    intruders, 111
    lymph node, 262
    t cells, 111, 114
infertility, 225-226, 274

infinite, 17, 50, 58, 64, 72, 76, 91-92, 97, 117, 123, 252-253, 268
inflammation, vi, 46, 48, 55, 79-80, 90, 105, 132, 175, 180, 191, 195, 236, 241
inhalation, 67, 90, 92, 103, 248
injury/trauma, 47
interstitial fluid, 68
intestinal flora, 181, 183, 186
intruders, 111
intuition, xi, xiv, 9, 15, 74, 164-165, 172, 218, 241, 254, 268
inversions, 36, 77, 235
involuntary, 49, 90, 227
ischial tuberosities, 32
ischium, 32-33
ishnaan, 80-81
Islam, 73

jalandhar bhand see neck lock
joints, 29-30, 37-40, 52, 55-56, 76, 180, 259
    joint capsule, 28, 39
    joint pain, 180
    synovial joints, 39
Judaism, 73

kapha, 22, 24, 105, 125, 196-197, 236
karma, vii, 37, 117, 188, 267-268
kidneys, 10, 92, 159, 187, 200-204, 206, 209-212, 214-216, 258, 266
    acid/alkaline and, 187
    adrenals and, 159
    camel pose and, 10, 200
    cleansing and, 215
    diaphragm and, 92
    electrolyte and, 214
    Kidneys(Chinese) and, 210-211
    urinary system and, 200-209
Kirtan Kriya, vi-vii, 132, 168, 252-253
kitcheree, see mung beans and rice
kriya, vii, 53, 90, 122, 150, 170, 241-242, 245, 250, 264-266, 268
    analysis, 241-251
    asymmetrical, 90
    by body system, 264-266
    deep relaxation and, 170
    definition, 268

Index

immunity, 122
Kirtan Kriya, vii, 252-253
nervous, endocrine connection, 170
Sat Kriya, 150
body system, 264-266
kundalini energy, 24, 36, 164-165, 208, 267-268
kyphotic, 35

labia, 220, 222
lactation, 222
Lakota, 73
large intestine (colon), 176-177
leadership, 14, 145, 198, 255
left brain, 133
leg lifts, 50, 122
legacy, 219, 233
liberation, 4, 13, 19, 50, 75
licorice, 171
Life Nerve Stretch, 147
lifestyle, 22, 24, 146, 148, 201, 225, 227-228, 231, 233
    Ayurvedic, 22
    celibacy, 148, 231
    Humanology, 24, 228
    nervous system, 146
    praanayam, 101
    reproduction and, 225, 227
    sexuality, 233
ligaments, 30, 33, 39, 41, 48, 204, 235
limbic system, 131
liver, 92, 161-162, 176, 178-179, 242, 249, 259
Liver, 52, 137, 174
locust pose, 234
long Deep Breathing, 101
lordotic, 35
love, vii, x, xiv, 6, 14, 35, 58, 61, 69-71, 75, 81-82, 98, 137, 141, 208, 233, 254, 264
lower back, 33, 35, 43-44, 187, 212-213, 235, 246
lower triangle, 13-14, 266
lumbar, 35-36
lungs, 62-64, 67, 84, 86-90, 94, 104, 139, 187, 226, 241, 243, 245, 254, 261-262
    Lungs (Chinese), 97-98, 120, 137
    diaphragm and, 45, 92

hands on exploration, 103
heart chakra and, 14, 69
ribcage and, 36-37
lymphatic system, 48-49, 114, 151, 249
    lymphatic fluid, 49, 68, 110, 114, 122, 233, 262
    lymph node, 262

macrophage, 271
magnesium, 55-56, 214, 236
mantra, xiv, 73, 81-82, 104, 109, 122-123, 142, 148, 150, 169, 216, 236-237, 245, 249, 251-252
masala, 149, 197
maya, 209, 268
meditation 72, 74-75, 138, 251, 252, 265
    Heart and, 74-75
    Neutral Mind, 72
    Seven Wave Sat Nam Meditation, 138, 265
    Kirtan Kriya, vi-vii, 132, 168, 252-253
    Meditation for Cold Depression 251
    Religion and, 73
    Seasons, appropriate meditations, 258-261
melatonin, 135, 154-155, 170, 274
memory cells, 112
menstrual cycle, 153, 222, 225
    moon cycle, 81, 102, 222
    menopause, 164, 210, 222
meridians, ix, 9, 20, 22, 25, 28, 52, 56, 101, 103, 174, 190, 211-212, 216, 247, 249, 268
    bodywork and, 56
    Breath of Fire and, 103
    chanting and, 148, 169
    Conception vessel, 213, 234
    definition of, 268
    elements and, 22, 256-257
    Gallbladder, 52, 137, 190, 218
    Governing vessel, 167
    Heart, 28, 60, 74-75, 77, 137, 244
    joints and, 52
    Kidney, 52, 137, 210-212
    Large Intestine, 28, 137, 190
    Liver, 52, 137, 174, 179, 190
    long deep breathing and, 101
    Lung, 52, 84, 100, 137

naadis, 20
Pericardium, 28
Spleen, 52, 108, 121, 137
Small Intestine, 137, 174
Stomach, 52, 60, 137, 190-191, 248
subtle anatomy and, ix, 9, 25
Triple Burner, 52
Urinary Bladder, 52, 137, 200, 204, 210, 211-212
Yogi Bhajan and, 9
mesoderm, 225
metaphysical anatomy, 9
milky oat seed, 80
mitochondria, 71
Moolbandh, see Root Lock
motility, 227
motor nerves, 136
mouth, 53, 79, 87-89, 94, 132, 148, 156, 169, 175-178, 197, 263
mouth breathing, 87-88
moving twists, 122
mucus, 54-55, 89, 94, 104-105, 176, 178, 211
mung beans and rice, 21, 195, 197, 215, 260
muscles, 29, 33-35, 41-46, 49, 53-54, 66, 140, 203, 242, 244, 246-248
    diaphragm, 92
    heart and, 71
    navel chakra and, 187
    nervous system and, 130, 134, 136, 140
    pelvic floor, 205, 208-209
    psoas, 28, 44-45, 245
    root lock and, 212-214
    secondary muscles of respiration, 94
    supplements and, 56
overuse,
    postural muscles and, 47
    secondary muscles of respiration and, 94
psoas, 28, 44-45, 245

nadis, 20, 150
navel,
    root lock and, 53-54, 212, 214
    Breath of Fire and, 102-103,
Navel (third) Chakra, 14, 137, 139, 159, 174, 187-188, 198, 254

Exploring Physical and Subtle Human Anatomy

Navel Point, 20, 36, 147, 208, 214, 224, 242-245, 251
neck, 35-36, 41, 77, 98, 101-102, 111, 120, 122, 126, 136, 155
    breathing and, 101-102
    lymph and, 111, 122
    Throat Chakra, 98
    vagus nerve, 136
neck lock, 53-54, 136, 138, 155, 162
Negative Mind, 18, 72, 206, 208-209, 268
nephrons, 203
nervous system 49, 95, 103, 128-149, 151, 153-154, 156-157, 159, 162, 169-170, 180-181, 185, 197, 207, 225-227, 251
    autonomic nervous system, 49, 95, 138-139
    central nervous system, 130
    deep relaxation and, 170
    digestion and, 49, 180-181, 185
    effect of breath, 95, 103
    endocrine system and, 151, 153-154, 156-157, 162, 170
    mantra, 169
    meditations for, 251
    musculoskeletal and, 49
    nerves, 25, 56, 128-130, 133-137, 140, 142, 147, 149, 194, 247
    neurotransmitters, 135, 138
    neuron, 134, 135, 138, 147
    parasympathetic nervous system, 137, 139-140, 180-181
    peripheral nervous system, 134-135
    sympathetic nervous system, 139-140
    vagus nerve, 78, 136-137, 140, 162, 244
neti pot, 106
nettle Leaf, 80
Neutral Mind, 18, 60, 72, 80-81, 268
nine holes, 204
nose breathing, 87, 94
nuchal ligament, 41

oil massage, 125
oil, 23, 57, 81, 105-106, 125-126, 149, 170, 195-196, 210, 236, 259-261
ojas, 133, 164, 232, 268
onion, 21, 148-149
oocytes, 221

optic nerve, 154, 156-157, 164, 168
oral hygiene, 78
osteoclast, 153
ovaries, 81, 155, 160, 167, 205, 218, 220-223, 227
oxytocin, 137, 152, 156

pain, 19, 25, 37, 39-40, 44, 48, 55-56, 69-70, 75, 119, 122, 134, 156, 180, 189, 198, 245
pancreas, 120, 155, 160, 162, 167, 176, 178, 260
parasympathetic nervous system, 137, 139-140, 180-181
pathogens, 94, 111-114, 116, 119-120
pectoral, 34, 52, 94
pelvis, 13, 28, 30, 32-33, 35, 39, 44, 52-53, 205, 208, 212-213, 221, 235, 254
    hands on exploration, 32
    pelvic floor muscles, 45-46, 205, 209, 212
    Pelvic opening, 33
penis, 220, 227
peppermint, 195, 225
peripheral nervous system, 134-135
permanent habits, 163
physical armoring, 34
physical barriers, 109-110, 114
Physical Body 17-18, 50-51, 99, 169, 188, 255
physical vessel, 3
pineal gland, 15, 133, 135, 154-155, 164, 168, 233, 241, 253-254
pineapple ginger juice, 105
pingala, 20, 87-88, 267-268
pitta, 22-23, 79, 105, 125, 197, 236
pituitary gland, 15, 88, 133, 156-157, 164, 168, 204, 212, 216, 233, 241, 253-254, 263, 265
plasma, 65, 68, 110-111
plow pose, 36, 138, 145, 235
polarity, 6, 18, 72, 210, 218, 220, 228, 230, 255
pomegranate black pepper tea, 105
Positive Mind, 18, 72, 208, 268
postural distortion, 47
postures
    arm swings, 77, 122, 147, 199, 254
    armpit postures, 147
    baby pose, 103, 147

    bear grip, 122, 244
    bow pose, 167, 212, 234
    bowing, 76, 147, 167
    bridge pose, 8, 77
    bundle rolls, 147
    butterfly stretch, 212
    camel pose, 10, 77, 100, 200, 212
    cobra pose, 42, 100, 138, 247, 42, 44, 52, 77, 100, 122, 138, 247
    Ego Eradicator, 82, 84, 100, 147, 189, 254
    fish fry, 147, 265
    frogs, 52, 167, 254
    Guru Pranaam, 147
    half wheel, 77
    inversions, 36, 77, 235
    leg lifts, 50, 122
    Life Nerve Stretch, 147
    locust pose, 234
    moving twists, 122
    plow pose, 36, 138, 145, 235
    rocking bow pose, 212
    Sat Kriya, 53, 122, 147, 150, 190, 234, 242, 266
    seated twists, 122
    shoulder shrugs, 53, 122, 167
    shoulder stand, 36, 52, 77, 122, 138, 235
    spinal flex, 100, 230, 234
    standing forward bend, 77
    static twist, 122
    Sufi Grind, 190
    triangle pose, 77, 128, 247
    windmill, 122
    yoga mudra, 77, 100
power struggles, 14
prana, ii, 253
praanayam, 37, 46, 74, 78, 79, 90, 91, 98, 101, 190
    Breath of Fire, 102
    children, 91
    definition, 268
    Heart and, 74, 78
    Left Nostril, 190
    Long Deep Breathing, 101
    ribcage, lungs, 37, 90, 98
    Sitali, 79
    stagnation and, 46

Index

Pranic Body, ii, 18-19, 99, 242, 268
prayer, xi, 19, 38, 72-73, 117, 124, 151, 177, 179, 223, 255, 268
pregnancy, 33, 45, 153, 156, 163, 221-226, 232, 235, 272-273
    womb, 221, 223, 225
progesterone, 153, 160, 222
prolapsed bladder, 205
proprioceptive, 41
prostate gland, 205, 215, 220, 227
psoas, 28, 44-45, 245
puberty, 37, 222, 227
pubic bone, 32, 42-43, 45-46

Radiant Body, 16, 18, 20, 128, 145, 243, 268
rectum, 53, 175-176, 178, 209, 212-213
red blood cells, 30-31, 79, 113-114
red marrow, 113
reflex arc, 41, 134
relaxin, 33
religion
    Christianity, 73
    Islam, 73
    Judaism, 73
    Lakota, 73
    Tibetan Buddhism, 73
reproduction, 13, 152-153, 160-161, 219, 222, 227, 230
reproductive system, iv, 14, 19, 206, 218-237, 258, 266
reptilian brain, 131
respiratory system, iii, 15, 19, 54, 84-107, 254, 264
    respiratory diaphragm, 45, 92
retina, 154
ribcage, 33, 36-38, 43-45, 92-93, 102-103
right brain, 128, 133
rocking bow pose, 212
Root (first) Chakra, 13, 46, 58, 82, 137, 159, 200, 206, 209, 216
Root Lock, 43-44, 46, 53-54, 205, 212-214, 234-235, 242, 258
rotator cuff, 33, 42

Sacral (second) Chakra, 13-14, 137, 218, 230-231, 234, 237

sacrifice, 37, 70, 253
sacrum, 13, 32, 35-36, 46, 230, 254
sadhana, 73-74, 125, 129, 131, 151, 179, 251, 264, 266
sangat, see community
Sat Kriya, 53, 122, 147, 150, 190, 234, 242, 266
sattvic, 223
scalenes, 94
scapula, 33
seat of the soul, 15, 155, 164, 254
seated twists, 122
serotonin, 138
service, v-vi, xi, 14, 61, 64, 69-72, 85, 99, 125, 233, 253-254
Seven Wave Sat nam Meditation, 138, 265
sexuality, 13, 218, 220, 222, 227, 230-232
    Sex characteristics, 160-161
    Sex hormones, 153, 236
    Sexual orientation, 220
shadow emotion, 11, 69, 254
shoulder shrugs, 53, 122, 167
shoulder stand, 36, 52, 77, 122, 138, 235
shoulders, 14, 34, 77, 94, 100-102, 158, 242, 247, 249, 254
shu points, 145, 248
single cell, 3
sinuses, 15, 87-88, 254
sit bones, 32, 45, 205
Sitali Praanayam, 79
skeletal muscle, 41, 66, 71
skull, 15, 30, 35, 37, 39, 41, 54, 134, 148, 169, 244, 254
sleep, 56, 74, 78, 143, 152-154, 161, 169-170, 185, 195
    Sleep-wake cycle, 154
small intestine, 52, 137, 174, 176-177, 259
smoking, 106
smooth muscle, 41, 65
Sodarshan Chakra Kriya, 147, 265
solar plexus, 14, 187, 242
solstice, 125, 208, 216, 253, 270
somatic nervous system, 140
soul 11, 13, 36-37, 51, 72-75, 97-99, 142-144, 155, 164, 223, 225, 233
    Cold Depression, 142-144
    grief, 97-99

heart center, 72-75
in the womb, 223, 225
Seat of, 155, 164
Soul contracts, 11
Subtle Body, 233
sperm, 164, 221-225, 227, 232
spinal cord, 35, 128, 130, 134, 136, 138, 247, 263
spinal flex, 100, 230, 234
spine, 28, 32, 35-36, 39, 44, 54, 79, 103, 134, 136-137, 145, 150, 203, 208-209, 211, 232, 242, 247-248, 250, 263-264, 268, 273
    cervical spine, 35-36
    cervical vertebrae, 35, 41, 254
    kyphotic, 35
    lordotic, 35
    lower back, 33, 35, 43-44, 187, 212-213, 235, 246
    lumbar, 35-36
    thoracic spine, 35
    vertebrae, 14, 35-36, 39, 41, 136, 254, 263
spirit, 21-22, 37, 72-74, 78, 97, 133, 144, 166-167, 172, 246, 250, 273
spiritual practice, 5, 51, 72, 91, 118, 129, 133, 151, 165, 223
Spleen, 52, 108, 110, 114, 120-122, 137, 179, 248-249, 260
stability, 13, 28, 31-33, 35, 37, 43, 45, 52-53, 152, 158, 169, 207, 209, 212
stagnation, 38, 46-47, 77, 89, 103, 259
standing forward bend, 77
static twist, 122
sternocleidomastoid, 42, 94
sternum, 36, 69
stomach, 92-93, 176-178, 260
    stomach acid, 114
    enteric nervous plexus, 138
    food quantity, 186, 192
Stomach Meridian, 52, 60, 137, 191, 248
stomach acid, 114, 177-178, 185
stress, vi, 34, 37, 56, 71, 78, 80, 95, 169,
    sdrenals and, 159, 201, 209
    Aura and, 188
    brain and, 131-132
    digestion and, 175
    Spleen and, 121

sympathetic nervous system and, 139-142
subconscious mind, 147, 262, 269
Subtle Body, vii, 19, 233, 244, 267
Sufi Grind, 190
sunlight, 55, 104, 188, 212, 216
sympathetic nervous system, 139-140
synovial joints, 39
systolic pressure, 67

T cells, 111, 114
tailbone, 13, 35-36, 209, 254
Tantric numerology, 17
tattvas, 21-22, 51, 142, 148-149, 169, 181, 249, 257-258, 267
Ten Light Bodies, iii, 15-17, 72, 165
    Arcline, 18-19, 108, 117-118, 232-233, 255, 268
    Aura, 11-12, 15, 18-19, 145, 165-166, 188-189, 199, 232, 243, 248, 253-255, 268
    Negative Mind, 18, 72, 206, 208-209, 268
    Neutral Mind, 18, 60, 72, 80-81, 268
    Physical Body 17-18, 50-51, 99, 169, 188, 255
    Positive Mind, 18, 72, 208, 268
    Pranic Body, ii, 18-19, 99, 242, 268
    Radiant Body, 16, 18, 20, 128, 145, 243, 268
    Soul Body, 16-17, 50
    Subtle Body, vii, 19, 233, 244, 267
tendon, 30, 33, 39, 41, 45, 48-49, 92, 259

testicles, 155, 161, 167, 218, 221, 227
testosterone, 37, 153, 160-161, 223, 227
therapeutic massage, 56
Third Eye (sixth) Chakra, 1 5, 156
    Third Eye Point, 15, 156, 168, 172, 190, 198, 245, 253
third ventricle, 133
thoracic cavity, 45
thoracic spine, 35
throat (fifth) chakra, 14-15, 84, 98-99, 107, 137, 244, 248
thymus gland, 14, 69, 81, 110, 113, 122, 155, 162, 167, 254
thyroid gland, 14, 81, 108, 155-156, 158, 167, 241, 254
Tibetan Buddhism, 73
tongue, 53, 78-79, 124, 132, 136, 148, 156, 169, 214, 243
tonic, 26, 79, 148, 180, 216
trachea, 14, 84, 86-87, 89, 158, 254
transformation, 14, 24, 38, 45, 52, 64, 76, 82, 133, 187, 223, 232, 234, 252, 260, 264-265
transit time, 183-185, 190
transverse abdominis, 44, 53, 212-214
trauma, 29, 47, 56, 93, 163, 231
Triangle Pose, 77, 128, 247
tribes, 109
turmeric, 55, 57, 149, 180, 196, 259, 271

universe, 3, 5, 21, 32, 64, 85, 90-93, 99, 117, 146-148, 152, 266-268
upper triangle, 13-14, 88
urethra, 46, 202, 204, 227

Urinary Bladder 137, 200, 205, 210-212,
Urinary system, iv, 13, 18, 200-216, 245, 258, 266
urine, 203-204, 211, 214, 227

vagina 213, 220-222, 227
vagus nerve, 78, 136-137, 140, 162, 244
vata, 22-23, 125, 196-197, 236
Vedic philosophy, 21
ventricles, 67, 164
    heart, 67
    brain, 164
venules, 65
vertebrae, 14, 35-36, 39, 41, 136, 254, 263
vitality, 1, 37, 50, 52, 63, 78, 90, 92, 95, 129, 175, 189, 191, 236, 253, 271
vitamin D, 55, 216, 258, 273
vocal cords, 14

waste, 50, 62-63, 65-66, 68, 85, 114, 177-178, 201-203, 268
water 156, 184, 192, 202-204
water *tattva*, 21, 181, 207-208, 210-212, 229, 256-257, 258
Wei Qi, 120
weight loss, 163
white blood cells, 63, 110-111, 113, 262
white matter, 134, 144
windmill, 122

yellow marrow, 113
yoga mudra, 77, 100

About the Authors

Nirmal Lumpkin, LMT, is a Level 2 Kundalini Yoga Practitioner and a Professional Trainer in the KRI Aquarian Trainer Academy. A massage therapist practicing in Saint Paul, Minnesota, Nirmal began her journey in the study of the human body and therapeutic wellness with extensive training in dance and Kundalini Yoga from a very early age. She earned a Bachelor of Fine Arts in Dance from State University of New York-Brockport and certification as a massage therapist at Northwestern Health Science University in Minnesota. Nirmal is an engaging and inspiring yoga teacher and trainer, specializing in *Physical and Subtle Anatomy and Postures.* In her work with students and clients, she helps them understand their own physical bodies as a means to deepening their practice of self-awareness and contemplation.

Japa K. Khalsa, DOM, is a Kundalini Yoga teacher and Associate Trainer in the KRI Aquarian Trainer Academy. She earned a Bachelor of Science from Northwestern University and completed her Master of Oriental Medicine degree at the Midwest College of Oriental Medicine in Chicago. Dr. Japa is a gifted integrative Doctor, combining traditional acupuncture with herbal and nutritional medicine, injection therapy, and energy healing. Her work with patients and students emphasizes optimal health and personal transformation through self-care and awareness of the interconnectedness of all life. Japa is a minister of Sikh Dharma and lives in New Mexico with her husband and son.

For more information, including teaching tools, curriculum and supplemental materials please see EnlightenedBodies.com.